T0254466

Promoting Healthy Behaviour

The new edition of this leading text is an essential guide to promoting healthy behaviour in a multi-cultural society, providing a holistic stance that integrates both physical and mental health and wellbeing.

With a comprehensive overview of the interplay between social class, gender, ethnicity and individual health differences, the book also looks at key lifestyle issues such as eating well, smoking, drinking alcohol and safe sex, as well as the mechanisms for behavioural change. Each chapter features engaging case studies, points for discussion and student activities. Updated since the COVID-19 pandemic, the new edition also discusses the effects of lockdowns on healthy behaviours.

An accessible and engaging text, the third edition of *Promoting Healthy Behaviour* will continue to be essential reading for both students and practitioners across nursing, public health and allied health professions.

Dominic Upton, Professor of Health Psychology and Pro Vice-Chancellor for the Faculty of Health, Charles Darwin University, Australia.

Katie Thirlaway, Professor of Applied Psychology and Dean of the Cardiff School of Sport and Health Sciences, Cardiff Metropolitan University, UK.

Promoting Healthy Behaviour

A Practical Guide to Physical Health and
Mental Wellbeing

Third Edition

Dominic Upton and Katie Thirlaway

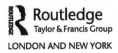
Routledge
Taylor & Francis Group

LONDON AND NEW YORK

Designed cover image: © Getty Images

Third edition published 2024
by Routledge
4 Park Square, Milton Park, Abingdon, Oxon, OX14 4RN

and by Routledge
605 Third Avenue, New York, NY 10158

Routledge is an imprint of the Taylor & Francis Group, an informa business

© 2024 Dominic Upton and Katie Thirlaway

First edition published by Pearson Education Limited 2010
Second edition published by Routledge 2014

British Library Cataloguing-in-Publication Data
A catalogue record for this book is available from the British Library

ISBN: 978-1-032-74850-4 (hbk)
ISBN: 978-1-032-13734-6 (pbk)
ISBN: 978-1-003-47123-3 (ebk)

DOI: 10.4324/9781003471233

Typeset in Sabon
by MPS Limited, Dehradun

Contents

Tables

Figures

Preface

Background to this book

In 2010, the first edition of this text was published in response to the growing recognition that health practitioners needed to respond to the challenges of preventable disease with more than just education and advice. During the 3 years between the first and second editions there were concerted efforts by governments and practitioners to encourage healthy lifestyles and prevent or delay the onset of so called 'lifestyle diseases'. Some initiatives showed promise whilst others were less successful but the real benefits of our efforts to improve our lifestyles are unlikely to be seen at a population for at least a decade. Consequently, it was time to update and reflect on what we have learnt since the first two editions of this book.

Given that nearly 15 years have passed since we conceived and started work on this book, there was much to reflect on and much has changed. However, much is the same. Indeed, the rationale for this book remains the same as the first edition: 'lifestyle diseases' Tony Blair (2006) are one of the major challenges facing the NHS. This is not a supposition put forward by us exclusively but by many others, including not least many of the former Prime Ministers during the era of this book's evolution. Gordon Brown suggested that with '..a rise in so-called "lifestyle diseases", the NHS finds itself with new challenges in supporting and caring for patients with long-term conditions' (7 January 2008: http://news.bbc.co.uk/2/hi/uk_news/politics/7175083.stm). Similarly, David Cameron (6 December 2011) hoped that although: '...old frontiers are conquered, new ones appear: lifestyle epidemics like obesity' (https://www.gov.uk/government/speeches/pm-speech-on-life-sciences-and-opening-up-the-nhs). His successor, Theresa May (21 May 2018) considered these choices to be significant: 'And we can all play our part – by making healthier lifestyle choices ourselves' (https://www.gov.uk/government/speeches/pm-speech-on-science-and-modern-industrial-strategy-21-may-2018). Boris Johnson, not surprisingly, had differing views which he expressed variably (see chapter 12) although his government did launch the Better Health national campaign encouraging individuals to make healthier lifestyle choices, by losing weight, getting active and quitting smoking with Boris Johnson commenting that one reason he had such a difficult time with COVID was a consequence of his lifestyle and he had a very common underlying condition: 'my friends, I was too fat.' Liz Truss had little time to focus or comment on 'lifestyle diseases' given her concentration on the economy. However, Rishi Sunak's signature lifestyle move was to ban a growing number of people from purchasing cigarettes and vapes by increasing the legal age at which this could be done (interestingly both Liz Truss and Boris Johnson indicated their unwillingness to support such a move).

Of course, politicians are not the only ones to have entered the debate: Opinion formers, academics and leader writers have all contributed to these deliberations, with increasing attention given to these diseases, whether this be within academia, social policy or the media. We and many others have long recognised the importance of psychology in the development of these lifestyle diseases and we wanted to ensure that appropriate psychological theory and practice were discussed and disseminated for use as part of the armoury available for health care professionals.

It has been appreciated for some time that poor lifestyles are associated with increasing health risks – at both an individual and a population level. Of course, such diseases are not distributed evenly across the population; there are certain sections of society that may suffer more than others. Hence, the influence of social class, gender and ethnicity should not be overlooked. It is essential that all health care professionals take into account these variables when discussing some of the approaches in this text. Furthermore, it is obvious that cognisance has to be taken of the individual differences when in a clinical situation; the personal characteristics and situation of the individual client can have a significant bearing on an individual's health and lifestyle. These characteristics may be related to their current situation or may be related to more cultural aspects. Moreover, there are differences between the individual countries of the UK, with certain behaviours and health and illnesses more prominent in some areas compared to others. There are also psychological variables that may be described as either 'risk' factors or 'protective' factors – 'personality' variables, self-efficacy or mood, for example.

Psychological models have attempted to integrate all of these social, demographic and psychological variables to predict behaviours and develop theoretically based interventions. This has been the fundamental foundation of this text. We have tried to demonstrate the value of these psychological models and how they can be used practically by health care professionals.

We see the role of psychology in lifestyle as of significant, if not of primary, importance. Similarly, we see the role of lifestyle in health and in illness as predominating and likely to become ever more important to the NHS in the coming decades. Indeed, the Foresight report described the 'obesity epidemic' as a problem comparable to climate change (Jones et al., 2007). Obviously, how these issues are going to be addressed is a matter of debate and potential solutions range from the theoretically driven to the more light-hearted. Lifestyle is an issue about which every commentator feels confident to express an opinion. For example, the stigmatisation of obese people (albeit in, one would assume, a humorous article) is not uncommon: 'Most obesity is a consequence of stupidity and indolence and not of some genetic affliction. It is a lifestyle choice which people would be less inclined to adopt if they knew we all hated them for it' (Liddle, 2008, with a thorough review of shaming of the obese in Cooper et al., 2023). In this text, we review some of the more serious and theoretically driven approaches, debate their value and discuss the potential ways that health care professionals can use these for the benefit of their patients and clients.

Overall, we hope that you find this edition useful and informative and a guide for your practice both now and in the future. It is geared towards health care professionals at any stage of their careers: those wishing to enter a health education/promotion, health (or social) care profession, those new to their particular role and those who have been engaged in professional practice for a number of years but wish to enhance their practice. It is not a manual of tips or a series of laws that have to be followed by all. There are some methods and guiding principles that we hope you will find useful, but this text is intended to be a series of thought-provoking chapters that will intrigue, stimulate and provoke, and hopefully enhance your practice for the benefit of your patients and clients.

The content of this book

We thought for some time about the content of this book – what should we include and what should be excluded? We also had advice from others who suggested additional material, but then others suggested other forms of behaviour that could be included. For example, should we include sleeping? After all, it is a behaviour and can affect health either positively or negatively. Similarly, others considered that we should include stress, which can impact both mental and physical health and contributes significant mortality through accidents. In the first book, we included a chapter on drug taking, but for the second edition we decided to concentrate on the five main behaviours that are the focus of the majority of health promotion activities.

We also knew the psychology that needed to be included. So what was the cause of our consternation? Why did we spend so much time discussing the content over well-brewed coffee (other than the obvious)? We appreciated at the outset that there was a possibility of considerable repetition within this text. Many of the behaviours discussed are underpinned by similar psychological variables and have been investigated within similar theoretical modes. After writing the first couple of chapters we recognised this and re-jigged the book to include the chapter on psychological concepts, which presents the information in a more coherent and sensible manner. We hope that this has removed considerable overlap, although we recognise that there are key psychological principles and models which will play a central part in many of the behaviours we discuss. For the second edition we have included new chapters that consider more carefully who is responsible for promoting lifestyle change, how we address inequalities and the implications of lifestyle change in different groups of people. For this third edition we have thoroughly updated all chapters across the text.

We should emphasise at the outset that this is not a book about smoking or obesity or psychological concepts *alone*. It is a book that attempts to cover a range of topics in an integrated framework. Hence, there are sections on social support, for example, that some may consider skimpy, and there are psychological factors and models that could have been included in many more chapters than currently presented. We have done this on purpose—we have not written a book that is dedicated to any one behaviour or any one approach. We obviously cannot compete with more narrowly focused texts for specific behaviours or models. However, we present an overview with a thematic connection between the chapters which we hope readers will find interesting, thought provoking and, most importantly, of practical use.

Chapter 1: Introduction to healthy behaviour

In this opening chapter we set the context within which health practitioners are working and individuals are making choices about how they behave. We look historically at the socio-cultural climate in which we all operate, considering how and why lifestyle diseases and related behaviours have become so pertinent for us in the twenty-first century. We also consider the political imperative to encourage individual responsibility for long-term health and we reflect on the environmental influences over twenty-first century lifestyles.

Chapter 2: Health promotion

In this chapter we introduce the concept of health promotion, health education and health literacy and where these various activities sit within Public Health. The chapter considers who is responsible for health promotion and how the health promotion priorities for a community are established.

Chapter 3: Health and health inequalities

Inequalities in health are apparent in practically all societies across the world. In the developed world, and in the UK in particular, these inequalities can be significant. This chapter explores these inequalities with a particular focus on socio-economic differences in health. Prior to this, however, a brief overview is provided on defining health, measuring health and measuring socio-economic and deprivation.

Chapter 4: Psychology in practice

In this chapter we describe a number of key psychological concepts that are of relevance to the topic of lifestyle and lifestyle change. The decision not to introduce specific theories but rather to introduce the key concepts that have consistently proved relevant for behavioural change is an attempt to bridge the gap between theory and practice. It is intended to make identifying the key aspects of research relevant to practice simpler. However, this is in no way intended to undermine the importance of theory, and the chapter highlights further reading for the interested reader.

Chapter 5: Eating well

In this chapter we explore eating and diet. The problems in providing a clear message of a 'healthy diet' are stressed, as are the issues surrounding the social environment's impact on diet. The governmental approaches to the 'obesity epidemic' are outlined and the role of psychological models in the development of appropriate interventions is stressed – ultimately, what the health care professional can do to promote healthy eating in those who are currently overweight, and how healthy eating can be promoted in the young.

Chapter 6: Being physically active

In this chapter we consider active and sedentary behaviours and how they are shaped by the lives we lead. Physical activity is the output side of the input–output energy equation and so is a key factor in the rising levels of obesity. The role of the obesogenic environment and how psychological interventions can work in often adverse environmental conditions are explored.

Chapter 7: Sensible drinking

Drinking is a popular component of many aspects of leisure in Britain. Drinking has adverse consequences for social and physical well-being. The changing nature of drinking patterns in the UK and in particular in women is described and discussed. Government policies to establish healthy drinking patterns in the young and promote healthy drinking in adults are outlined and the role of psychological interventions to support healthy drinking and deter deleterious drinking is evaluated.

Chapter 8: Quitting smoking

The health consequences of smoking are well established and well known throughout the population—smoking can have a significant impact on morbidity and mortality. However, approximately a quarter of the population still smoke and this has a significant impact on both the individual and the country's health. Given the significant impact that smoking has on the health of the nation, there has been extensive research into smoking and much of this has a psychological nature. In this chapter, the psychological variables and models that have been applied to smoking and, more importantly, how they can be used to promote smoking cessation are discussed.

Chapter 9: Sexual health

The safe sex message is being promoted in order to reduce the spread of sexually transmitted diseases. Sexual behaviours are not simply a consequence of physiological drives, but there are social, emotional and cultural (to name but three) variables that influence such behaviour. Within these broader influences the psychological factors have to be appreciated and developed. These psychological models and how they can be applied to promote safer sex are discussed. Importantly, safer sex is discussed within a pleasure-promoting context rather than a fear-inducing one.

Chapter 10: Specific conditions

Increasingly it is acknowledged that healthy lifestyles are as relevant (if not more so in some cases) for individuals diagnosed with chronic conditions as they are for individuals with no diagnosed condition. Recommending and supporting lifestyle change for individuals with a chronic condition requires health practitioners to consider any particular risks and associated amendments to standard advice that different conditions indicate. For some conditions there are specialist lifestyle support courses available. This chapter considers four different chronic conditions: Type 2 diabetes, coronary heart disease, mental health, and chronic obstructive pulmonary disease.

Chapter 11: Special populations

Although approaches to lifestyle behaviour change are common across the population, there are specific groups that require targeted interventions. These groups are numerous across the population but this chapter will explore three specific groups: those with a learning difficulty, those in prison, and the elderly. To a large degree, these were selected at random but are there to exemplify the skills, attributes and targeted interventions required to alter unhealthy health behaviours.

Chapter 12: Conclusion

This final chapter attempts to draw together the diverse behaviours discussed in the previous chapters and identify the key similarities and differences in the various behaviours we have considered. It is crucial for health practitioners to recognise which psychological techniques are effective across all behaviours in order to enable them to deal more effectively with the various prevention and promotion targets they are required to meet. This final chapter also tries to look ahead and identify what else we need to know to make our interventions more effective.

For each of these chapters we have included a selection of the following features:

- *Learning objectives:* What you will find in this book, so that you can navigate your way through the text and know what to expect and what you can achieve.
- *Case study:* We provide a brief case study that highlights some key principles to be discussed later in the chapter. In some of these you are asked to take the role of the individual practitioner dealing with the client and we hope that this will highlight issues that you may face in practice (or have faced), whether this be as a qualified or student health care professional. We hope that the case study will raise questions and issues that we address later in the chapter.
- *Introduction:* The introduction follows the case study – we hope that the case study has whetted your appetite and you will begin to appreciate during the chapter the importance of the case study and how it relates to the chapter content.
- *Applying this to...:* At stages throughout the chapter a box highlights how the principles discussed in the text can be applied to the case study.
- *Applying research in practice:* In the chapter, empirical research studies are presented throughout to demonstrate the evidence base of the suggested techniques. More detail on a couple of these is provided in these boxes.
- *Working with others:* Each chapter will consider the other professionals who may also be involved with or could support you in your health promotion activities
- *Key points:* At the end of chapter the key points will be summarised.
- *Discussion points:* These act as points for discussion – they relate either to all of the chapter content or to the case study highlighted at the outset.

We hope you are interested and engaged in this book and that it leads to an enhancement of your personal and professional skills. Overall, we hope that it leads to an improvement in healthy behaviours in your client group and goes some way to reducing the immense health problems associated with a poor lifestyle currently evident in the UK today.

References

Blair, T. (2006). Speech on healthy living. *The Guardian*, 26 July. Available at: http://www.guardian.co.uk/society/2006/jul/26/health.politics (accessed 30 November 2009).

Cooper, F., Dolezal, L., & Rose, A. (2023). *COVID-19 and shame: Political emotions and public health in the UK [Internet]*. London (UK): Bloomsbury Academic. Chapter 4, I was too fat: Boris Johnson and the fat panic. Available from: https://www.ncbi.nlm.nih.gov/books/NBK592723/

Jones, A., Bentham, G., Foster, C., Hillsdon, M., & Panter, J. (2007). *Tackling obesities: Future choices – Obesogenic environments – Evidence review*. London: United Kingdom Government Foresight Programme, Office of Science and Innovation.

Liddle, R. (2008). Laugh at the lard butts – But just remember Fatty Fritz lives longer. *Sunday Times*, 27 January.

Acknowledgements

Both of us have spent our careers research and teaching in health psychology and during the preparation of the third edition of this text it has been salutary to reflect on the valuable part research and education has played in understanding and changing behaviour. We have done our best to curate the wealth of research available into a series of practical chapters that could assist and develop an individual professional's practice. The material we are presenting here reflects the work and contribution of not only psychologists but colleagues from health care, medicine, sociology, philosophy, and policy. We have tried to encompass the literature from both an academic and a practitioner basis. We would like to thank the researchers, clinicians and policy makers for the contributions they have made to the current knowledge base.

On a more personal level, several key colleagues have acted as researchers and reviewers for us and have contributed their time, effort and opinions with vigour and frankness, much improving this third edition. Particular thanks should go to Professor Diane Crone and Dr Lowri Edwards (for KT) and to Rebecca Mursic (DU). We want to thank all our colleagues at Cardiff Metropolitan University (for KT) and Charles Darwin University (for DU) for their support and advice as we have been working on this project.

Many thanks also to our long-suffering Publishers who have been very patient as we slowly worked our way through the process of updating the chapters. There have been a number of significant changes to evidence and policy in the decade since the second edition which we have wanted to do justice to our third edition.

Finally, we would like to thank our family and friends for providing tea and sustenance during the inevitable manic periods. Mark & Penney, Francesca, Rosie, Gabriel, Anna, Hetty and Keir have all played their part in ensuring we got to the end of the book with our health intact.

1 Introduction to healthy behaviour

LEARNING OBJECTIVES

At the end of this chapter you will:

- Recognise how the concepts of lifestyle diseases and lifestyle behaviours have arisen.
- Understand the health behaviours central to the development and progression of chronic diseases.
- Recognise why lifestyle change is so complex and difficult.
- Recognise the multiple influences on lifestyle choice.
- Understand the challenges for health professionals involved in health promotion.

Health professionals and particularly primary care practitioners have health promotion and disease prevention as a central aspect of their role. This book is about this central element of a health care professional's role. Although lifestyle change should be a key part of *all* health professionals' role, and this has been recognised for many decades, in recent years its importance has moved higher up the policy hierarchy. In 2006, the then prime minister of the UK, Tony Blair called for 'lifestyle change' to relieve the pressure on the National Health Service (BBC News, 2006): the prime minister suggested that 'failure to address bad lifestyles was putting an "increasing strain" on the health service'. The COVID-19 infection might have heralded a shift in focus from prevention to protection but it was soon apparent that obesity and lack of physical fitness were significant factors in how ill people became with the infection.

Eluned Morgan, the Welsh Health Minister, repeated the call for people to practise health behaviours to protect the NHS in the winter of 2022/23 as the NHS struggled to respond to the challenges of the post-pandemic winter of flu, COVID and other respiratory diseases exacerbated by staff shortages and strikes over pay (Wales Online, 2023). Whilst lifestyle change wasn't going to resolve the acute crisis of the winter of 2022/23 the underlying principle of preventing ill-health and relieving the pressure on the health service remains a consist political message, but seldom supported by the resourcing necessary to generate significant, impactful change.

The impact of this cross-party political rhetoric and our increasing understanding of the role of lifestyle in health, has been significant. Many health professionals now provide the patients and clients who come into their clinics with expert advice about lifestyle

DOI: 10.4324/9781003471233-1

behaviours and health. The frustration and disillusionment that are felt when patients fail to follow advice and go on to develop chronic diseases that could possibly have been avoided have been influential on this textbook. This frustration is frequently articulated by health professionals involved in treating the major lifestyle diseases of the twentieth century. In 2009, Professor Wiseman, medical and scientific adviser for the World Cancer Research Fund, said:

> *This means that we are now more sure than ever before that by limiting the amount of alcohol they drink, maintaining a healthy weight and being physically active women can make a significant difference to their risk. We estimate over 40% of breast cancer cases in the UK could be prevented just by making these relatively straightforward changes.*
>
> Wiseman (2009)

Lifestyle change is a tantalising solution to the chronic ill-health that is the scourge of modern societies. It is such a cheap, effective, non-toxic, low-risk solution to the rising incidence of heart disease, diabetes, chronic back pain, cancers and many other conditions that it can seem incredible that we have not been able to deliver widespread population change. This book does not present a solution to effect instant population-wide uptake of health advice but it does explain why changing lifestyle behaviours is so difficult for so many people and not quite as straightforward as Professor Wiseman suggests. Furthermore this book points the reader in the direction of techniques and interventions proven to have at least some success in increasing the likelihood of successful behavioural change. Finally, in writing this third edition of this textbook we are more convinced than ever that lifestyle is not solely or even primarily a matter of individual choice. It is significantly shaped by the socio-political and environmental contexts in which we live.

So what are the key health behaviours that the government would like us to change? The word lifestyle is used confidently by health professionals, the media, and individuals but what does it mean and which health behaviours are included under its umbrella? Initially, the medical profession started to refer to 'lifestyle diseases' to reflect the role that lifestyle choices play in certain diseases. Doyle (2001) suggested that the six major lifestyle diseases are coronary heart disease, stroke, lung cancer, colon cancer, diabetes and chronic obstructive pulmonary disease. The rationale for their inclusion is that they 'trace mainly to imprudent living' (Doyle, 2001).

Interestingly, few authors would call sexually transmitted diseases 'lifestyle diseases', although they are clearly entirely a result of behavioural choices with none of the genetic component that plays a part in the six major lifestyle diseases identified by Doyle (2001). Sexually transmitted diseases are more usually defined as infectious diseases (Migchelsen et al., 2022), an important distinction for clinicians but perhaps less so for primary care and community-based practitioners interested in public health.

In between an 'imprudent lifestyle' (Doyle, 2001) and the development of lifestyle diseases are a number of 'precursor' conditions. High cholesterol, high blood pressure and obesity are risk factors for the development of a number of the aforementioned lifestyle diseases. The distinction between these precursors, the diseases they predict and the behaviours that are associated with them is often blurred. They are often presented as diseases *per se* and interventions are prescribed by the medical profession. The Department of Health (2010) categorises high blood pressure as a cardiovascular disease. Obesity is frequently referred to using disease parameters. For instance, the phrase 'obesity epidemic'

(Gard & Wright, 2005) is common and suggests that obesity is a disease and furthermore that it is somehow catching! Consequently, obesity is considered a lifestyle disease by some authors whereas others categorise it as lifestyle behaviour (Doyle, 2001).

The behaviours that are usually cited as being involved in the aetiology of lifestyle diseases are poor diet, lack of physical activity, cigarette smoking (Doyle, 2001; Blaxter, 1990; Egger et al., 2011) and excess drinking (Burke et al., 1997; Blaxter, 1990).

Sexual practices are also often described by public health professionals as health and/or lifestyle behaviours (Wardle & Steptoe, 2004). Despite not being directly linked to what clinicians refer to as lifestyle diseases, sexual practices nevertheless are still considered by most public health practitioners to be an aspect of lifestyle worthy of both concern and intervention (Egger et al., 2009; Wardle & Steptoe, 2004). Furthermore, sexual practices are a clear cause of preventable and treatable diseases. Consequently, the promotion of safer sex is also included in this book.

During the first 2 decades of the twenty-first century the unhealthy lifestyles that predominate in Western societies have been presented by the media as a new and modern crisis. Stories about drunken young women, rising levels of obesity and Type 2 diabetes are no longer restricted to the health pages but frequently take the front pages of national papers and make the lead story of television news bulletins. However, it is important to recognise that people have been drinking too much and eating the wrong things for many centuries. In Victorian times there were many gin addicts and in Elizabethan times diets were poor and dangerous levels of drinking were widespread (Plant & Plant, 2006). Perhaps the main difference between then and now is the level of understanding we have. We have a better *scientific* understanding of the relationship between our lifestyle and our health than previous generations. Nevertheless, as long ago as Roman times, the importance of a moderate lifestyle was recognised. For example, Pythagoras suggests that 'No man, who values his health, ought to trespass on the bounds of moderation, either in labour, diet or concubinage' and Hippocrates that 'Persons of a gross relaxed habit of body, the flabby, and red-haired, ought to use a drying diet ... Such as are fat, and desire to be lean, should use exercise fasting; should drink small liquors a little warm, should eat only once a day, and no more than will just satisfy their hunger' (cited in Haslam, 2007, p. 32). The connection between obesity and angina was emphasised in 1811 by Robert Thomas who wrote: 'It is found to attack men much more frequently than women, particularly those who have short necks, who are inclinable to corpulency, and who at the same time lead an inactive or sedentary life ... he should endeavour to counteract disposition to obesity, which has been considered a predisposing cause' (Thomas, 1811).

It was towards the end of the eighteenth and during the nineteenth century that lifestyle approaches to health in Western societies were subsumed in the battle to control infectious diseases. Developing industrial societies and their new, crowded, urban ways of living promoted the spread of infectious diseases such as smallpox and scarlet fever (Scambler, 2018). In reality, better sanitation, nutrition and living conditions led to the decline of infectious diseases, but at the same time as these public health measures were being instigated; doctors were simultaneously starting to understand that diseases such as smallpox and measles were caused by single infectious agents. Vaccines were developed against these, and people were protected from the associated diseases. Antibiotics to treat bacterial infections were discovered and on the back of these major discoveries the biomedical principle that all disease can be traced to specific causal mechanisms emerged and dominated the practice and development of medicine over the next century (Scambler, 2018). Many would argue that the biomedical model of disease remains the underlying principle behind the majority of medical practice in Western societies. However, in actuality, a number of models of disease and health (such as genetic, environmental and lifestyle models) influence medical practice and public health initiatives; it is just that the biomedical model usually takes prominence.

Infectious diseases declined throughout the twentieth and twenty-first centuries and in some cases have been completely eradicated. Nevertheless, epidemiologists and researchers who specialist in biosecurity and public health had been anticipating a major new viral infection and monitoring of new infections and risk analysis is continuous (UK Health Security Agency, 2023; Maxman, 2021). History is clear on this; more than six distinct influenza pandemics and epidemics have struck in just over a century. Ebola viruses have spilled over from animals 25 times in the past 5 decades. Basic surveillance needs to improve globally if we are going to see emerging infections early enough to contain them. According to the 2019 Global Health Security Index 70 countries are sorely lacking in the capacity to detect emerging epidemics and 130 countries have health systems that would be inadequate in an outbreak. Drug companies developed vaccines in record time during COVID-19 but there was still a long period when public health measures such as masks and isolation were the only available response.

Despite the COVID pandemic the major health problems for modern developed societies are still the chronic or so-called 'lifestyle diseases' identified by Doyle (2001). These chronic conditions are complex and cannot easily be traced to specific causal mechanisms. They are influenced at a number of levels—biologically, psychologically and sociologically. That is to say, the genes we inherit and the environment we inhabit are central to whether we go on to develop a chronic disease. Pivotal to the genetic and environmental circumstances of an individual is the way they respond to their environment and to their biological make-up. One individual may recognise that diabetes 'runs' in their family and make active choices to try to prevent it. Another with the same understanding of their family history may decide that it is inevitable that they will develop the disease and continue with damaging health choices. Similarly, one person may use smoking as a coping strategy to deal with the adverse environmental circumstances they find themselves in whereas the next may use exercise as a coping strategy. In this text we recognise that the socio-cultural circumstances in which an individual finds themselves can severely limit their lifestyle choices but we argue that usually some level of choice remains. This text explores how to encourage positive lifestyle change whilst recognising that the biological and environmental circumstances of each individual will vary enormously and have a large role to play in the degree of volitional choice each person has.

The biomedical model of disease is often characterised as curative but also has a preventative remit, albeit one that is frequently focused on vaccination or the avoidance of a specific causal organism. Chronic diseases are not generally something that you catch; rather they are a long-term response to stressors such as poor diet, lack of exercise, excess alcohol, high blood pressure, poverty or environmental hazards. Consequently, the lifestyle model of disease, first promoted by the Greeks/Romans, is once again taking precedence and influencing health policy. Interestingly, one impact of COVID-19 has been to increase measures to improve the health of the population, reduce obesity and increase physical fitness in order to make people more resilient to the symptoms of the infection (So & Kwon, 2022).

A lifestyle model of disease is very focused on prevention. Lifestyle changes are clearly still pertinent once a disease is diagnosed and can slow the progress of the disease and reduce complications, but fundamentally the principle of lifestyle change is to prevent disease. This can be viewed as a threat to the medical profession and to commercial companies that make a profit from curing disease. However, lifestyle approaches have their own commercial spin-offs, and the proliferation of private gyms and diet products is a visible sign of the commercial potential of a lifestyle approach to health and disease prevention.

Lifestyle approaches to health, whilst having the potential to generate profit for commercial operators, are attractive to governments because of the potential to shift the responsibility for health from the government to the individual. In this way, whilst some can see a way to profit from lifestyle approaches to health, the government can see a potential low-cost solution to health care. Many policy documents emphasise the role of individual choice in health-related behaviour and stress personal responsibility. There is a danger that this approach can be seen as a 'way out' for governments who can fairly cheaply provide individuals with the information they need to make informed choices about their lifestyle and leave them to get on with it. However, this is a short-sighted approach because when such tactics don't work the NHS is increasingly 'burdened' with the job of treating people who have developed chronic diseases. Indeed, many commentators remain concerned about the lifestyle approach to disease, arguing that by emphasising individual choice the huge social factors involved in inequities in health can be ignored.

It is certainly true that early responses to the evidence that chronic diseases are influenced by behaviour did focus on knowledge-based health promotion campaigns that left the individual to change their behaviour. However, the evidence from decades of educational health promotion is that it doesn't produce lifestyle change. Consequently, public health policy makers at all levels have made position statements about expanding the medical definition of 'lifestyle' to take into account the social nature of lifestyle behaviour (Ashton & Seymour, 1988; Bruce, 1991; Armstrong, 1993, cited in Hansen and Easthope, 2007). 'New public health', as it has been described, aims to discard health education initiatives in favour of enhancing people's life skills and creating supportive environments (McPearson, 1992; Ashton & Seymour, 1988). 'New public health' operates with a biopsychosocial understanding of health which requires education and lifestyle modification to be part of general public policy, the workplace and education, not restricted to health promotional campaigns (O'Conner and Parker, 1995, cited in Hansen & Easthope, 2007). The lifestyle model of disease, rather than being individualistic, can at its best enable individuals to take control of their health and influence policy to enable them to do so. The importance of supportive environments in promoting behavioural change has been emphasised recently by the impressive impact of the public smoking ban on rates of heart attacks, reduced by 10% in England and 14% in Scotland (Nursing Times, accessed 2009).

If we are to move away from a health promotion approach to lifestyle behaviour towards developing people's 'life skills', then a sound basis in the psychology of behavioural change will be necessary. To move from providing knowledge to improving the ability to change requires a psychological approach. We need to work with people within their current socio-economic resources whilst pressuring governments to provide the resources to enable change.

As recognised by the World Health Organisation (1986, 2021), lifestyle is more than simply an individual choice. The way we live is dictated by our economic and cultural circumstances (Frieden, 2010). Health lifestyle theory views health lifestyles as the intersection of 'life chances' and 'life choices' (Mollborn et al., 2020).

Indeed, the use of the term 'lifestyle change' reflects the importance of socio-demographic factors in health behaviour change rather better than the term 'health promotion'. Ethnicity, sex, gender, age, socio-economic circumstances and cultural groups all interplay to influence the way we choose to behave (Blaxter, 1990; Short & Mollborn, 2015; Mollborn et al., 2020). The evidence for socio-demographic influences on lifestyle choices is irrefutable (Craig & Mindell, 2008; Short & Mollborn, 2015; Mollborn et al., 2020).

The UK government and, more recently, the devolved institutions of Wales, Scotland and Northern Ireland have been collecting demographic mortality and morbidity data for some time, enabling comparisons between the health and health behaviours of different demographic and socio-economic groups. Each of these UK institutions has commissioned surveys on a continuing basis to enable comparisons between behaviours over time and to monitor health targets. The demographic data collected in each survey includes sex, age and socio-economic class. Each of these will be explored in the coming section to detail how these demographic factors can influence health and well-being so that the health care professional is able to recognise and understand the influence that some of these variables exert.

Both biological sex and gender are related to health and health outcomes, but it is generally accepted that gender has more of an influence than biological sex on lifestyle choices. Indeed, the gender influence on health is primarily mediated through lifestyle choices. Many studies confuse the terms sex and gender. Sex refers to the physical differences between people who are male, female or intersex. A person typically has their sex assigned at birth based on physiological characteristics, including genitalia and chromosome composition. Gender is how a person identifies. People may identify with the sex they were assigned at birth or with none at all. Gender identities include transgender, nonbinary and gender neutral. Gender also exists as a social construct with gender norms, so some behaviours may be considered appropriate for or indicative of sex and gender (Short & Mollborn, 2015).

A female born between 2018 and 2020 has a life expectancy of 82.9 years, a male 79 years (http://www.ons.gov.uk; accessed February 2023). Men and women also have different morbidity rates. Females are less likely to suffer from cardiovascular disease and more likely to suffer from breast cancer than males. Prostate cancer is a solely male disease as females do not have a prostate gland. Male and female differences in morbidity and mortality are influenced by biological sex (physiological and hormonal differences) but also by gender and gender role casting (Annandale & Hunt, 2000). The difference in male and female mortality rates is diminishing and this is generally held to be due to changing gender roles in Western societies rather than to biological factors, although early menarche may play a part in the rising prevalence of some female hormonally linked cancers. The relationship between gender and health is complex, with mortality differences favouring women but disparities in many morbidities favouring men. The influence of gender over health is mediated through the lifestyle choices that men and women make. However, Mollborn et al. (2020) have concluded that there are more variations in health lifestyle behaviours within genders than between; there are high levels of change across ages and the intersection of gender with age and socio-economic status is important.

Age is different from every other demographic variable in that the majority of us will experience old age. There are clear differences in health and health outcomes between different age categories and, unlike sex/gender differences, a large factor will be physiological changes over the lifespan rather than cultural expectations about age-related behaviour. Nevertheless, cultural expectations of how people of different ages should behave do play a role in the way that, for example, teenage mothers approach their pregnancies and older people participate in exercise and sport. Furthermore, even though presumably we must all hope to become older, older people experience considerable discrimination, which has implications for their health and well-being and for their lifestyle choices (Scambler, 2018; AgeUK, 2018). Hence, it is important to explore the impact of the cultural influences of age on lifestyle and health and this will be addressed in each of the lifestyle behaviour chapters.

Socio-economic is a broad term encompassing many variables and is assessed using a range of different factors. Social class, income, work, housing, and physical and social environments have all been found to influence our health directly and also indirectly through their influence on lifestyle choices (Doyle, 2001). The definition of social class adopted by this text has been provided by the seminal Black Report (Townsend & Davidson, 1989), which first clearly stated the link between health and social class in modern society:

Segments of the population sharing broadly similar types and levels of resources, with broadly similar styles of living and (for some sociologists), some shared perception of their collective condition.

In essence, different classes have differential power to access material resources: homes, cars, white and electronic goods, etc.

Explanations for behavioural choices are both contentious and politically sensitive. In 1989, Townsend and Davidson recognised that there were a number of explanations for differing levels of health in different sections of society. The key most plausible explanations are a materialist explanation and a behavioural explanation. Simply, a materialist explanation suggests that most of the class differences in health can be explained by the environmental circumstances in which individuals find themselves. A behavioural explanation suggests that most of the class differences in health can be explained by the choices that individuals make. At first sight, these explanations would seem to argue for different causes of disease but actually the distinction is more subtle. To use late-onset diabetes as an example, a behaviourist explanation would argue that a proportion of the class difference in diabetes morbidity can be explained by what individuals choose to eat. A materialist explanation does not refute the claim that diet is a major cause of late-onset diabetes but questions the degree of choice that individuals actually have about the food that they eat. More recently, Kraft and Kraft (2021) have argued that low socio-economic status is associated with increased levels of many types of acute and chronic stressors such as job insecurity, poor housing quality, heavy traffic and criminality. Under stress it is more difficult for people to practise healthy behaviours, as coping mechanisms are often unhealthy and focused on short-term gains rather than the longer-term gains of making healthy behavioural choices (Kraft & Kraft, 2021). Another way of considering behavioural choices is in terms of individual or collective responsibility. In the first case, the right of individuals to do as they wish with their own lives is emphasised; in the second, the inability of individuals to exert control over their environment is considered key (Blaxter, 1990). At first sight, a lifestyle model of health would appear to operate within behaviourist or individualistic explanations for lifestyle choices. However, for these authors the use of the term lifestyle behaviours rather than health behaviours is a deliberate attempt to recognise the role of socio-environmental factors in decisions individuals make about behaviours that impinge on their health. The challenge for health practitioners is to identify how to enable individuals to make positive changes to their lifestyle within the socio-economic circumstances in which they live. Kraft and Kraft (2021) would argue we have to address the stressors in people's lives if they are going to have any chance to be future-oriented and make healthy choices rather than choosing behaviours that help them cope with their acute stress. Even if we recognise that social and environmental circumstances are an integral aspect of lifestyle choice, we shouldn't rule out the possibility of effective behavioural change within those parameters. Clearly, a blanket-style approach to lifestyle change is unlikely to be successful and lifestyle interventions must be tailored to the circumstances in which individuals find themselves.

One popular way of describing the role of the environment in behavioural choice is to refer to obesogenic environments. The common use of the term obesogenic environment reflects the widening acceptance of the role of factors external to the individual in the development of obesity. The complexities of what contributes to an obesogenic environment are not well understood. We know that roads and cars promote sedentary modes of travel through their ease and convenience and discourage active transport by being a danger to pedestrians and cyclists, but cars also enable people to travel to leisure activities that support health and well-being. We understand that the easy availability of high-calorie food and the increasing portion size in restaurants promote over-eating of the 'wrong' types of food, but there is far greater availability of healthy food choices as well. Other factors such as shift working, alcohol and drug consumption, and media output all contribute to an obesogenic environment. The key to what makes an environment obesogenic would seem to be understanding and influencing the cultural responses we make to that environment (Jones et al., 2007).

Lifestyle behaviours have multiple functions; they are not simply or even primarily health focused. Lifestyle behaviours play a key role in developing and maintaining social relationships. They can be mood enhancing or a way of coping with stressful circumstances. Lifestyle behaviours are often pleasurable. Furthermore, the roles they play in our lives change during the lifespan. Lifestyle behaviours are all under some degree of volitional control, although the amount of control individuals have over their lifestyle choices is debatable and likely to vary a lot between people. The term lifestyle reflects that these are behaviours we do regularly and probably habitually. Negative lifestyle behaviours have most of their positive consequences in the present and most of their negative outcomes in the future. Any lifestyle behavioural change intervention consequently requires individuals to be future orientated. When you start to consider the complexity of lifestyle behaviours it becomes apparent why change is not as straightforward as it first appears.

It is true that, to some extent, the rise in chronic diseases is a reflection of the success of modern health care and social reform in that more people live long enough to experience the chronic conditions associated with old age. However, there is considerable evidence that, in addition, people take less exercise (Department of Health, 2011), drink more alcohol (HM Government, 2012), are less safe in their sexual practices (Center for Disease Control, 2007) and eat poorer diets (Fox & Hillsdon, 2007) than they did in previous recent generations. Smoking is the only lifestyle behaviour where incidence is declining, although a considerable minority of the population continue to smoke (Cancer Research UK, 2012). It is important to try to understand why unhealthy lifestyles have become so widespread, particularly since Western societies seem to be exporting these deleterious practices to developing nations (Wagner & Brath, 2011).

The lifestyles of societies are constantly evolving and will change in response to modernisation and social reform. We can see this in the different patterns of lifestyle choices in countries at different stages of modernisation and with different cultural norms (WHO, 1986). Life in modernised societies is easier and requires less physical effort than it did in previous generations (Department of Health, 2011; Fox & Hillsdon, 2007). Employment is more likely to be sedentary, housework is less demanding and far fewer people are physically active in the process of travelling. There is no evidence that people are less active in their leisure time than they were in previous generations, but because the majority of physical activity is now leisure, people's total physical activity has declined (Department of Health, 2004). The increase in cheap fast-food outlets, high-calorie snacks and ready-prepared meals all contribute to the poorer diets we eat today (Myslobodsky, 2003; Blouin et al., 2009). Alcohol has become considerably cheaper and is more readily available (Plant & Plant, 2006; Babor et al., 2010). Cultural acceptance of heavy drinking remains a stable facet of British life but there is some evidence that young people aged between 16 and 24 are less likely to drink than previous generations (MacLean et al., 2021). It is probably in terms of sexual behaviour that cultural expectations have altered most dramatically, with sex outside marriage and children out of wedlock virtually normalised in secular society (Schubotz et al., 2003). There are many positives from a more liberal attitude towards sex. It has enabled better education and communication about safe sex, empowering some women to control their sexual destinies and consequently protect themselves from sexual infection and unwanted pregnancy.

Beck (1990) coined the phrase 'risk society' to acknowledge that we live in a world where perceptions of risk are heightened, and the identification and management of risk are a major concern at all levels of society. Risk assessment in the workplace is now a legal requirement. Similarly, in schools and colleges all activities must be risk assessed, which may result in a reduction of school trips if procedures to mitigate the risk cannot be simply and cheaply instigated. Alongside risk assessment has emerged the concept of informed consent. Many professionals, health practitioners included, must ensure that they have the informed consent of an individual before embarking on a treatment programme or other intervention. All these procedures combine to create the impression that we live in a high-risk environment, when in reality we are probably safer from environmental hazards and disease than at any previous point in history. The perception of a high-risk environment is further perpetuated by the media who bombard us with 'risk' stories. Stories about crime, environmental and health risks dominate the media because they meet key news agendas in that they are negative and often sensational: 'Drinking a glass of wine a day increases your risk of breast cancer by 6%'. Lifestyle risks such as the risk of breast cancer from alcohol consumption are just some of a range of risks that we need to manage daily. For many people, the best way to deal with the plethora of risk messages that they receive on a daily basis is to ignore them (Thirlaway & Heggs, 2005).

Lifestyle behaviours are embedded in daily life. There are four aspects to most people's lives: sleeping, travelling, occupation and leisure (Buckworth & Dishman, 2002). However, it is impossible to describe a typical 24 hours for someone working in the UK. The complexities of modern life in terms of work patterns and outside responsibilities mean that fewer and fewer people work a 9-to-5 day. However, if you consider an average night's sleep to be about 8 hours, the average working day to be 8 hours and an average journey to and from work to be an hour then there are about 7 hours left a day for leisure and/or caring and household responsibilities. Obviously, many people will take longer to travel to work, sleep for longer or less, and have greater or fewer responsibilities outside of work, but most people will have some time each day that is not taken up with travelling, work, caring or sleeping. Many people work for longer than 8 hours at a time. People in the UK work some of the longest hours in Europe (TUC, 2019). Many people work fewer but longer days each week, e.g., those in the police force and nursing. Shift work is common, and it is associated with unhealthy lifestyle choices (Folkard et al., 2005; Lowden et al., 2010). Probably one of the major changes in daily living in the UK has been the increase in parents with young children who work (Office for National Statistics, 2011). This means that people are busy with household responsibilities outside of work that may previously have been completed during the day. In summary, given that the physically active nature of housework and shopping has reduced (Department of Health, 2004) and that there has been a reduction in time available for physically active pursuits, it is not surprising that changes in the pattern of a 'normal' day have had consequences for both lifestyle and health.

While we are travelling, we could be physically active, we could eat or smoke. However, smoking was banned in all public places, including public transport vehicles, in the UK in 2007. This is the first major piece of legislation for many years that pertains to volitional lifestyle behaviour and initially evidence emerged that the public ban had a significant positive effect on heart attack rates in the UK (Nursing Times, accessed 2009). In 2016, a Cochrane review concluded that the introduction of legislative smoking bans leads to improved health outcomes. The clearest outcome is from reduced admissions for acute coronary syndrome (Fraser et al., 2016).

For the majority of people, the trip to work, school or college is the most frequent journey. A minority of people take the opportunity to walk or cycle to their place of work or study, but the majority will drive or use public transport. Most adults do some walking, 71% of adults in England walk once a week (Hirst, 2020). The Department for Transport (2020) reported after increases in miles walked a year between 2015 to 2019 the annual miles walked fell in 2019 to 205 miles. Cycling miles also dropped in 2019 after gradually increasing since 2002. However, despite some gains in cycling distances since 2002, only 11% of people in the UK cycle and whilst walking is common for short journeys rates drop off when the journey is longer than a mile (Hirst, 2020). The UK continues to report some of the lowest levels of walking and cycling in Europe, ranking 11th (out of 28) in 2013.

Work and caring for relatives are the primary occupations for most people and most jobs these days are predominantly sedentary (Department of Health, 2004; Heron et al., 2019). Similarly, most caring roles do not involve physical activity, although they can require heavy lifting. At work, most people will eat at least one meal and the quality of available food will influence the food choices. Evidence about the relationship between the proximity of fast-food outlets to the workplace and what people eat is mixed (van Rongen et al., 2020). There is little evidence about the influence of on-site food provision in the workplace on food choice, although the healthy workplace initiatives in Scotland (Scotland Health Improvement Agency, accessed 2009) and Wales (Welsh Assembly Government, accessed 2009) were designed to improve on-site food choice. The majority of work on on-site provision of food has been carried out with children. Prior to 2006, unhealthy food choices have dominated school food sales in the UK but the impact of new nutritional standards in schools in September 2006 have resulted in significant improvements in the nutritional content of school lunches (Spence et al., 2013).

Whilst drinking alcohol at work is extremely rare, the workplace culture of drinking outside of working hours has been found to be significantly related to both drinking with work colleagues and non-work-related drinking (Delaney & Ames, 1995; Barrientos-Gutierrez et al., 2007). The establishment of healthy drinking norms in the workplace could have beneficial effects for drinking both with work colleagues and more widely.

Patterns of leisure activity have changed dramatically with the development of sedentary activities such as watching television, using computers and the myriad of electronic game consoles available. The relationship between time spent in such sedentary leisure activities and reductions in time spent in physically active leisure pursuits has been, and still is, the subject of much concern, particularly in children (Department of Health, 2011). At the same time, the number of health clubs and gyms has proliferated and a small increase in the proportion of people taking leisure-time physical activity has been reported (Department of Health, 2004). Television cookery programmes are popular but it would seem that watching cookery programmes rather than actually cooking is the popular leisure pursuit! Other popular leisure activities such as going to the cinema are associated with unhealthy food availability and large portion sizes. Similarly, recent studies have highlighted the increase in portion sizes of meals served in restaurants (Steenhuis & Vermeer, 2009). Hence, leisure activities themselves can lead to an increase in unhealthy lifestyles.

Conclusion

The world we live in is both the safest yet and a highly risky place, and probably the biggest risk to health, for most people, is the lifestyle choices that they make. However, most of us continue to be concerned about dramatic risks such as aeroplane crashes but continue to ignore the far more likely risks associated with a lifetime of smoking, eating and drinking too much and remaining sedentary. Education has little impact on people's failure to respond to risk. Choices about eating, drinking, smoking or physical activity are possible, although not for everyone in every context. Enabling choice, supporting choice, empowering choice is what all health practitioners want to achieve, and understanding how best to do this is what this book is about.

Key points

- The major lifestyle diseases are coronary heart disease, stroke, lung cancer, colon cancer, diabetes and chronic obstructive pulmonary disease.
- Unhealthy lifestyles have arisen as a response to modern society.
- We understand the risks associated with unhealthy lifestyle behaviours probably better than at any other time in history but we still fail to make appropriate changes to our behaviour.
- Lifestyle change is more difficult for some people than others, depending on their socio-demographic and environmental circumstances.
- Lifestyle behaviours are complex, which makes instigating change similarly complex and difficult.

Discussion points

The success of the ban on smoking in public places has made some commentators suggest that we should ban certain types of unhealthy food. What are the complications involved in banning certain food stuffs?

To what extent should lifestyle change be an individual choice or imposed on people through policy and legislation?

Practising an unhealthy lifestyle is more common in people living in deprivation. How can we make healthy lifestyles more accessible to all?

References

AgeUK. (2018). Ageism and age equality (Great Britain): Policy position paper. www.ageUK.org.uk

Annandale, E., & Hunt, K. (2000). Gender inequalities in health. Buckingham: Open University Press.

Ashton, J., & Seymour, H. (1988) The new public health: The Liverpool experience. Milton Keynes: Open University Press.

Babor, T. F., Caetano, R., Casswell, S., Edwards, G., Giesbrecht, N., Graham, K., ... & Rossow, I. (2010). Alcohol: No ordinary commodity: Research and public policy: Research and public policy. Oxford: Oxford University Press

Barrientos-Gutierrez, T., Gimeno, D., Mangiane, T. W., Harrist, R. B., & Amick, B. C. (2007). Drinking social norms and drinking behaviours. Occupational and Environmental Medicine, *64*, 602–608.

BBC News. (2006). Blair calls for lifestyle change. www.news.bbc.co.uk

Beck, U. (1990). Risk society: Towards a new modernity. London: Sage.

Blaxter, M. (1990). Health and lifestyles. London: Sage.

Blouin, C., Chopra, M., & van der Hoeven, R. (2009). Trade and health 3: Trade and the social determinants of health. Lancet, *373*(9662), 502–507.

Bruce, N. (1991) Epidemiology and the new public health: Implications for training. Social Science and Medicine, *32*(1), 103–106.

Buckworth, J., & Dishman, R. (2002). Exercise psychology. London: Human Kinetics.

Burke, V., Milligan, R. A., Beilin, L. J., Dunbar, D., Spencer, M., Balde, E., & Gracey, M. P. (1997). Clustering of health-related behaviours among 18 year old Australians. Preventative Medicine, *26*, 724–733.

Cancer Research UK. (2012). Percentage of population who smoke. Available at: http://www.cancerresearchuk.org/cancer-info/cancerstats/types/lung/smoking/lung-cancer-and-smoking-statistics#history

Center for Disease Control. (2007). Healthy Youth! Sexual Risk Behaviours. Available at: http://www.cdc.gov/HealthyYouth/sexualbehaviors/index.htm (accessed 20 December 2007).

Craig, R., & Mindell, J. (2008). Health survey for England 2006. Volume 1: Cardiovascular disease and risk factors in adults. London: The Information Centre.

Delaney, W. P., & Ames, G. (1995). Work team attitudes, drinking norms and workplace drinking. Journal of Drug Issues, *25*, 275.

Department of Health. (2010). Our health and wellbeing today. London: Department of Health.

Department of Health. (2011). Start active, Stay active: A report on physical activity for health from the four home countries' Chief Medical Officers. London: Department of Health.

Department of Health. (2004). At least five a week: Evidence on the impact of physical activity and its relationship to health. London: Department of Health.

Department for Transport. (2020). Gear change: A bold vision for cycling and walking. London: DfT Publications. www.gov.uk/dfdt.

Doyle, R. (2001). Lifestyle blues. Scientific American, *284*, 30.

Egger, G. J., Binns, A. F., & Rossner, S. R. (2009). The emergence of "lifestyle medicine" as a structured approach for management of chronic disease. Medical Journal of Australia, *190*(3), 143.

Egger, G. J., Binns, A., & Rossner, S. (2011). Lifestyle medicine: Managing diseases of lifestyle in the 21st century. Australia: McGraw-Hill Education.

Folkard, S., Lombardi, D. A., & Tucker, P. T. (2005). Shiftwork: Safety, sleepiness and sleep. Industrial Health, *43*, 20–23.

Fox, K. R., & Hillsdon, M. (2007). Physical activity and obesity. Obesity Reviews, *8*(Suppl. 1), 115–121.

Fraser, K., Callinan, J. E., McHugh, J., van Baarsal, S., Clarke, A., Doherty, K., & Kelleher, C. (2016). Legislative smoking bans for reducing harms from secondhand smoke exposure, smoking prevalence and tobacco consumption. Cochrane Reviews. Doi: 10.1002/1465185 8.CD005992.pub3

Frieden, T. R. (2010). A framework for public health action: The health impact pyramid. Journal Information, *100*(4), 590–595.

Gard, M., & Wright, J. (2005). The obesity epidemic: Science, morality and ideology. London: Routledge/Taylor & Francis Group.

Hansen, E., & Easthope, G. (2007). Lifestyle in medicine. London: Routledge.

Haslam, D. (2007). Obesity: A medical history. Obesity Reviews, *8*(Suppl. 1), 31–36.

Heron, L., O'Neill, C., McAneney, H., Kee, F., & Tully, M.A. (2019). Direct healthcare costs of sedentary behaviour in the UK. Journal of Epidemiology and Community Health, *73*, 625–629.

HM Government. (2012). The government alcohol strategy. London: The Home Office. Available at: http://www.homeoffice.gov.uk/publications/alcohol-drugs/

Hirst, D. (2020). Briefing paper 8615: Active Travel: Trends, policy and funding. www.parliament.uk/commons-librarypapers@parliament.uk@commonslibrary

Jeffery, R. W., Baxter, J. E., McGuire, M. T., & Linde, J. A. (2006). Are fast food restaurants an environmental risk factor for obesity? International Journal of Behaviour, Nutrition and Physical Activity, *3*, 2.

Jones, A., Bentham, G., Foster, C., Hillsdon, M., & Panter, J. (2007). Tackling obesities: Future choices – Obesogenic environments – Evidence review. London: United Kingdom Government Foresight Programme, Office of Science and Innovation. Crown Copyright.

Kraft, P., & Kraft, B. (2021). Explaining socioeconomic disparities in health behaviours: A review of biopsychological pathways involving stress and inflammation. Neuroscience and Biobehavioural Reviews, *127*, 689–708. Doi: 10.1016/j.neubiorev2021.05.019

Lowden, A., Moreno, C., Holmbäck, U., Lennernäs, M., & Tucker, P. (2010). Eating and shift work-effects on habits, metabolism and performance. Scandinavian Journal of Work, Environment and Health, *36*(2), 150–162.

Maxman, A. (2021). Has COVID taught us anything about pandemic preparedness? News Feature *Nature* www.nature.com

MacLean, S. J., Pennay, A., Caluzzi, G., Holmes, J., & Torronen, J. (2021). Why are young people drinking less than their parents' generation did? The Conversation.

McPearson, P. D. (1992). Health for all Australians. In H. Gardner (Ed.), Health Policy. Melbourne: Churchill Livingstone.

Migchelsen, S., Sonubi, T., Ratna, N., Harb, A. K., Enayat, Q., Anderson, A., Charles, H., Green, F., Dunn, J., Shaw, D., Walker, S., Sinka, K., Folkard, K., Mohammed, H., & Contributors. (2022). *Sexually transmitted infections and screening for Chlamydia in England*. London: UK Health Security Agency.

Mollborn, S., Lawrence, E. M., & Hummer, R.A. (2020) A gender framework of understanding Health lifestyles. Social Science and Medicine, *265*. 10.1016/j.socscimed.2020.113182

Myslobodsky, M. (2003) Gorurmand savants and environmental determinants of obesity. Obesity Reviews, *4*, 121–128.

Nursing Times. (2009). www.nursingtimes.net (accessed 2009).

Office for National Statistics. (2011). Social Trends. Mothers in the labour market 2011. Newport ONS.

Plant, M., & Plant, M. (2006). Binge Britain. Oxford: Oxford University Press.

Scambler, G. (Ed.). (2018). Sociology as applied to medicine, 7th Ed. London: Bloomsbury Publishing

Schubotz, D., Simpson, A., & Rolston, B. (2003). Towards better sexual health: A survey of sexual attitudes and lifestyles of young people in Northern Ireland. Research Report. Belfast: FPA in Partnership with the University of Ulster.

Scotland Health Improvement Agency. Health improvement agency. http://www.healthscotland.com/ (accessed 23 November 2009).

Short, S. E., & Mollborn, S. (2015). Social determinants and health behaviours: Conceptual frames and empirical advances. Current Opinion in Psychology, 5, 78–84.

Steenhuis, I. H., & Vermeer, W. M. (2009). Portion size: Review and framework for interventions International Journal of Behavioral Nutrition and Physical Activity, 6, 58.

Spence, S., Delve, J., Stamp, E., Matthews, J. N. S., White, M., & Adamson, A. J. (2013). The impact of food and nutrient-based standards on primary school children's lunch and total dietary intake: A natural experimental evaluation of government policy in England. PLoS ONE, 8(10), e78298.

So, B., & Kwon, K. H. (2022). The impact of physical activity on well-being, lifestyle and health promotion in an era of COVID-19 and SARS-CoV-2 variant. Postgraduate Medicine, 134(4). 10.1080/00325481.2022.2052467

Thirlaway, K. J., & Heggs, D. (2005). Interpreting risk messages: Women's responses to a health story. Health, Risk and Society, 7, 107–121.

Thomas, R. (1811). The modern practice of Physic. New York: Collins and Co.

Townsend, P., & Davidson, N. (1989) Inequalities in health: The black report. Harmondsworth: Penguin.

TUC. (2019). British workers putting in longest hours in the EU. www.TUC.org.uk

UK Health Security Agency. (2023). Guidance: Emerging infections: How and why they arise. www.gov.uk

Van Rongen, S., Poelman, M. P., Thornton, L., Abbott, G., Lu, M., Kamphuis, C. B. M. Verkooijen, K., & de Vet, E. (2020). Neighbourhood fast food exposure and consumption: The mediating role of neighbourhood social norms. International Journal of Behavioural Nutrition and Physical Activity, 17(61). Doi: 10.1186/s12966-020-00969-w

Wagner, K. H., & Brath, H. (2011). A global view on the development of non communicable diseases. Preventive Medicine, 54(Suppl), S38–S41.

Wardle, J., & Steptoe, A. (2005). Public health psychology. The Psychologist, 18, 672–675.

Wales Online. (2023). 'Exercise more to save the Welsh NHS' says health minister. www.walesonline.co.uk

Wardle, J., & Steptoe, A. (2004). Health-related behaviour: Prevalence and links with disease. In A Kaptein & J Weinman (Eds.), Health Psychology (pp. 21–51), Oxford: Blackwell Publishing.

Welsh Assembly Government (accessed 2009). http://new.wales.gov.uk/topics/health/improvement/healthatwork/corporate-standard/?lang=en

Wiseman, M. (2009). www.wcrf-uk.org

World Health Organisation (Health Education Unit). (1986). Lifestyles and health. Social Science in Medicine, 22, 117–124.

World Health Organisation. (2021). Designing cities for health: How to change urban environments for the better? News Release. www.who.int

2 Health promotion

Case Study

Jemma is a secondary school Physical Education (PE) teacher working in a school in the suburbs of a large city. The secondary school has a Free School Meals (FSM) percentage that is above the national average and is considered a deprived area with a low socioeconomic status. Over the past few years Jemma has become increasingly concerned about the health, wellbeing, and physical activity levels of the pupils in her school. Very few pupils walk to school; the majority are dropped off in a car or bus. She is aware that there are a sizeable number of pupils (particularly girls) who do not enjoy PE lessons who are also sedentary at break and dinner time. Another concern is the diet of the pupils across the whole school. Jemma knows that many of the pupils in her school are living in poverty and often come to school hungry. In a recent school project about food, the majority of pupils reported disliking fruit and vegetables and nearly half were reluctant to try any during the project. Over the past decade, there has been a noticeable increase in pupil referrals to mental health and wellbeing services. All teaching assistants in her school have undertaken emotional literacy support assistant (ELSA) training, to better support young people's wellbeing. Finally, there has been a significant increase in the use of e-cigarettes by pupils across all year groups, with vape

DOI: 10.4324/9781003471233-2

detectors being fitted in all school toilets to try and minimise this health concern. Jemma and her colleagues in the school would like to try and promote healthy behaviours including healthy eating, physical activity, improved wellbeing, and reduction of vaping in their school, but recognise for many families living on low incomes that diet and physical activity are hard to prioritise. Jemma has been tasked with exploring what support there is in their area for promoting a healthier school. She has been asked to draw up a proposal for an intervention to present to the school governors. Jemma is now looking for advice from the local public health team, sport development department and the local education authority about what interventions might be feasible and sustainable for the school to adopt.

Introduction

The World Health Organization (WHO) in 1986 defined health promotion as:

The process of enabling people to increase control over, and to, improve, their health.

WHO (2023)

There are two elements to health promotion: the **process** of empowerment and the **aim** of improving health. In theory, the process of empowerment leads to improvements in health, but we need to recognise that this assumes that individuals and communities wish to improve their health. The WHO Ottawa Charter for Health Promotion in 1986 is still considered the 'gold standard' for health promoters worldwide who wish to improve health and reduce inequalities. However, the opportunities to transfer these principles into practical solutions have been largely missed (Thompson et al., 2018). The charter identifies health promotion action areas:

1 Build health public policy
2 Create supportive environments
3 Develop personal skills
4 Strengthen community action
5 Re-orient health services

WHO (1986)

Health promotion is about improving the health of communities as a whole and that of the individuals within those communities. Communities can be defined by their geographical, demographic or cultural characteristics. So a particular city council may decide to promote active transport in their city and target all the inhabitants. Alternatively, a charity such as Diabetes UK may decide to promote walking to the diabetic community. Often the aim may be to reach a particular community of individuals, but the intervention may be at the level of the community, individualised or indeed a combination of both types of strategies.

It is important to recognise that health promotion, for the WHO, should be focused on reducing health inequalities. At the 1988 WHO International Conference on Health Promotion, a target to reduce health inequalities by 25% by the year 2000 was set. By

2005, it was clear that this target had not been achieved, and the WHO set up the Commission on Social Determinants of Health to marshal the evidence on what can be done to promote health equity and to foster a global movement to do better (WHO, 2008). The latest target is to close the gap in a generation. In 2020, WHO reiterated its commitment and focus on inequalities and social determinants of health with strategic objective 7:

Address the underlying social & economic determinants of health through policies and programmes that enhance health equality and integrate pro-poor, gender-responsive, and human rights-based approaches

WHO (2020)

The global focus on reducing health inequalities through health promotion is reflected in all UK policy. In 2021, the UK government set up the Office for Health Improvement and Disparities to focus on:

… levelling up health disparities to break the link between background and prospects for a healthy life.

Office for Health Improvement and Disparities (2023)

The strategies of all the four UK government bodies responsible for health promotion: Public Health England (2020), Public Health Wales (2022), Public Health Scotland (2022) and Department of Health, Social Science & Public Safety (2014) reflect a similar commitment to reducing inequalities. For example, Public Health England states that:

… . we work to narrow the health gap. There is still a huge disparity in the number of years lived in poor health between the most and least deprived people across the country. Many conditions also take a disproportionate toll on minority communities. Our work aims to reduce these unjust and avoidable inequalities in health outcomes.

Public Health England (2020)

It is sobering to reflect that, instead of reducing health inequalities through our health promotion policies, strategies, interventions, and practice over the past three decades, the evidence suggests we have made no inroads on health equalities and in some areas, inequalities may be widening. A recent bulletin from the Office of National Statistics (2022) reported that from 2018 to 2020 both sexes have seen statistically significant increases in the inequality in life expectancy at birth between 2015 and 2017. Equally concerning is the gap in disability-free life expectancy between people living in the least and most deprived areas which in England was 17.6 years for men and 16.8 years for women (Office of National Statistics, 2022). Gaps in disability-free life expectancy of similar magnitude persist across the whole of the UK and the implications for health and social care are starting to impact dramatically as seen by the reporting of the pressures on the NHS during the winter of 2022/23 (Kings Fund, 2023). It has been argued that rather than reducing health inequalities, health promotion interventions can increase them. Those who are more affluent and have a higher level of formal education are more likely to modify their diets, give up smoking and increase levels of physical activity than are the less affluent with lower levels of formal education (Buck & Frosini, 2012). In 2012, Buck and Frosini in a report for the Kings Fund described how engagement with unhealthy lifestyle behaviours was decreasing but that these reductions have been seen mainly among those in higher socioeconomic and educational groups. They found that people with no qualifications were more than five times as likely as those with higher education to engage in all four *poor* behaviours in 2008, compared with only three times as likely in 2003.

Health promotion is not solely or even predominantly focused on lifestyle behaviours but also includes issues such as: accident prevention, road safety, immunisation against infectious disease, food safety, support for individuals with learning disabilities to live in the community and supporting patients in adhering to medical advice and treatments (WHO, 2009). Health promotion has previously been described as having two main activities (Shriven, 2017):

1 Providing services for people who are ill or who have a disability
2 Positive health activities which are about personal, social and environmental changes aimed at preventing ill health, developing healthier living conditions and lifestyles

However, this distinction can create an artificial divide between people who are disabled or have a diagnosis of an illness and those who are currently free from disability or a diagnosed condition. Having a disability does not necessarily lead to ill health and many people with disabilities and chronic conditions are interested in leading healthy lifestyles (Kroll et al., 2006; Heggdal et al., 2023). Many people with a diagnosed chronic condition would describe themselves as healthy and are committed to preventing any deterioration of their health (Hobbis et al., 2011). Individuals with Type 2 diabetes are a good example of this. They have a diagnosis of an illness that in itself may not impact their quality of life particularly during the early stages (Department of Health, 1999). Indeed, it may require no medical treatment and may be managed solely through lifestyle modification. However, they are a community who are at high risk of developing other associated diseases that arise from the damage that high levels of circulating blood glucose can cause to cells (see Chapter 10, Special Conditions) and are an important group for health promotion to target as many health gains are possible through lifestyle modification (Herman et al., 2015).

Health promotion is a complex activity and clarity about its precise meaning and the role of related activities such as health education, health improvement, health protection and health prevention are not consistently defined or understood. The WHO in 2012 described health promotion as involving a combination of health education activities and the adoption of healthy public policies and their diagrammatic representation of the relationship between the major health concepts is a useful starting point for under-standing what health promotion involves (WHO, 2012).

Health improvement

Public Health generally works across three areas: health improvement, service improve-ment and health protection and health promotion is involved in all three. The focus of this book, which is lifestyle behaviours, is very clearly health improvement and across the UK the words promotion and improvement are used interchangeably. It is clear though that lifestyle behavioural change could deliver improvements in health and longer life expectancy whereas other more protective health promotion activities such as vaccina-tion schemes are more about maintaining health.

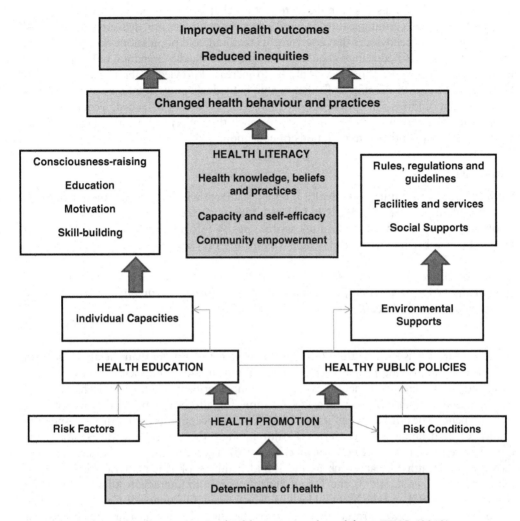

Figure 2.1 Relationship between major health concepts adapted from WHO (2012).

Health education

Health education activities are a central strategy to achieve the goals of health promotion. Health education has been defined by the WHO (2012) as:

> *Consciously constructed opportunities for learning involving some form of communication designed to improve health literacy, including improving knowledge and developing life skills which are conducive to individual and community health.*
>
> WHO (2012)

Health education, at its broadest and best, involves educational, motivational, skill-building and consciousness-raising techniques (Figure 2.1). However, too often it is solely educational and too focused on communicating risks and benefits which is now well established to have little influence on lifestyle change (Thirlaway & Upton, 2009;

Whitehead, 2001). As discussed in the introductory chapter of this book, decades of health education and risk communication-focused interventions have not delivered the targeted changes in lifestyle behaviours that governments required, and populations needed. In 2012, the WHO argued that education should not be limited to the dissemination of health-related information. Its purpose should not only be to increase knowledge about personal health behaviour but also to develop skills that enable individuals and communities to engage in activities that address the physical, psychological, behavioural, social, economic, and environmental determinants of their health. As such the concept of health education is far broader than many other interpretations of education.

Health literacy

Similarly to Health Education, Health Literacy is a term with no one accepted definition; it is an evolving concept (Rudd, 2015). Health Literacy is frequently defined as the ability to obtain, process, understand and use written health information. However, the WHO (2012) takes a broader view and defines Health Literacy as:

> *The cognitive and social skills which determine the motivation and ability of individual to gain access to, understand and use information in ways which promote and maintain good health.*

> WHO (2012)

Health Literacy is seen by the WHO (2012) as something more than the ability to read and write. By improving people's access to health information, and their capacity to use it effectively, health literacy is viewed as crucial to empowerment (Figure 2.1). Defined in this way, improved Health Literacy is a key outcome for any health promotion activity but measurement of health literacy in its broadest WHO conception is a challenge. Despite the challenges in defining and measuring Health Literacy there has been an extraordinary growth of research in this area (Nutbeam et al., 2018). There are now a plethora of available measures of Health Literacy such as the Rapid Estimate of Adult Literacy in Medicine (REALM) (Davis et al., 1993), the Test of Functional Health Literacy in Adults (TOFHLA) (Parker et al., 1995) and the Mental Health Literacy Scale (O'Connor & Casey, 2015). The REALM is a 66-item word recognition and pronunciation test that measures the domain of vocabulary. The TOFHLA measures reading fluency. Neither of these measures attempts to assess general health knowledge; which is clearly an aspect of the WHO definition of health literacy. However, as Rudd (2015) reminds us, poor literacy skills however measured, predict health outcomes. Rudd (2015) has argued that too much focus has been placed on improving the health literacy of individuals at the expense of ensuring health materials are readable by all sections of the intended audience:

> *We cannot continue to allow the proliferation and dissemination of poorly developed and ill designed health materials and messages.*

> Rudd (2015)

The literacy skills of the audience and the communication skills of professionals both need addressing and the responsibility for understanding the message cannot sit solely with the recipients. The conceptual idea that health literacy can empower individuals and enable them to improve their health rather than it simply being a proxy measure of broader social deprivation that is the causal factor in poorer health outcomes is a popular and attractive idea (Muscat et al., 2016). However, the relationship between improving Health Literacy and reducing health disparities is yet to be clearly demonstrated (Mantwill et al., 2015).

Social capital

Social Capital is a concept developed to formalise and acknowledge the role that the cultural norms and informal networks that exist in communities can play in the economic viability and health of communities. It was defined by the Government Performance and Innovation Unit in 2002 as:

> *The networks, norms, relationships, values and informal sanctions that shape the quantity and co-operative quality of a society's social interactions.*
>
> Performance and Innovation Unit (2002)

Building Social Capital may be one way of empowering communities to improve their health and for the WHO it is a key aspect of health literacy (Figure 2.1). Shared values and normative beliefs can shape the way that health promotion is perceived and understood by individuals within different communities. The potential that building Social Capital offers for using community and civic pathways to promote and improve health has been promoted by some as a useful means of tackling inequalities in health (Morgan & Swann, 2004; Dauner et al., 2015).

Understanding what Social Capital is and how to measure it in communities is difficult (Agampodi et al., 2015). Communities are hard to define; they are fluid and perceived differently by the various individuals within them. Many people are members of more than one community. Furthermore, different professional groups view Social Capital differently, measure it differently and will try and build it within communities differently as well. So policy makers and political scientists may view Social Capital in terms of activism and wish to promote activism within communities. Whereas, teachers, social workers, community workers and sociologists may take a more structural view looking at the networks and community groups that exist within a defined community. Psychologists, tend to take a more individualised view of Social Capital focusing on the relationships that people have been able to establish within a community. Agampodi et al. (2015) reviewed the methods available to measure Social Capital in low and middle-income countries and concluded that more individual constructs of Social Capital such as trust, social cohesion, and a sense of belonging had a positive association with measured health outcomes. The links between social relationships, social support, social isolation and health are well established across many different communities (Kumar et al., 2012; Uchino, 2009; Agampodi et al., 2015; Dauner et al., 2015) but community-level interventions to improve Social Capital are often focused on local resource improvement or the development of community groups and the way these feed an individual's social support networks is not well understood (Morgan & Swann, 2004; Agampodi et al., 2015).

Social marketing

Social Marketing was first named and introduced in the 1970s by Kotler and Zaltman (1971). In their seminal paper, Kotler and Zaltman (1971) argue that marketing concepts and techniques that are commonly used to sell commodities and goods may be effectively applied to promote health and social change in areas such as driving safely and family planning. Since its introduction, social marketing has been defined as:

> *A process that applies marketing principles and techniques to create, communicate, and deliver value in order to influence target audience behaviours that benefit society as well as the target audience.*

Cheng et al. (2010, p. 2)

Although similar in principle to traditional marketing methods, Social Marketing is different because it is used to achieve specific behaviour change for the good of society as well as the target group whose behaviour it is aiming to influence. Its focus is to enable, encourage and support behavioural change and/or maintenance and this will often involve the development or re-structuring of services to support and facilitate this change (Coutinho Da Silva & Mazzon, 2016; French et al., 2009). Its efficacy as a framework for behaviour change interventions has been demonstrated across a range of behaviours (Stead et al., 2007; Carin & Rundle-Theile, 2014; Fujihira et al., 2015). Social Marketing has the potential to achieve behavioural change across different contexts and levels of influence, including the individual, environment and wider policy levels (Stead et al., 2007). Its utility as an approach to behaviour change is therefore diverse. Andreasen (2002) established six benchmark criteria for social marketing (Table 2.1). Research has shown that employing all six benchmark criteria offers the greatest potential to change behaviours, but few interventions use all six (Carin & Rundle, 2014; Fujihira et al., 2015).

The fourth social marketing criteria (Table 2.1) makes reference to the principles derived from commercial marketing, in particular the marketing mix strategies, otherwise termed the 4Ps:

Table 2.1 Benchmark criteria for social marketing

Social marketing criteria

1 **Behaviour change** – the intervention seeks to change behaviour and has specific measurable behavioural objectives.
2 **Consumer research** – formative research is conducted to identify consumer characteristics and needs. Interventions are pre-tested with the target group.
3 **Segmentation and targeting** – different segmentation variables are used, and a strategy tailored to the segments.
4 **Marketing mix** – the intervention must consist of communications plus at least one other of the four 'P's' – Product, Price, Place, Promotion.
5 **Exchange** – the intervention considers what will motivate people to engage voluntarily with the intervention and offers them something beneficial in return, either tangible or intangible.
6 **Competition** – the intervention considers the appeal of competing behaviours (including the current behaviour) and includes strategies to decrease competition.

Source: Adapted from Andreasen (2002).

1 Product (e.g., condoms; quit smoking kits; screening tests; breastfeeding practice)
2 Price (e.g., monetary cost; time or effort; risk of embarrassment/disapproval)
3 Place (distribution of product)
4 Promotion (e.g., advertising; public relations; personal selling; public service announcements)

Kotler and Lee (2008) explain that social marketing aims to influence the target audience's behaviour in four different ways:

1 *Accepting* a new behaviour (e.g., joining a gym)
2 *Rejecting* a potential undesirable behaviour (e.g., unsafe sex)
3 *Modifying* a current behaviour (e.g., increasing daily fruit and vegetable consumption)
4 *Abandoning* an established undesirable behaviour (e.g., quitting smoking)

Social Marketing has been used extensively in health promotion programmes both at national and international levels. In the UK, campaigns that have applied social marketing to increase the adoption of healthy behaviours for target populations have included the Change4life campaign, which aimed to reduce childhood obesity by eating well and moving more (Department of Health, 2009); Food Dudes, which aims to increase fruit and vegetable consumption in primary school-aged children (Horne et al., 2009); and England's National Marketing Strategy for Tobacco Control (2007–2010).

Cheng et al. (2010) have clearly outlined how the principles and techniques within Social Marketing have been successfully applied in practice over the years. These broadly include:

1 Health promotion-related behavioural issues:
   Obesity; teen pregnancy; tobacco use; breastfeeding; sensible drinking
2 Injury prevention-related behavioural issues:
   Domestic violence; drink driving campaigns; seatbelt use
3 Environmental protection-related behavioural issues:
   Waste recycling; water conservation; air pollution from cars
4 Community mobilisation-related behavioural issues:
   Organ donation; blood donation; childhood immunisation
                              Kotler and Lee (2008) in Cheng et al. (2010, p. 3)

However, care must be taken when designing health promotion campaigns using Social Marketing techniques because it is possible to unintentionally reach a different audience and/or change behaviour in an unexpected direction. One example of this is a sensible drinking campaign aimed at young adults that, rather than encouraging heavy drinkers to drink less, encouraged light drinkers to drink more (Wechsler et al., 2003). More about this intervention can be found in Chapter 7, Sensible Drinking.

Who delivers health promotion?

The simplest but perhaps least helpful answer to this question is everyone. The health of the public is the concern of the whole of society and all members of society have a stake in the health of the Nation, Communities or Groups to which they belong. Indeed it is this philosophy of health being the responsibility of everyone within a community that has driven the interest in Social Capital and its relationship to health. The sharing of beliefs, knowledge and skills is crucial to the lifestyle decisions individuals make and the habits they develop. Every individual within a community or group will contribute to that shared understanding whether it is teaching boy scouts how to play hockey or introducing friends or family to a new food at a meal. However, formal health promotion activities in the UK, as they do in many other countries, come under the remit of Public Health. The WHO defines Public Health as:

All organised measures (whether public or private) to prevent disease, promote health and prolong life among the population as a whole

WHO HQ (accessed 2023)

Public health works in three spheres (Griffiths et al., 2005; Sin, 2020):

Health Improvement (inequalities, education, housing, employment, family/community, lifestyles, surveillance and monitoring of specific diseases and risk factors)

Improving services (clinical effectiveness, efficiency, service planning, audit and evaluation, clinical governance, equity)

Health protection (infectious diseases, chemical and poisons, radiation, emergency response, environmental health hazards)

It is clear that whilst health promotion may be relevant in all three spheres, lifestyle behavioural change, which is the focus of this book, falls predominantly in the sphere of health improvement.

Health promotion and health improvement both require a wide range of competencies and are multi-disciplinary activities involving people from many professions and backgrounds. In essence there are four levels of involvement in health promotion/improvement (see Figure 2.2).

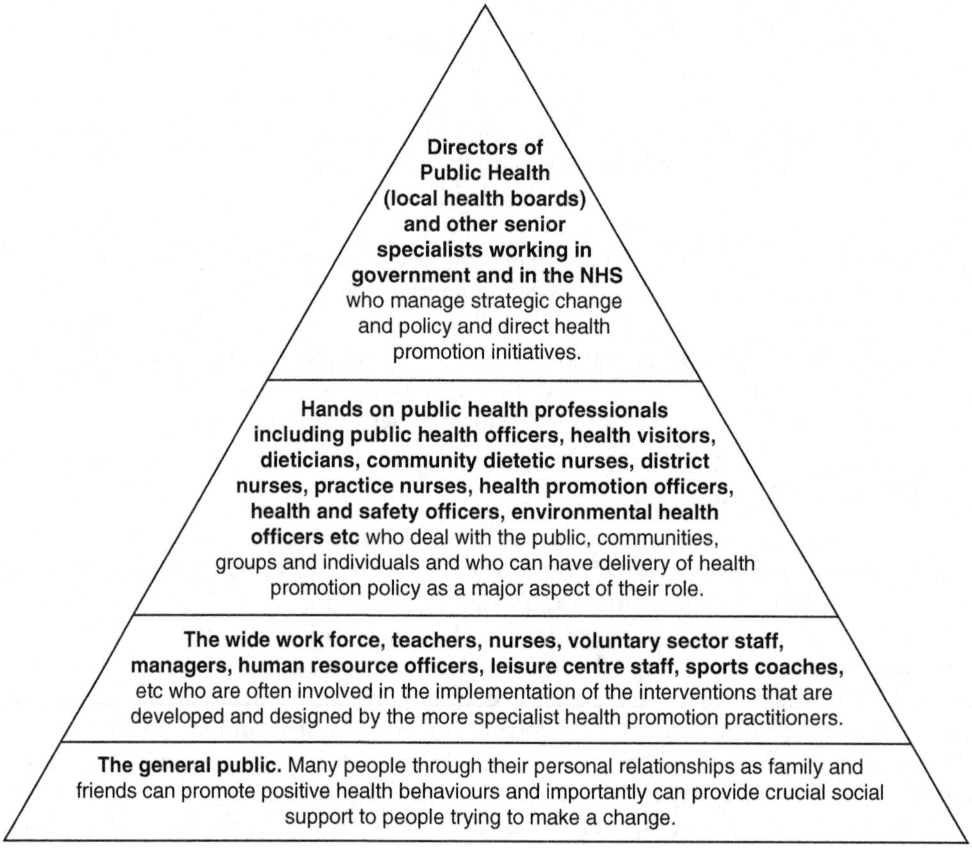

Directors of Public Health (local health boards) and other senior specialists working in government and in the NHS who manage strategic change and policy and direct health promotion initiatives.

Hands on public health professionals including public health officers, health visitors, dieticians, community dietetic nurses, district nurses, practice nurses, health promotion officers, health and safety officers, environmental health officers etc who deal with the public, communities, groups and individuals and who can have delivery of health promotion policy as a major aspect of their role.

The wide work force, teachers, nurses, voluntary sector staff, managers, human resource officers, leisure centre staff, sports coaches, etc who are often involved in the implementation of the interventions that are developed and designed by the more specialist health promotion practitioners.

The general public. Many people through their personal relationships as family and friends can promote positive health behaviours and importantly can provide crucial social support to people trying to make a change.

Figure 2.2 People involved in public health.

There are a relatively small number of Public Health Specialists at the top of the Health Promotion Triangle who are involved in the strategic development and funding of health promotion activities within their regions. They will usually have at least an advanced qualification in Public Health and are often, although not exclusively, originally medical practitioners. The next level of practitioners who deliver or manage health promotion activities may include specialist public health practitioners or health promotion officers but will also include other health professionals with a significant interest in public health such as community dieticians, health visitors and district nurses. Finally, there are many other non-health professionals who have the opportunity to get involved with and deliver health promotion interventions, such as teachers like Jemma. The final level is the community members themselves whose impact, either positively or negatively, on health promotion can be considerable.

Many health professionals during the course of their career recognise that they have become focused on the health promotion aspects of their role and are interested in pursuing this aspect of their work. Although there have been attempts to create a clear pathway to professional registration for public health practitioners the whole system approach to public health and health promotion was difficult simplify whilst staying relevant to the broad range of practitioners involved in public health.

The UK Public Health Register was established in 2003 and provides a regulatory body for public health specialists and practitioners. It is currently voluntary, but it provides registrants, who perhaps may not be able to register with other more specialist professional bodies, with a regulatory body who can give their professional work a 'kite' mark of approval. It also recognises the range of relevant professional routes towards a public health-related professional registration (Figure 2.3).

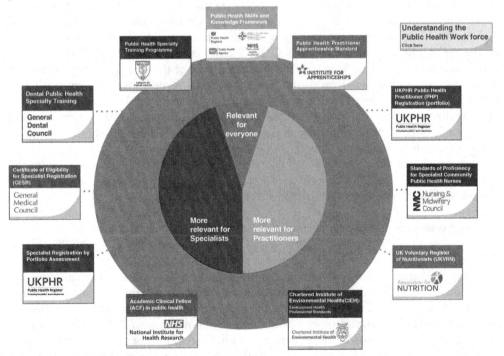

Figure 2.3 Infographic showing competency frameworks and professional Standards in Public Health including routes to professional registration (UKPHR Public Health Register, accessed 2023).

The Faculty of Public Health is the professional body for Public Health practitioners whilst the UK Public Health Register manages the regulation of practitioners and the protection of the public from any malpractice from its registrants (UKPHR.org accessed 2023). This division between the regulatory body and the professional body is standard practice within many health professions. The Health and Care Professions Council (HCPC) is the statutory regulatory body for many health care professionals for whom registration is mandatory, such as physiotherapists, podiatrists, psychologists, dieticians. Each profession also has a discipline-specific professional body. In 2023, the statutory regulation of public health practitioners seems unlikely.

Applying this to Jemma

Jemma has recognised that as a teacher, she can play a role in health promotion. She is now looking for advice and support from more specialist practitioners to inform her approach.

Delivering and evaluating health promotion/improvement interventions

In theory the process of empowerment leads to improvements in health. However, giving people the resources, the knowledge, skills and environment doesn't always lead to a change in behaviour and/or a measurable health gain. Sometimes empowerment can take decades to deliver an improvement. For example promoting eating fruit at break time instead of crisps, sweets and chocolate in schools may lead to a reduction in levels of Type 2 diabetes in the population but not for three or four decades after the intervention was implemented. Alcohol consumption in young people aged 16 to 24 is lower than in previous generations (Health Survey for England, 2020; Welsh Health Survey, 2020; Health Survey (NI), 2021; Scottish Health Survey, 2020) but the impact of this change of behaviour will not be seen for at least two decades and currently alcohol-related hospital admissions and deaths are increasing due to the alcohol consumption habits of adults through their lives who are now in their 40s and 50s (Office of National Statistics, 2021). Often health promotion is assessed by far shorter-term targets of changes in health-related behaviour and/ or improvements in illness and disease within targeted populations.

The term Health Gain emerged in policy documents in the late 1980s as governments and policy makers started to be interested in measuring the effectiveness of their policies and associated interventions. Health Gain has been defined as:

A measured improvement in the health of a person or a population.

NICE (2023)

How you define an improvement in health status is a key element of evaluation of health promotion interventions. Increasingly, the efficacy of interventions is being questioned and if funding depends on clear demonstration of benefit the outcome measure for improvement becomes crucial. Many empowerment-focused activities that enable people, but do not force or persuade individuals, are not able to demonstrate changes in primary measures of health status (such as weight loss, reduction in blood pressure, or reduction in diagnosis of disease) within the available time for evaluation.

Consequently, it is important to measure aspects of health status that are more likely to change in a shorter time frame but are known to predict better health in the longer term. The process of health improvement may be lengthy and the final outcome of better physical health may be very long term so we may need to measure outcomes that we know are likely to occur during the process. Within behavioural change you can argue that there are a range of relevant 'process' measures (Table 2.2). So for example if you introduce a school policy of fruit only at break times you are unlikely to see changes in weight in the children but could demonstrate an increase in the required behaviour.

Applying this to Jemma

When Jemma evaluates her intervention, behaviour change will probably be the most appropriate measurement in a population of school children. Measuring fitness or weight in school-aged children is a contentious issue as it is highly personal, potentially stigmatising information. Furthermore, changes in these criteria are unlikely to be evident in the short to medium term (Table 2.2).

Public Health Specialists such as directors of public health are responsible for the strategy direction of health promotion within their region. Guided by national strategy they will decide how resources will be allocated within their region. Ideally, their planning should be guided by strategic assessment of the needs of the particular communities within their region as well as by national targets. One particular technique promoted to help policy makers and practitioners plan their health promotion activities is a Health Needs Assessment (HNA). It is only one of several similar approaches. Other approaches are: Health Impact Assessment (HIA), Integrated Impact Assessment (IIA) and Health Equity Audit (HEA). Although there are similarities in these approaches, a key difference is their starting point. HNA starts with a population and assesses their health needs with a view to developing an intervention. In this way it is in line with the WHO aim of empowering communities to improve their health by ensuring that they are involved in the decisions about what is appropriate for their community.

Health needs assessment

HNA is a systematic approach to understating the needs of a population and can be used as part of a commissioning process so that the most effective support for those in the greatest need can be planned and delivered (Public Health England, 2017). Health needs can be as follows:

1 Perceptions and expectations of the profiled population (felt and expressed needs)
2 Perceptions of professionals providing the services
3 Perceptions of managers of commissioner/provider organisations, based on available data about the size and severity of health issues for a population, and inequalities compared with other populations (normative needs)
4 Priorities of the organisations' commissioning and managing services for the profiled population, linked to national, regional or local priorities (corporate needs).

Adapted from Cavanagh and Chadwick (2005)

Table 2.2 Potential outcome measures for a health promotion activity using example of a 'bike to work scheme'

	Promotional activity	Knowledge outcome (time scale: immediate)	Psychological outcome (time scale: short term)	Behavioural outcome (time scale: short term)	Physiological change outcome (time scale: medium to long term)	Disease outcome (time scale: long term)
Example	Bike to work scheme by city council: Includes information leaflets, tax-free bike purchase schemes and building of more cycle lanes and parking facilities.	Better understanding of value of physical activity. Knowledge about local facilities Increased Health Literacy	Reduction in stress from physical activity. Increase in self esteem Improvement in self efficacy Better mental health Increased Health Literacy (depending on measurement)	Increase in physical activity Reduction in sedentary time	Increase in aerobic fitness Increase in strength Reduction in weight	Lower levels of lifestyle related diseases

A good HNA will involve comparing and balancing these different needs when selecting priorities for action. The information can then be used as a basis for bringing about change through negotiation with stakeholder groups (Cavanagh & Chadwick, 2005). Often a health challenge will be identified centrally, such as reducing the prevalence of obesity in the population, and then a Health Needs Assessment will identify potential strategies and interventions that would be helpful within a specific population. In 2005 NICE (Cavanagh, Chadwick & National Institute for Health & Clinical Excellence) produced guidance for effective HNA which identified five steps in the process (Table 2.3).

Table 2.3 Five steps for an effective health needs assessment

Step 1
Getting started
What population?
What are you trying to achieve?
Who needs to be involved?
What resources are required?
What are the risks?
Step 2
Identifying health priorities
Population profiling
Gathering data
Perceptions of needs
Identifying and assessing health
conditions and determinant factors
Step 3
Assessing a health priority
for action
Choosing health conditions
and determinant factors
with the most significant
size and severity impact
Determining effective and
acceptable interventions
and actions
Step 4
Planning for change
Clarifying aims of intervention
Action planning
Monitoring and evaluation strategy
Risk-management strategy
Step 5
Moving on/review
Learning from the project
Measuring impact
Choosing the next priority

Source: Adapted from Cavanagh, Chadwick & National Institute for Health and Clinical Excellence (2005).

HNA can provide a clear protocol for planning and delivering health promotion work that can be adapted to a wide range of behaviours. By starting with the population it takes a client-centred perspective from the outset. However, a comprehensive HNA requires considerable resourcing that is often not available within health promotion budgets. Nevertheless, much of the good practice identified by NICE (2005) (Table 2.3) can still be applied even if the funds for a full HNA are not available. Consulting with stakeholders, agreeing priorities and planning for action are key aspects of the HNA that can be applied to smaller-scale projects with limited funding to improve the outcomes of the project

---

Applying this to Jemma

Whilst Jemma has not carried out a HNA she has identified a health priority for pupils in her school. She now needs to determine effective and acceptable interventions and actions and start to plan for change.

Whilst taking an HNA approach to health promotion has many advantages often health promotion activities are more top-down activities with health promotion officers responding to policy directives and government targets. However, health promotion can also be localised and driven by the particular interests of a well-motivated individual or organisation. For example, in Wales Diabetes UK Cymru have supported screening events through local pharmacies in order to reach the 50,000 undiagnosed diabetics predicted to be currently living in Wales.

Individual level interventions

There are numerous individualised and family-focused health promotion interventions to try and improve the health of people in the UK. Some of these are standardised, evaluated UK-wide interventions others are localised and access to schemes will vary significantly depending on where you live. There are pluses and minuses to both locally derived health promotional activities and more standardised initiatives; with the latter usually being evidence-based and evaluated and the former being more tailored and specific to the local community. Some programmes have been developed within the public sector and others within the private sector. It is then down to local funding bodies which may be the NHS, a local authority or third sector organisations to decide whether to fund particular programmes. For example both standardised and local programmes are available on lifestyle for individuals with Type 2 diabetes and there is more about these programmes in Chapter 10, Specific Conditions.

To demonstrate the range of health promotion/improvement initiatives that can co-exist in any one area this text will use the NHS Better Health website in the UK (www. nhs.uk) as an example. Better Health has four areas: lose weight, quit smoking, get active, drink less. Each area has a free app (the get active area has two) to provide health education and support self-regulation. For example, as part of the get active area of the site Better Health Site there is a link to the Couch to 5k App (A running programme for absolute beginners) and the Active 10 App which records every minute of walking, tracks steps, helps set goal, demonstrates achievements and provides tips to boost activity. It provides links to three other websites: Couch to Fitness (couchtofitness.com), This Girl Can (thisgirlcan.co.uk) and Join the Movement (sportengland.org). There are health education materials in a number of formats and links to nationwide providers such as leisure centres, online instruction and classes and private gyms. Better Health is an attempt to bring the range of activities together in a whole systems approach where the government policy and health education supports more local initiatives. In the lose weight area there are links to the NHS weight management pathways in primary and secondary care where more local and bespoke initiatives maybe available and may vary in different health boards.

The NHS Couch to 5 K programme is a 9-week scheme consisting of three runs a week which trains novice runners to run continuously for 30 minutes. The accompanying free podcast series is one of the most popular podcasts in the UK. Bates (2013) set up a group version of the programme and found that all the participants increased their weekly physical activity and lost weight over the 9 weeks.

The Mind, Exercise, Nutrition, Do it programme (MEND) is a multi-component, community-based childhood obesity intervention that has been well evaluated and utilised widely in the UK (Sacher et al., 2010; Skouteris et al., 2016). The programme is based on evidence-based principles of education, skills training and motivation and involved sessions about behavioural change, nutrition education and physical activity. It involves intensive twice weekly 2-hour sessions with small groups of children who are obese and their carer/s. All MEND leaders are required to attend a 4-day training programme to ensure consistency of delivery and the programme provides all the handouts, manuals and teaching aids.

The children involved in the evaluation of MEND by (Sacher et al., 2010) were aged between 8 and 12 and attended the 9-week programme with at least one parent or carer. See research into practice (Box 2.1).

The exercise referral scheme is a UK-wide individualised health promotion scheme delivered locally and has been adapted in different communities to suit local requirements and facilities. Individuals can be referred by a health practitioner from primary or secondary care to the exercise referral scheme. Initially, clients were referred predominantly to gyms where they were given between 10- and 16-week tailored gym programme and free access to the local facilities for that period. The scheme has now expanded considerably and there are a range of referral programmes that individuals can

---

Box 2.1   Research into Practice

Randomised Controlled Trial of the MEND program: A family-based community intervention for childhood obesity. (Sacher et al., 2010)

The aim of this study was to evaluate the effectiveness of the Mind, Exercise, Nutrition, Do it (MEND) Programme.

One hundred and sixteen obese children (BMI > or = 98th percentile) were randomly assigned to the MEND intervention or waiting list control (6-month delayed intervention). Parents and children attended 18 2-hour group educational and physical activity sessions held twice weekly in sports centres and schools, and were then given a 12-week free family swimming pass.

Participants in the intervention group had a reduced waist circumference z-score (−0.37; $P < 0.0001$) and BMI z-score (−0.24; $P < 0.0001$) at 6 months when compared to the controls. Significant between-group differences were also observed in cardiovascular fitness, physical activity, sedentary behaviours, and self-esteem. At 12 months, children in the intervention group had reduced their waist and BMI z-scores by 0.47 (P < 0.0001) and 0.23 (P < 0.0001), respectively, and benefits in cardiovascular fitness, physical activity levels, and self-esteem were sustained.

High-attendance rates (86%) suggest that families found this intensive community-based intervention acceptable. Other large controlled trials for example (Skouteris et al., 2016) are reporting similar positive findings.

be directed towards, including a number of outdoor 'green activities'. The period of the scheme is acknowledged to be rather short and the scheme is keen to explore longer support periods or perhaps a less intense on-going support package. In 2014, NICE produced the Exercise Referral Scheme Guidance which recommended that exercise referral schemes should not be funded for people who are sedentary but otherwise well. Commissioners should only fund exercise referral schemes for people who are sedentary and have an existing health condition. All funded interventions must be based on good behavioural change principles, as outlined in the NICE Behavioural Change: individual approaches NICE public health guidance 54 (NICE, 2014).

So the individualised health promotion activities across the UK are a mixture of standard programmes that different government bodies may or may not choose to adopt and locally generated schemes sometimes funded by government, sometimes by lottery funding and sometimes by national and/or local charities. This is the case across all aspects of health promotion/health improvement. Alongside the individualised health promotion/improvement activities that are happening in the community will be more specialised, individualised health promotion delivered by health care practitioners in one-to-one settings either in primary or secondary care. Health service interventions are often only initiated once individuals have clearly identified health or behavioural problems such as morbid obesity, an alcohol dependency, Type 2 diabetes, or other lifestyle-related conditions. One of the challenges for health promotion is to try and direct health promotion resources away from secondary care settings and those with health problems into the community to try and prevent the currently well ever needing the services of secondary care. Regardless of health condition the considerable pressures from secondary care for resources to care for the currently ill can often limit the resources available to attempt to prevent the condition arising in the first place.

Applying this to Jemma
An individualised programme such as MEND is not really what Jemma is looking for. Jemma is hoping for a whole school approach to improving the eating and physical activity habits of all children in the school rather than identifying particular children with a problem, such as weight.

Community-level interventions

Community-level interventions in the UK may be delivered by the Department of Health across the UK. Alternatively, some maybe Scottish, English Welsh or Northern Ireland only initiatives or more localised still. Many interventions will sit under the umbrella of a wide-scale promotional campaign. UK-wide campaigns are often media based;

traditionally involving television advertising and poster campaigns. However, internet-based campaigns and initiatives are increasing with the Change4life intervention, recently re-branded as healthier families being the most high-profile example of a campaign where the internet is a central communication tool. Change4life was launched in 2009 and was aimed at parents with school-aged children. In 2021, it was brought under the Better Health Brand and re-named healthier families. Its purpose has been to:

> *Inspire a social movement, though which government, the NHS, local authorities, business, charities, schools, families and community leaders can all play a part in improving children's diets and physical activity levels*
>
> Healthy Families (2023)

Change4life was a social marketing-based campaign to reduce childhood obesity. The main website had a number of messages and also linked users to a range of national and local initiatives to support healthy eating and physical activity. Croker et al. (2012) reviewed the campaign through surveying 1,419 families. They concluded that the campaign materials increased awareness of the campaign but had little impact on attitudes or behaviour. They concluded that the campaign targeted a broad range of behaviours and perhaps lacked a clear focus. The aim of Change4life was to prevent obesity but no mention of obesity was made in any of the materials. Despite claiming to be based on Social Marketing principles it is unclear whether all of the 6 principles of social marketing were adhered to (Croker et al., 2012).

Better Health is a national campaign launched by the UK government in July 2020 (Public Health England, 2020). It was launched to encourage individuals to make healthier life choices and to respond to the evidence that obese people were significantly more likely to become seriously ill with coronavirus than people with healthy BMIs (Hussain et al., 2020). It is an example of a complex intervention that is housed on a website (Better Health, 2023) but also interacts with and introduces its users to a range of other national and local initiatives. It includes mobile applications, online support groups, virtual fitness videos and offers with organisations who provide weight loss, fitness and other health plans. The responses to the Better Health campaign have been mixed with Sport England 2020 and the British Heart Foundation welcoming measures to tackle obesity, such as the 9 pm watershed on fast food adverts. However, there has also been negative coverage from eating disorder organisations who felt the focus on weight loss and calorie counting would be detrimental to people with eating disorders. Talbot and Branley-Bell (2022) analysed the content of original tweets about the Better Health Campaign and concluded the campaign was problematic due to its lack of consideration for mental health and the wide-societal factors that contribute to obesity. The perceived 'fat-shaming' approach was a particular concern.

Another example of a UK-wide complex intervention is the January 2013 'smoking causes genetic mutations' campaign. In January 2013, the Department of Health launched its new 2.7 million campaign to encourage people to stop smoking. The campaign involved television adverts that focus on the fact that smoking causes genetic mutations. According to the Department of Health (http://www.dh.gov.uk/health/2012/12/smoking-health-harm/ accessed January 2013):

The health harms message focuses on the fact that every 15 cigarettes smoked causes a
mutation that can lead to cancer and aims to increase motivation to quit.

DoH (accessed 2013)

This is another interesting campaign. It doesn't actually present a new risk of smoking but focuses on our better understanding of how smoking causes disease. It utilizes some unpleasant images of mutations growing on cigarettes and appears to hope that informing people that smoking damages your health through genetic mutation will be a motivating risk factor. However, there is limited evidence to suggest that using genetic risk information will be any better at promoting lifestyle change than non-genetic risk information (Davies & Thirlaway, 2012). On the positive side, the informational campaign is not stand alone and is supported by clearly signposted free quit-smoking kits that are available in local pharmacies. In the autumn of 2012, pharmacies were pre-warned of the new campaign and asked to order their quit-smoking kits in advance. Furthermore, local public health teams and smoking cessation clinics were primed to provide the motivational and behavioural support to any new clients that the campaign brings to their doors. For example: The NHS Stop Smoking Service is a national network of advisers who provide professional support during the first few weeks that an individual attempts to stop smoking. There are regional variations in how these advisers work (www.nhs.uk/Livewell/smoking, accessed January 2023). One criticism of mass media campaigns is that they are not targeted at the most 'at risk' communities and that its message may not reach smokers from more deprived communities who are most likely to smoke.

UK-wide health improvement campaigns such as 'Better Health' have the potential to reach and influence the least deprived more effectively than the most deprived and thereby improve the overall health of the nation whilst failing to address health inequalities. Conversely however, targeting interventions at the most deprived communities can also fail to be effective and universal approaches do not stigmatise particular groups in society.

Other community-level interventions can be at school or organisational level. An intervention that has been very successful at increasing the fruit and vegetable consumption of primary school-aged children is the Food Dudes Healthy Eating Programme (Horne et al., 2009; Marcano-Oliver et al., 2021). It is an evidence-based programme based on the known determinants of children's food preferences:

1 rewards
2 role modelling
3 repeated tasting

Role modelling of eating fruit and vegetables is provided by a video series introducing the Food Dudes who are cartoon characters and are the 'good guys' in battle with the bad guys General Junk and his Junk Punks. Children are rewarded for trying fruit and vegetables each time they try them which encourages repeated tasting. Rewards include stickers, stationery and lunch boxes all with Food Dude characters depicted on them. The Food Dude programme provides all the materials for schools and will start the intervention off with an intensive introduction. All the studies carried out on the programme so far show increases in children's fruit and vegetable consumption which in some cases generalised to the home setting. The increases in consumption were greatest in those that ate the least initially and another good outcome reported in some studies from the programme is that unhealthy snacks reduced as fruit and vegetable intake increased (Horne et al., 2009). In 2021 Marcano-Oliver *et al.* found that children's consumption of fruit, vegetables, vitamin C & E increased while total energy consumption, fat saturated fat and sodium intake decreased after their school participated in the Food Dudes programme. No such changes were seen in the control school (Marcano-Oliver et al., 2021). Programmes like Food Dudes can be targeted at particular schools and so could be targeted at more deprived communities and perhaps contribute to reducing inequality. More about the Food Dude programme can be found in Chapter 5 Eating Well.

Applying this to Jemma

Jemma found reports of the Food Dudes programme through her city council healthy living network that she joined on the recommendation of her local public health team. Jemma is keen to get involved and thinks the programme may work in the context of her school for her Year 7 and 8 pupils. She is interested in working with the school's linked primary schools to develop a partnership to address eating well.

Working effectively with others

Promoting lifestyle change is usually a multi-disciplinary undertaking and can be a top-down activity when public health practitioners attempt to deliver a policy through localised initiatives and need to get various different professionals involved. Alternatively health promotion can be a bottom-up activity when individuals or organisations attempt to improve the health of their particular community and look towards policy and health promotion specialists to support them in their endeavour.

Within health and social care services a multi-disciplinary team has been defined as:

> *a group of health and care staff who are members of different organisations and professions (e.g., GPs, social workers, nurses) that work together to make decisions regarding the treatment of individual patients and service users. MPTs are used in both health and care settings.*
>
> NHS England Transformation Directorate (2023)

Multi-disciplinary and multi-agency working involves appropriately utilising knowledge, skills and best practice from multiple disciplines and across service provider boundaries, e.g., health, social care or voluntary and private sector providers to redefine, re-scope and reframe health and social care delivery issues and reach solutions based on an improved collective understanding of complex patient need(s) (NHS England, 2014).

In some literature the terms inter-disciplinary or inter-professional are used. Inter-disciplinary has been defined as:

> *The sharing of exclusive knowledge with the professional team*
>
> Welsh Government (2011)

In practice the term multi-disciplinary team (MDT) is used to describe very many different structures, practices and groups. The MDT can be a permanent group of staff from different professions all employed by the same organisation and based in the same physical space where the multi-disciplinary working is often integrated in to the day-to-day working and where team meetings to discuss one patient or one project are frequent and regular. Alternatively, it can be a group of professionals who regularly work together from different organisations. In this instance more formal meetings are often required to bring people from different locations and organisations together. Finally, informal discussions between two or more professionals can be referred to as a multiple disciplinary team meeting.

Multi-disciplinary working is perhaps easiest to deliver effectively in health care settings such as specialist units where consultants, nurses, physiotherapists, psychologists, dieticians, social workers etc are all located in one physical area. Whilst successful teams are not assured through the sharing of geographical space it is far easier to communicate and to establish a common purpose and established agreed methods of delivery when everyone is located together (Heitkemper et al., 2008).

Whilst multi-disciplinary working may be easier in on-site settings it is equally important for community-based health promotion (Tzenalis & Sotiriadou, 2010). As we increasingly recognise how many factors interact to influence the lifestyle choices that individuals make; building a supportive physical, cultural and socioeconomic environment in which the population can live and work healthily cannot be the responsibility of one group, or indeed solely the province of government health departments. What is essential for effective health promotion is collaboration across different health care professionals, government agencies and public or private sectors (Tzenalis & Sotiriadou, 2010). Slowly, we can see governments in the UK responding to the challenge of multi-disciplinary, multi-sector health promotion. Active transport policies are joint Department of Health and Department of Transport initiatives. The full impact of environmental and cultural change initiatives may not be seen for many years, but they are an encouraging step towards supporting change in the population.

It is acknowledged within the literature on multi-disciplinary working that certain factors are key if a group of different professionals are going to come together and create a high-performing MDT (Tzenalis & Sotiriadou, 2010; Welsh Government, 2011). The key factors consistently reported across the literature are as follows:

1 Good communication, which can be facilitated by the use of a common language and an avoidance of discipline-specific jargon
2 Good leadership
3 Effective administration
4 An identified key worker

These four factors enable the three core capabilities for multi-disciplinary working to be achieved:

1 Successful multi-disciplinary meetings
2 Co-ordinated assessment and planning
3 Integrated systems and practices

Frequently reported barriers to successful multi-disciplinary working include: a lack of commitment at senior level, professional rivalry, competing budgets and sharing of data (Tzenalis & Sotiriadou, 2010; Welsh Government, 2011).

Health promotion activities are sometimes delivered by MDTs that do indeed have meetings, an identified leader and administrative support. Frequently, these teams may come together to deliver a particular initiative, such as a new advice booklet for newly diagnosed diabetics, and then disband. Task-specific groups are sometimes referred to as 'Task and Finish Groups'. However, health promotion is often delivered by a diverse group of professionals who seldom get the opportunity to meet and so cannot function as a traditional MDT. For example; an individual with Type 2 diabetes could receive advice about their lifestyle from their GP, their practice nurse, the community dietician, the community diabetic nurse, the exercise professional in the leisure centre or the community pharmacist depending on the resources available in their community. These professionals are unlikely to get together to discuss a co-ordinated prevention strategy for that individual so the likelihood of the individual receiving conflicting advice is high. The key factors that apply to more traditional multi-disciplinary working can still apply:

1 Effective communication between professionals (even if it is virtual rather than face-to-face and around general principals of advice rather than individual patient prevention plans)
2 A clear leader for diabetes prevention in each area
3 A key worker who facilities the referral of the patient to all the other potential lifestyle support practitioners
4 Effective administration that supports the sharing of data between practitioners

---

Applying this to Jemma

Jemma is most likely to achieve her aim of improving the healthy eating habits and physical activity levels of the pupils in her school if she has the support of the whole school and the wider community. So if her local public health team are running healthy school initiatives or funding the Food Dudes initiatives she will be able to apply to get involved in the schemes they are supporting. She could also investigate any continuing professional development opportunities to increase her understanding of how to promote health in her school.

As for any project her aim is most likely to be realised if she takes a strategic and planned approach and follows as far as is possible the guidelines for a Health Needs Assessment. If she involves the relevant stakeholders: children, parents and staff from the outset and plans her intervention including their perceptions of needs then she stands a greater chance of success. Careful planning and on-going evaluation using realistic outcome measures give any intervention the best chance of success.

Conclusion

Health promotion is a wide-reaching umbrella that encompasses a large range of different behaviours and a large range of diverse initiatives from very large-scale media-driven campaigns to very localised small-scale schemes. The role of the various public health agencies is to support the diversity of initiatives that all undoubtedly have a role to play in the health of the nation and to try to ensure that its wide and diverse workforce is as well-trained and up-to-date as possible. National public health bodies play an important role in trying to take public health and health improvement outside of traditional health settings, to move the activity further 'upstream' and encourage non health practitioners to get involved in promoting health behaviours. Schools, workplaces and all organisations that interact with the public have a role to play in supporting behavioural change and public health bodies can provide valuable expertise and resources to support them.

Key points

- Health promotion has the reduction of health inequalities as central ambition but often health promotion activities whilst improving the health of the nation as a whole are least effective in the most deprived.
- Health education and health literacy can be interpreted as about knowledge and ability to comprehend and communicate about health. However, the WHO and most public health organisations conceptualise them more broadly to include aspects of motivation and empowerment.
- Health promotion activities are frequently complex interventions that are hard to evaluate as their benefits may be realised decades after the intervention. Consequently, it can be challenging to demonstrate the effectiveness of an intervention and to justify its funding. More innovative and process-orientated evaluations are required.
- Health promotion is a multi-disciplinary activity often requiring the co-operation and collaboration of non-health professionals and organisations. Working effectively across disciplines and with non-health organisations has the potential to deliver health benefits but can be controversial if it involves organisations that produce or promote unhealthy products.
- Health promotion activities do not often deliver short-term tangible benefits to physical health but the beneficial impact that they may have over the course of the lifespan may be considerable.

Discussion points

- Should health promotion be targeted at specific groups such as overweight children or people at high risk of developing diabetes or are more community-wide interventions to encourage general healthy behaviours more appropriate?
- What sort of evidence would you require about the effectiveness of a health promotion intervention in order to utilise it in your practice?
- How important is it to include significant others in any intervention to change an individual's behaviour?

Further resources

www.UKPHR.org
http://www.fph.org.uk/what_is_public_health
BetterHealth www.nhs.uk

References

Agampodi, T. C., Agampodo, S. B., Glozier, N., & Siribaddana, S. (2015). Measurement of social capital in relation to health in low and middle income countries (LMIC): A systematic review. Social Science and Medicine, *128*, 95–104. Doi: 10.1016/j.socscimed.2015.01.005

Andreasen, A. R. (2002). Marketing social marketing in the social change marketplace. Journal of Public Policy Marketing, *21*(1), 3–13.

Bates, S. (2013). NHS couch to 5K programme. British Medical Journal Blogs. www.blogs.bmj.com (accessed 2023).

Better Health. (2023). www.nhs.uk (accessed 2023).

Buck, D., & Frosini, F. (2012). Clustering of unhealthy behaviours over time: Implications for policy and practice. London: The Kings Fund.

Carin, J. E., & Rundle-Theile, S. R.(2014). Eating for the better: A social marketing review (2000–2012). Public Health Nutrition, *17*, 1628–1639.

Cavanagh, S., Chadwick K., & National Institute for Health and Clinical Excellence. (2005). Health needs assessment a practice guide. London: NICE.

Cheng, H., Kotler, P., & Lee, N. (2010). Social marketing for public health: Global trends and success stories: Global trends and success stories. Jones & Bartlett: Learning.

Coutinho Da Silva & Mazzon. (2016). Developing social marketing plan for health promotion. International Journal of Public Administration, *38*(8), 577–586. Doi: 10.1080/01900692.2015.1023447

Croker, H., Lucas, R., & Wardle, J. (2012). Cluster-reandomised trial to evaluate the "Change for Life" mass media/social marketing campaign in the UK. BMC Public Health, *12*, 404.

Dauner, K. N., Wilmot, N. A., & Schultz, J. F. (2015). Investigating the temporal relationship between individual-level social capital and health in fragile families. BMC Public Health, *15*, 1130. Doi: 10.1186/s12889-015-2437-3

Davies, L., & Thirlaway, K. (2012). Effect of genetic explanations of type 2 diabetes on patients' attitudes to treatment efficacy. Journal of Diabetes Nursing, *16*(4), 132–139.

Davis, T. C., Long, S. W., Jackson, R. H., et al. (1993). Rapid estimate of adult literacy in medicine: A shortened screening instrument. Family Medicine, *25*, 391–395.

Department of Health. (1999). National service framework for diabetes standards. London Department of Health.

Department of Health, Social Sciences & Public Safety. (2014). Making life better: A whole system strategic framework for public health 2013–2023. Belfast: Department of Health, Social Sciences & Public Safety.

Department of Health. (2009). Change4life principles and guidelines for promotion. London: Department of Health.

French, J., Blair-Stevens, C., McVey, D., & Merritt, R. (2009). Social marketing and public health: Theory and practice. USA: Oxford University Press.

Fujihira, H., Kubacki, K., Ronto, R., pang, B., & Rhundle-Thiele. (2015). Social marketing physical activity interventions among adults 60 years and older: A systematic review. Social Marketing Quarterly, *21*(4), 214–229. Doi: 10.1177/1524500415606671.

Griffiths, S., Jewell, T., & Donnelly, P. (2005). Public health in practice: The 3 domains of public health. Public Health, *119*, 907–913.

Healthy Families. (2023). www.nhs.uk (accessed 2023).

Health Survey England. (2020). Health Survey for England 2019: Adult health-related behaviours. NHS Digital.

Health Survey (NI). (2021). Health Survey (NI): First results 2020/21. Public Health Information and Research Branch, Information Analysis Directorate.

Heggdal, K., Stepanian, N., & Hamilton Larsen, M. (2023). Health care professionals' experiences of facilitating patient activation and empowerment in chronic illness using a person-centred and strengths-based self-management program. Chronic Illness, *19*(1), 250–264. Doi: 10.1177/17423963211065006

Heitkemper, M., et al. (2008). The role of centers in fostering interdisciplinary research. Nursing Outlook, *56*(3), 115–122.

Herman, W. H., Ye, W., Griffin, S. J., Simmons, R. K., Davies, M., Khunti, K., Rutten, G. E. H. M., Sandbaek, A., Lauritzen, T., Borch-Johnson, K., Brown, M. B., & Wareham, N. J. (2015). Early detection and treatment of type 2 diabetes reduce cardiovascular morbidity and mortality: A simulation of the results of the Anglo-Danish study of intensive treatment in people with screen-detected diabetes in primary care (ADDITION-Europe). Diabetes Care, *38*(8), 1449–1455.

Hobbis, S., Hendry, L., Sanders, L., & Thirlaway, K. (2011). Retirement and lifestyle behaviours: A thematic analysis. Health Psychology Update, *20*(2), 2–8.

Horne P. J., Hardman C. A., Lowe, C. F., Tapper, K., Le Noury, J., Madden, P., Patel, P., & Doody, M. (2009). Increasing parental provision and children's consumption of lunchbox fruit and vegetables in Ireland: The food dudes intervention. European Journal of Clinical Nutrition, *63*, 613–618.

Hussain, A., MAhawar, K., Xia, Z. et al. (2020). Obesity and mortality of COVID-19. Meta-anaylsis. Obesity Research and Clinical Practice, *14*(4), 295–300.

Kotler P., & Lee N. R. (2008). Social marketing: Influencing behaviours for good (3rd ed.). Thousand Oaks, CA: Sage Publications.

Kotler, P., & Zaltman, G. (1971). Social marketing: An approach to planned social change. The Journal of Marketing, *35*, 3–12.

Kroll, P., Jones, G. C., Kehn, M., & Neri, M. T. (2006). Barriers and strategies affecting the utilisation of primary preventative services for people with physical disabilities: A qualitative inquiry. Health and Social Care in the Community, *14*(4), 284–293.

Kumar, S., Calvo, R., Avendano, M., Sivaramakrishnan, K., & Berkman, L. F. (2012). Social support, volunteering and health around the world: Cross-national evidence from 139 countries. Social Science and Medicine, *74*(5), 696–706.

Mantwill, S., Monestel-Umana, S., & Schulz, P. J. (2015). The relationship between health literacy and health disparities: A systematic review. PLoS ONE, *10*(12), e0145455. Doi: 10.1371/journal.pone.0145455

Marcano-Olivier, M., Sallaway-Costello, J., McWilliams, L., Horne, P. J., Vikto. S., & Erjavec, M. (2021). Changes in the nutritional content of children's lunches after the Food Dudes healthy eating programme. Journal of Nutritional Science, *10*(40), 1–10.

Morgan, A., & Swann, C. (2004). Introduction: Issues of definition, measurement and links to health. In A. Morgan & C. Swann (Eds.), Social capital for health: Issues of definition, measurement and links to health. Health Development Agency.

Muscat, D. M., Smith, S., Dhillon, H. M., Morony, S., Davis, E. L., Luxford, K., Shepard, H. L., Hayen, A., Comings, J., Nutbeam, D., & McCaffery, K. (2016). Incorporating health literacy in education for socially disadvantaged adults: An Australian feasibility study. International Journal for Equity in Health, Doi: 10.1186/s12939-016-0373-1

NHS England. (2014). MDT Development – working toward an effective multidisciplinary/multiagency team. NHS England.

NHS England - Transformation Directorate. (2023). www.transform.england.nhs.uk (accessed 2023)

NICE. (2023). Glossary: www.nice.org.uk (accessed 2023)

NICE. (2005). Health needs assessment: A practical guide www.nice.org.uk

NICE. (2014). Physical activity: Exercise referral schemes. Public Health Guideline 54 www.nice.co.uk

Nutbeam, D., McGill, B., & Premkumar, P. (2018). Improving health literacy in community populations: A review of progress. Health Promotion International, *33*, 901–911. Doi: 10.1093/heapro/dax015

O'Connor, M., & Casey, L. (2015). The mental health literacy scale (MHLS): A new scale-based measure of mental health literacy. Psychiatry Research, *229*, 511–516.

Office for Health Improvement and Disparities. (2023). www.gov.uk (accessed 2023).

Office of National Statistics. (2021). Quarterly alcohol-specific deaths in England and Wales: 2001 to 2019 registrations and quarter 1 (Jan to Mar) to quarter 4 (Oct to Dec) 2020 provisional registrations. Census 2021.

Office of National Statistics. (2022). Statistical bulletin: Health state life expectancies by national deprivation deciles, England: 2018 to 2020. Office for National Statistics. ONS.gov.uk

Parker, R. M., Baker, D. W., Williams, M. V., & Nurss, J. R. (1995). The test of functional health literacy in adults (TOFHLA): A new instrument for measuring patient's literacy skills. Journal of General Internal Medicine, *10*, 537–541.

Performance and Innovation Unit. (2002). Social capital: A discussion paper. Performance and Innovation Unit.

Public Health England. (2017). Workplace health needs assessment: How to use the assessment and HNA questions. London: Public Health England. www.gov.uk

Public Health England. (2020). Public health England strategy 2020–25. London: Public Health England.

Public Health England. (2020). Major new campaign encourages millions to lose weight and cut COVID-19 risk. UK Government. Available at: https://www.gov.uk/government/news/major-new-campaign-encourages-millions-to-lose-weight-and-cut-covid-19-risk (accessed January 2023).

Public Health Scotland. (2022). A Scotland where everybody thrives. Public Health Scotland's three-year plan 2022–2025. Glasgow: Public Health Scotland.

Public Health Wales. (2022). Public health Wales: Our strategic plan 2022–2025. Cardiff: Public Health Wales: NHS Wales.

Rudd, R. E. (2015). The evolving concept of health literacy: New directions for health literacy studies. Journal of Communication in Health Care, *81*, 7–9. Doi: 10.1179/1753806815Z.000000000105

Sacher, P., Kolotourou, M., Chadwick, P. M., Cole, T. J., Lawson, M., Lucas, A., & Singhal, A. (2010). Randomised controlled trial of the MEND program: A family-based community intervention for childhood obesity. Obesity, *18*(S1), S62–S68.

Scottish Health Survey. (2020). Scottish health survey 2019. The Scottish Government, www.gov.scot

Shriven, A. (2017). Ewles & Simnett's promoting health: A practical guide (7th Edition). London: Elsevier.

Sin, J. (2020). Public health: Three Key domains in: Commissioning and a population approach to health services decision-making. Oxford University Press. 10/1093/oso/9780199884032.001. 0001

Skouteris, H., Hill, B., McCabe, M., Swinburn, B., & Busija, L. (2016). A parent-bsed intervention to promote healthy eating and active behaviours in pre-school children: Evaluation of the MEND 2–4 randomised controlled trial. Paediatric Obesity, *11*(1), 4–10. Doi: 10.1111/ijpo.12011

Stead, M., Gordon, R., Angus, K., & McDermott, L. (2007). A systematic review of social marketing effectiveness. Health Education, *107*(2), 126–191.

Talbot, C. V., & Branley-Bell, D. (2022). #BetterHealth: A qualitative analysis of reactions to the UK government's better health campaign. Journal of Health Psychology, *27*(5), 1252–1258. Doi: 10.1177/1359105320985576

The Kings Fund. (2023). Is the NHS in crisis? Kingsfund.org.uk (accessed 2023).

Thompson, S. R., Watson, M. C., & Tilford, S. (2018). The Ottawa Charter 30 years on: Still an important standard for health promotion. International Journal of Health Promotion and Education, *56*(2), 73–84. Doi: 10.1080/14635240.2017.1415765.

Thirlaway, K. and Upton, D. (2009). The Psychology of Lifestyle: Promoting Health Behaviour. London: Routledge.

Tzenalis, A., & Sotiriadou, C. (2010). Health promotion as multi-professional and multi-disciplinary work. International Journal of Caring Sciences, *3*(2), 49.

Uchino, B. N. (2009). Understanding the links between social support and physical health: A lifespan perspective with emphasis on the separability of perceived and received support. Perspectives on Psychological Science, 4(3), 236–255.

Wechsler, H., Nelson, T., Lee, J. E., Seibring, M., Lewis, C., & Keeling, R. P. (2003). Perceptions and reality: A national evaluation of social norms marketing interventions to reduce college students heavy alcohol use. Journal of Studies of Alcohol, 64, 484–494.

Welsh Government. (2011). Multi disciplinary working: A framework for practice in Wales. Cardiff: Welsh Government.

Welsh Health Survey. (2020). National survey for Wales 2019/20. Welsh Government.

Whitehead, D. (2001). Health education, behavioural change and social psychology: Nursing's contribution to health promotion? Journal of Advanced Nursing, 34(6), 822–832.

WHO. (2023). Health promotion: www.who.int (accessed 2023).

WHO. (2008). Closing the health gap in a generation: Health equity thought action on the social determinants of health. World Health Organisation.

WHO. (2009). Milestones in health promotion: Statements from global conferences. World Health Organisation.

WHO. (1986). Ottawa Charter for health promotion. Geneva: World Health Organisation.

WHO. (2012). Health education: Theoretical concepts, effective strategies and core competencies. World Health Organisation.

WHO. (2020). Promoting health and reducing health inequalities by addressing the social determinants of health. Denmark: World Health Organisation, Regional Office for Europe.

3 Health and health inequalities

LEARNING OUTCOMES

At the end of this chapter, you will be able to:

- define health inequality.
- understand the nature of health inequalities and the factors that contribute towards them.
- understand the measurements of health.
- demonstrate an understanding of the measurement of socio-economic status (SES) and how it relates to health status.
- appreciate the complexity of tackling health inequalities.
- understand the psychological, social and policy basis of tackling health inequalities.

Case Study

Dave is a 43-year-old manual labourer who was born, grew up and now lives in one of the most deprived areas of Wales. Dave had a poor attendance at secondary school and did not manage to pass any of his General Certificate of Secondary Education (GCSE) exams. Once he finished school at 16, he had no inspiration to gain a career and spent most of his time with his friends, watching TV and playing computer games. At 23, Dave began working as a manual labourer and has stayed in the trade on and off ever since.

Dave lives at home with his elderly mother (his father, a heavy smoker, died of lung cancer when Dave was 26) and has a 2-year-old daughter called Kelly. Dave does not maintain much contact with the mother of his child; therefore, he rarely visits his daughter. He spends much of his spare time with his friends in the local pub (he drinks heavily, particularly on weekends). While at the pub, he regularly goes for a cigarette with friends.

Since the age of 14, Dave has been a heavy smoker and occasionally takes drugs. Dave has always been in a smoking environment; his father and mother smoked throughout his childhood. His mother continues to be a heavy smoker. Dave has not visited the dentist since he was 25. Dave recently visited his general practitioner

DOI: 10.4324/9781003471233-3

(GP) due to experiencing tightness in his chest, mainly when undertaking physical activity at work. He has since been diagnosed with angina. Dave is concerned about the pain he is experiencing in his chest and wants to understand how he can help relieve the pain and improve his health.

Applying this to Dave

Consider Dave's situation. How does his environment, behaviour and overall situation affect his health?

Introduction

Health inequality refers to the variation in health outcomes and mortality rates between individuals, usually dependent on some demographic variable (e.g., socio-economic class, gender or ethnicity). Although various factors create health inequalities, this chapter will mainly focus on socio-economic differences—one of the major barriers to a long and healthy life expectancy. The discrepancy in life expectancy or health status outcomes may result from many factors, such as income level, environment, health behaviours, lifestyle choices and their complex inter-relationships. The strategic review of health inequalities post-2010—the Marmot Review (Marmot, 2010)—concluded that there is a vital need to reduce preventable health inequalities. Marmot suggested that health inequalities should be tackled in every social class, not just in the most disadvantaged communities. Making such changes and reducing the gap in health inequalities would benefit society as a whole. Furthermore, reducing the gap is a matter of social justice and a necessity to make society fairer for all. As stated by Marmot (2010), 'health inequalities that are preventable by reasonable measures are unfair. Putting them right is a matter of social justice'.

A decade after the seminal Marmot Review, a follow-up study was published titled 'Health Equity in England: The Marmot Review 10 Years On' (Marmot, 2020). This subsequent analysis underscored the concerning reality that health inequalities in England not only persisted but, in certain instances, had deteriorated over the past 10 years. Therefore, the 2020 report called for a reinvigorated commitment to tackling health disparities. A series of recommendations were proposed to achieve this, including allocating resources for early years support, enhancing working conditions and wages, and employing community-based and place-based strategies to foster healthier living environments.

Inequalities exist throughout the world and are apparent within all developed countries. Indeed, there are differences between European countries—the greatest inequalities appear in Hungary and Poland and the least in certain areas of Spain (Mackenbach et al., 2008). However, in recent decades, Western Europe has observed increasing relative inequalities in mortality between lower and higher socio-economic groups. However, due to overall declines in mortality among both lowly and highly educated groups, absolute inequalities have often decreased. Despite the financial crisis (2007–2008), no short-term effect on health inequalities has been observed at the population level in Western Europe (Mackenbach et al., 2018). This can be attributed to strong ongoing trends and protective living conditions that reduced the effect of health risks on a large scale.

Conversely, Eastern Europe experienced a sharp rise in relative and absolute inequalities in mortality since the early 1990s. Remarkably, recent years have demonstrated a reversal in mortality trends among lowly educated individuals in several Eastern European countries due to declines in mortality from various causes. This change has been attributed to policy improvements, although mortality levels among the lowly educated remain high (Mackenbach et al., 2018).

Compared to the United States, trends in health inequalities have been more favourable in Western Europe. European health care systems may play a role in constraining inequalities in mortality. However, follow-up studies are necessary to determine the long-term effect of recession and austerity on health inequalities (Forster et al., 2018).

Overall, life expectancy in the United Kingdom (UK) has improved year-on-year (see Table 3.1), although there is still some inequity between males and females. Although life expectancy is improving overall, health inequalities are still apparent between different societal groups. For example, while the most recent evidence suggests that all-cause mortality is declining overall, suicide rates are increasing due to the economic recession, indicating that health inequalities continue to affect the most vulnerable populations systemically (Mackenbach et al., 2018). Thus, it is still evident that the lower the social group you are in, the lower your life expectancy and healthy life expectancy will be (see Table 3.2).

Table 3.1 Life expectancy at birth: By sex and country (2008–2020)

Year	Males England	Females Wales	Scotland	NI	England	Wales	Scotland	NI
2008–2010	78.31	77.51	75.8	76.97	82.33	81.66	80.32	81.43
2009–2011	78.71	77.83	76.2	77.4	82.67	82.01	80.61	81.84
2010–2012	79.01	78.07	76.5	77.69	82.83	82.09	80.74	82.12
2011–2013	79.21	78.17	76.77	77.99	82.96	82.19	80.89	82.29
2012–2014	79.35	78.4	77.05	78.25	83.05	82.28	81.06	82.29
2013–2015	79.37	78.41	77.1	78.29	83.06	82.26	81.14	82.27
2014–2016	79.46	78.43	77.06	78.51	83.1	82.35	81.14	82.29
2015–2017	79.48	78.32	76.98	78.44	83.1	82.28	81.05	82.3
2016–2018	79.55	78.31	77.01	78.66	83.18	82.33	81.07	82.38
2017–2019	79.67	78.51	77.13	78.74	83.33	82.33	81.13	82.54
2018–2020	79.33	78.29	76.79	78.65	83.12	82.09	81.01	82.38

Source: Office for National Statistics (2021) National life tables—life expectancy in the UK: 2008 to 2020.

Table 3.2 Life expectancy and healthy life expectancy in years at birth by social class, 2001–2003 (England)

Social class	Males LE	HLE	Females LE	HLE
Professional (I)	80.2	76.7	85.5	80.0
Managerial & technical/intermediate (II)	78.9	73.9	82.8	76.6
Skilled non-manual (IIINM)	78.4	73.0	82.2	75.5
Skilled manual (IIIM)	76.4	69.3	80.6	71.9
Partly skilled (IV)	75.9	68.1	79.9	70.8
Unskilled (V)	73.5	64.2	78.7	68.6
England	77.1	70.7	81.3	73.7

Source: White and Edgar, 2010.

Defining and measuring social class

Societal research seldom considers society as a whole; usually, it considers the position of a group (or groups of people) within society. In this way, individual members of society can be categorised into different groups.

Some types of stratification are easy to apply (e.g., age bands), whereas others are more difficult and contentious to define (e.g., social class). Although there are several ways of stratifying society, this chapter will explore social status in detail.

The definition of social class was provided in the seminal Black Report (Townsend & Davidson, 1982), which clearly stated the link between health and social class in modern society. This definition is used for social class in this chapter. Social class is defined as 'segments of the population sharing broadly similar types and levels of resources, with broadly similar styles of living and (for some sociologists), some shared perception of their collective condition'.

In essence, different classes have differential power to access material resources (e.g., homes, cars, white goods and electronic goods) (Notten & Kaplan, 2021). There are several different methods for measuring social class.

The subjective method simply asks which social class people think they are in. Although this has been used in the past, there are some problems with this approach since it lies too much on self-perception rather than any objective measure of social class. By contrast, the objective method uses various measures, such as occupation, car ownership, unemployment, income, postcode and education. All of these indicators can be objectively measured, and these measures have been used most frequently in research.

Both of the two most widely used measures are based on occupation: the Registrar General's Standard Occupation Classification (renamed the 'Social Class based on Occupation') and the Socio-economic Groups. Although both of these methods have been supplanted by another method, which will be discussed later, it is worth outlining these older methods since much of the previous research has relied on them—particularly the Registrar General's classification system—and many health care workers still use it as a shorthand for classifying people (ONS, 2023).

The Social Class based on Occupation measurement was employed in the census from 1901 until relatively recently. It was based on the occupation of the individual head of the household (usually defined as the man—it was defined in less enlightened times!), who was classified into one of six groups:

- Class I: Professional (e.g., lawyer, doctor, university professor)
- Class II: Intermediate (e.g., farmer, nurse, office manager, health care professional)
- Class III(NM): Skilled non-manual (e.g., cashier, secretary)
- Class III(M): Skilled manual (e.g., machine fitter, miner, bus driver)
- Class IV: Partly skilled (e.g., postman[sic], traffic warden)
- Class V: Unskilled (e.g., labourer, messenger, window cleaner)

The Socio-economic Groups system was developed to overcome some of the difficulties associated with the Registrar General's classification system. The Socio-economic Groups system increased the number of categories into which individuals could be assigned. It was not based on status; rather, it was based on similar occupations:

- Employers and managers in central and local government, industry, commerce—large establishments
- Employers and managers in central and local government, industry, commerce—small establishments
- Professional workers—self-employed
- Professional workers—employees
- Intermediate non-manual workers
- Junior non-manual workers
- Personal service workers
- Foreman and supervisors—non-manual
- Skilled manual workers
- Semi-skilled manual workers
- Unskilled manual workers
- Own account workers (other than professional workers)
- Farmers—employers and managers
- Farmers—own account
- Agricultural workers
- Members of the armed forces
- Occupation inadequately described

However, this system was rather subjective and offered little more than being an extension of the Registrar General's classification system. As can be appreciated from the listed categorisations, it becomes difficult to classify individuals without jobs, such as the unemployed, retirees and students. A new government social classification system was developed to overcome these difficulties: the National Statistics Socio-economic Classification (NS-SEC). This new classification method was used in the 2001 Census and continues to be used today (ONS, 2023). The NS-SEC is an occupation-based classification system, but it has rules to cover the whole adult population (see Table 3.3). For further information on best practices for conceptualising and assessing social class outside the British system, see the review by Diemer et al. (2013).

Indices of multiple deprivation

More recently, the focus has shifted from SES to measures of deprivation. Deprivation is a broad concept that has many dimensions. It refers to a range of problems arising from

Table 3.3 The National Statistics Socio-Economic Classification (NS-SEC)

The National Statistics Socio-Economic Classification analytic classes	
1	Higher managerial and professional occupations
	1.1 Large employers and higher managerial occupations
	1.2 Higher professional occupations
2	Lower managerial and professional occupations
3	Intermediate occupations
4	Small employers and own account workers
5	Lower supervisory and technical occupations
6	Semi-routine occupations
7	Routine occupations
8	Never worked and long-term unemployed

a lack of resources or opportunities that we might expect to have access to in our society (Welsh Government, 2019). It encompasses a wide range of domains: health, education, employment, housing, income, access to services and community safety. As the term suggests, multiple deprivation collectively refers to these different types or domains of deprivation. Each country in the UK has its own index of multiple deprivation that it uses to measure relative deprivation for small geographical areas within that country (see Table 3.4). This index can identify and understand how deprivation is distributed across a country so that policies, funding and resources can be targeted to the most deprived or disadvantaged areas (Scottish Government, 2020).

As demonstrated in Table 3.4, each country's indices of multiple deprivation (IMD) comprises domains or categories. These domains are used to calculate an overall relative measure of deprivation for small geographical areas within each respective country in the UK. Each domain within the index is given a percentage score, which is calculated to establish the relative importance of that domain as an aspect of deprivation (Welsh Government, 2019). For example, higher percentage scores, or 'weightings', have greater importance than domains that have lower weightings. Table 3.4 clearly shows that domains with the greatest weighting across all indices are income and employment. This indicates that income and employment are the two most important aspects of deprivation, relative to the other domains, across all four IMDs.

The indices detailed in Table 3.4 are not homogenous; consequently, it is difficult to accurately compare deprivation across England, Wales, Scotland and Northern Ireland. The weightings and indicators used to construct each deprivation domain differ across indices. For example, the living environment/housing domain is weighted differently across the four home countries (see Table 3.4). A weight of 9.3% is attributed to this domain in the English Indices of Deprivation 2019. This score is calculated from indicators measuring poor housing quality, lack of central heating, air quality and road traffic accidents. By comparison, the 2017 Northern Ireland Multiple Deprivation Measure (NIMDM) applies a weight of 5.0% to the living environment domain for (Northern Ireland Statistics and Research Agency, 2017). To complicate comparisons further, the indicators used to construct this measure differ from those used in the English index. The indicators used to construct the living environment domain in the NIMDM are: decent home standard, housing health, safety rating system, homelessness acceptances and a local area problem score (Abel et al., 2016).

Table 3.4 Deprivation domains and their relative weightings for each constituent country in the UK

Domains	England 2010 Weight	Scotland 2012 Weight	Wales 2011 Weight	Northern Ireland 2010 Weight
Income	22.5%	28%	23.5%	25%
Employment	22.5%	28%	23.5%	25%
Education	13.5%	14%	14%	15%
Health	13.5%	14%	14%	15%
Access/barriers to services	9.3%	9%	10%	10%
Living environment/ housing	9.3%	2%	5%	5%
Crime/community safety	9.3%	5%	5%	5%
Physical environment	Not measured	Not measured	5%	Not measured

Adapted from Payne and Abel (2012).

Other factors also limit the direct comparability of the indices in Table 3.4. The differing timescales and the fact that the data do not refer to the same year affect the direct comparison of data. Furthermore, the 2019 Welsh Index of Multiple Deprivation has eight separate domains of deprivation, including the physical environment domain. By contrast, the English Indices of Deprivation 2019 (Ministry of Housing, Communities & Local Government, 2019), Scottish Index of Multiple Deprivation 2020 (Scottish Government, 2020) and NIMDM (Northern Ireland Statistics and Research Agency, 2017) have just seven. Finally, each index is developed according to national policy, and these policies can differ across each constituent country. These differences are perhaps even more pronounced since devolution has evolved.

Many people are familiar with SES, and it would be an oversight not to explain briefly how this compares to IMD. Although standard economic and social measures, such as income, household expenditure and occupation are included, other factors may be relevant to this measurement, such as education, financial security and subjective perceptions of social status and social class (American Psychological Association, 2017). Perhaps the most striking difference between IMD and SES is that IMD measures relative deprivation at the small area level, while SES measures social and economic status at the individual or household level. The IMD also includes much broader environmental measures of deprivation, such as crime, housing and access to services. These domains extend beyond the standard income, education and employment measures used to calculate SES.

Health inequalities related to sex and ethnicity

The relationship between sex and health has been explored in several different ways depending on how health is defined and measured. In terms of mortality, the life expectancy of men and women in various countries is presented in Table 3.5. There is a consistent difference between men and women, with women consistently living longer than their male counterparts. This is true from poorer countries with low life expectancies (e.g., Nigeria) to richer countries (e.g., France) with higher life expectancies (see Global Health Observatory, 2022). Further, the COVID-19 pandemic has revealed significant inequalities in the distribution of cases and deaths across different sociodemographic profiles. Vulnerable populations—including those who are economically disadvantaged, elderly and who have underlying health conditions—are disproportionately affected. While there are very few sex-related differences in the number of COVID-19 cases globally, males in every age group are more likely to die from COVID-19 than females, except for people older than 80 years.

Table 3.5 Life expectancies by country

County	Male life expectancy	Female life expectancy
France	75.9	83.5
Albania	67.3	74.1
Denmark	74.8	79.5
USA	74.6	79.8
Canada	77.2	82.3
Nigeria	48.0	49.6
China	69.6	72.7

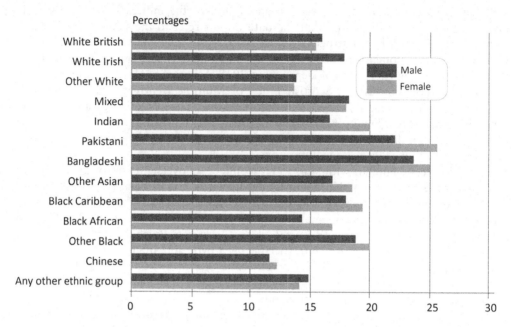

Figure 3.1 Age-standardised limiting long-term illness: by ethnic group and sex, April 2001, England and Wales.

The UK data also support this view, with women living longer than men. Figure 3.1 demonstrates the differences in life expectancy between men and women since the start of the century (Office for National Statistics, 2023). The life expectancy of both men and women has increased by some 3 years over the previous years—an impressive rate of improvement—and this looks like it is continuing.

Also presented on the graph is 'healthy life' expectancy, an important fact that accounts for quality of life and health of the individuals concerned. Again, this figure has improved considerably over the 20-year period. Gender differences in the health of males and females have been widely acknowledged. Data from the Office for National Statistics (2022) highlight this trend, reporting that a larger proportion of females live into their 80s and beyond compared to males. In 2020, the percentage of females in the 90–94-year age group was approximately 65.4%, and the percentage of males in the 90–94-year age group was approximately 34.6% (Office for National Statistics, 2022).

Applying this to Dave

Dave is male; his 'macho behaviour', such as drinking excessively, smoking and drug taking, can all affect his health.

There are also differences in health between ethnic groups. The health outcomes of Irish Traveller, Bangladeshi and Pakistani communities are the worst compared to other groups across various indicators. Data and analysis from the UK 2021 Census (ONS, 2023) showed that among the groups surveyed, individuals who identified as 'White: Gypsy or Irish Traveller' had the highest percentage of individuals reporting 'very bad' health. Notably, despite their relatively young age—with an average age of 27 years—individuals who identified as Bangladeshi within the 'Asian, Asian British, or Asian Welsh' category reported poorer health than expected. The census data show that people who identified as 'Mixed or Multiple ethnic group' of 'White and Asian' and those who identified as 'African' within the 'Black, Black British, Black Welsh, Caribbean or African' category reported the highest levels of 'very good' health.

Of recent relevance, ethnic minority communities have also experienced a disproportionate effect of COVID-19, with higher infection and mortality rates compared to the white population. While factors such as geography, deprivation, occupation, living arrangements and pre-existing health conditions account for some of the excess mortality risk, they do not explain it all. Consequently, some ethnic minority groups now have higher overall mortality rates than the white population due to COVID-19.

In April 2011, Pakistani and Bangladeshi men and women in England and Wales reported the highest rates of poor health and limiting long-term illness, while Chinese men and women reported the lowest rates. Figure 3.1 shows the percentages of people in different ethnic groups suffering from poor health and limiting illness in 2001. Some specific conditions are also noted to be higher in certain ethnic groups:

- South Asian people are reported to have high rates of heart disease and of hypertension.
- Black Caribbean people are reported to have high rates of hypertension but not heart disease.
- All ethnic minority groups are reported to have high rates of diabetes but low rates of respiratory illness (Raleigh & Holmes, 2021).

Health inequalities—Determinants of health

There are many models and frameworks used to explain the determinants of health in relation to inequalities within society—for example, the Field Model of Health and Wellbeing (Evans & Stoddart, 1990) and the Rainbow Model (Dahlgren & Whitehead, 1991). Dahlgren and Whitehead (1991) consider a socio-ecological theory and emphasise the relationship between the individual, who has fixed factors such as age and sex, and their environment, which is changeable. The model comprises several layers that orientate around the individual (see Figure 3.2):

- individual lifestyle factors (e.g., the decision to smoke and drink alcohol)
- social and community networks (e.g., social relations and support)
- living and working conditions (e.g., unemployment and housing)
- general socio-economic, cultural and environmental factors.

If health inequalities are to be successfully tackled, all contributing avenues—from the individual to the societal—must be explored and addressed.

Lifestyle behaviours—such as smoking, drinking alcohol, using drugs, engaging in risky sexual behaviour and a lack of exercise—influence health and health inequalities (Short & Mollborn, 2015). Specific chapters on smoking cessation, alcohol reduction and the promotion of exercise exist in this book, so those factors will be considered in passing rather than in detail here. However, it is worth noting that there tends to be a

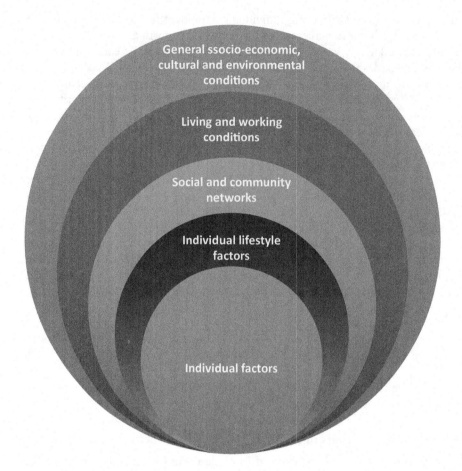

Figure 3.2 Social determinants of health rainbow.

relationship between individual poor lifestyle factors and SES (although this general-isation covers a complex relationship in some areas). For example, Wardle and Steptoe (2003) showed that boys and girls from more deprived neighbourhoods were more likely to have tried smoking, eat a high-fat diet and be overweight. Girls living in more deprived areas were also less likely to eat five servings of fruit and vegetables or exercise during weekends. Most differences persisted after controlling for ethnicity. A clear deprivation gradient emerged for each risk factor.

Smoking's relation to socio-economic class is well known. For instance, the data in Table 3.6 show that individuals in a manual job role are more than twice as likely to smoke than those in a non-manual job role. This emphasises the social gradient in smoking and the population more likely to suffer the health consequences of the behaviour.

Cancer is one of the conditions linked to smoking and is one of the main conditions linked to health inequalities (Marmot, 2020). Evidently, targeting smoking behaviour in the most deprived neighbourhoods would improve health status. However, this may not just be about targeting individuals but about addressing systematic inequalities in society and providing support for those in the most deprived areas of the UK, the argument

Table 3.6 Percentage of individuals smoking cigarettes in 2010

Socio-economic classification	Men	Women	Total
Managerial and professional	14	12	13
Intermediate	20	20	20
Routine and manual	29	28	28
Total	21	20	20

Source: General Lifestyle Survey, Office For National Statistics

being that people smoke because of their environment. Therefore, improving their environment will help reduce unhealthy behaviours.

One particular issue that requires fundamental consideration is the normative culture of differing socio-economic groups. Our social and community networks consist of various individuals, including friends, peers and family members. We learn the behaviours that others close to us exhibit through observation, imitation and modelling. Hence, it is possible that risky health behaviours and behaviours that have adverse health consequences are learned from significant others. Consequently, unhealthy behaviour begets unhealthy behaviour.

For example, research suggests that peer influence and peer norms are important factors in adolescents' sexual behaviour (Peçi, 2017), and the perceived behaviour of peers, rather than peer approval, has been linked to adolescents' risky sexual online behaviour. Further, in a study by Widman et al. (2016), 78% of participants provided riskier responses in the simulated chat room than in their private responses. Gender was the most robust predictor of this change, with boys being more susceptible to peer influence than girls. Additionally, there were significant interactions, indicating that boys with later pubertal development and African American boys exhibited greater susceptibility to peer influence. Once such behaviours have been adopted, they are socially reinforced by those around us who also display the same behaviours, such as smoking, drinking and drug use (see specific chapters for details).

Our living and working conditions can also significantly affect our health. From the obvious—working as a miner or in a steel foundry can potentially be more damaging to health than working in an office due to the inherent risks of the workplace—to the less-obvious psychological factors. For example, a review of more than 200 reports of research exploring the stress hormone cortisol found that the key factors are the unavoidable 'threats to the social self'—those threats to self-esteem and social status (Dickerson & Kemeny, 2004). People who are 'lower on the social hierarchy' and receive 'signals of rejection' from the rest of society are more likely to be stressed and ill.

Following the recent economic troubles, unemployment is a key concern that can also affect health. In December 2022, approximately 1.3 million individuals in the UK were jobless, resulting in an unemployment rate of 3.7%. This is the lowest rate since the 1970s (Office for National Statistics, 2023). It is well documented that unemployed individuals have higher rates of poor health (Maynou & Saez, 2016), which may be related to lower income, a lack of social support gained through working (Rözer et al., 2020) or the clear signals of rejection from the rest of society (Janlert & Hammarström, 2009).

All these factors must be considered when attempting to address health concerns. If there are health inequalities, the task is magnified. To take one such example, in the UK Department of Health's report on reducing infant mortality (Department of Health, 2010c), several key recommendations were made that crossed multiple boundaries (and these still apply today):

- improving access to services among different ethnicities
- improving poor housing conditions and overcrowding, which may play a role in sudden infant death syndrome
- optimising infant and maternal nutrition, including reducing maternal obesity and promoting breastfeeding
- reducing maternal smoking since smoking in pregnancy increases infant mortality by about 40%
- reducing teenage pregnancy because infant mortality rates are 60% higher in this age group than in 20–39-year-olds.

Recently, the US Department of Health and Human Services announced investments of more than $20 million to address the maternal health crisis and reduce disparities in maternal and infant health (U.S. Department of Health and Human Services, 2022). The funding aligns with the Biden–Harris Administration's commitment to prioritising equity and reducing maternal and infant health disparities. These funds will be used to support community-based doulas, rural obstetric care, state task forces targeting maternal health disparities and investments in infant health equity. The goal is to:

- improve maternal and birth outcomes
- expand and diversify the workforce caring for pregnant and postpartum individuals
- increase access to obstetric care in rural communities
- support states in tackling inequities in maternal and infant health.

From individual behaviours (e.g., reducing smoking and teenage pregnancies) to community and environmental actions (e.g., reducing poor housing conditions), the importance of a coordinated approach is evident.

Applying Research in Practice

Disparities in mortality among 25–44-year-olds in England: a longitudinal, population-based study (Kontopantelis et al., 2018). This study examined the growing north-south divide in mortality rates among adults aged 25–44 in England since the mid-1990s. Between 2014 and 2016, there was an annual excess of 627 deaths among women and 1,177 deaths among men in the north. The investigation identified drug misuse, alcohol misuse and cardiovascular disease as the primary factors contributing to this disparity, while male suicide and female cancer rates also played significant roles.

The researchers analysed regional data and discovered that most northern regions had higher mortality rates than southern regions, with London experiencing the lowest mortality rates. The study concluded that addressing this divide will require targeted initiatives that tackle the underlying causes and improve health services while also considering the complex historical concentration of power, wealth and opportunity in London. The mortality gap highlights the persistence of social inequalities in health, particularly among young and middle-aged adults in different regions of England.

Applying this to Dave

It might be suggested that Dave's social and community networks influence his smoking behaviour. He has been surrounded by people who smoke, including his parents and friends, all his life. Therefore, his living conditions, environmental factors and social networks all contribute to the maintenance of this behaviour. Dave will need more support if he attempts to quit smoking, as he is regularly surrounded by that behaviour.

Assessment of health

Assessing health reliably and robustly is important when investigating and considering health inequalities. The most cited definition of health is that provided by the World Health Organization (WHO) (WHO, 1946): 'health is a state of complete physical, mental and social wellbeing and not merely the absence of disease or infirmity' (Peng-Keller, Winiger and Rauch, 2022, p. 265).

The WHO definition was first conceptualised just after the Second World War and emphasises that peace and health are inseparable. Further, it clearly stated that disease and infirmity cannot be isolated from subjective experience, and any definition of health must include a social and psychological dimension.

The definition sets a high standard, but does anybody actually achieve this high status? Regardless, the definition provides something that countries and local communities should aspire to; therefore, it can be extremely useful as a guide and prompt for development. However, others have argued that the WHO definition is merely a definition of happiness rather than health (Saracci, 1997) and that this has important consequences in allocating resources for 'proper' health care. Of course, modern research recognises that although an important interplay exists between happiness and health, they are not conceptually synonymous (Diener et al., 2017). The WHO definition has not been revised since it was first conceptualised in 1946 and, as mentioned, has become the byword for health in health care practice in the twenty-first century (Svalastog et al., 2017). Notwithstanding this, the measurement of health is just as problematic. Given the central role these play in resource allocation, target setting and achievement, these definitions are worthy of further note.

Mortality statistics

One way of measuring health is to simply count the number of people who die in a particular area or in a particular month or who are from a particular group. This approach allows a comparison of rates from group to group (e.g., between men and women), from area to area (e.g., between Edinburgh and Cardiff) or from period to period (e.g., from the nineteenth century to the present day). That area, group or time with the highest death rate is, obviously, the unhealthiest. Since death rates have been collected from the mid-nineteenth century to the present day, it is possible to investigate several important factors.

Initially, the figure was just totalled, giving the crude death rate. This could then be used to provide an overview of the death rate over time (since we also know the country's population at the time), allowing a simple overview of, say, XX per 1,000 (the death rate in 2013). Data can then be collected and analysed at the basic level, and we can compare area, group or time (see Table 3.7).

This information can provide some useful, comparable information. For example, there is some variation in mortality rates between the constituent countries of the UK. In 2010, Scotland had the highest mortality rates for both males and females (785 and 552 deaths per 100,000 population, respectively), while England had the lowest rates for males and females (638 and 456 deaths per 100,000 population, respectively). Northern Ireland has experienced the largest mortality decline since 1980 for both males (51%) and females (43%). By contrast, males and females in Scotland have shown the smallest mortality rate declines over the last 30 years, at 44% and 35%, respectively.

Table 3.7 Death rates by year

Year	Male deaths	Female deaths
1990	277336	287510
1991	277582	292462
1992	271732	286581
1993	279302	299210
1994	266829	284951
1995	272709	293193
1996	269825	293182
1997	266164	291888
1998	264202	289233
1999	263166	290366
2000	256698	281179
2001	253608	278890
2002	254390	280966
2003	254433	284718
2004	245208	269042
2005	243870	269123
2006	240888	261711
2007	240787	263265
2008	243014	266076
2009	238062	253286
2010	237916	255326
2011	234660	249707
2012	240238	259093
2013	245585	261205
2014	245142	256282
2015	257207	272448
2016	257811	267237
2017	262678	270575
2018	267960	273629
2019	265300	265541
2020	308069	299853
2021	297989	288345

However, there are problems with this approach: the death rate in Bournemouth may be quite high, but it might be lower in Amersham. This is not because Bournemouth is a particularly unhealthy place to live. Rather, it is a place where people go to retire; hence, it is bound to have a higher death rate. Crude death rates ignore the fact that many different factors affect the death rate (e.g., an individual's sex, age or previous health). Due to these problems, crude death rates are rarely used when sensitive statistics are required.

Standardised mortality ratios

The standardised mortality ratio (SMR) compares the mortality rate for the whole population with that of a particular region or group (the so-called 'index population'), expressed as a ratio. Thus, the observed death rate is divided by the expected rate (derived from the index population) and then multiplied by 100.

SMRs are calculated to compare death rates from a single cause (e.g., heart attacks, breast cancer) between geographical areas or different groups (according to sex, class, ethnicity, etc.). The SMR for deaths from a particular disease is calculated by expressing the actual number of deaths in the group of interest in the index area as a ratio of the expected number of deaths in the standard population data. Sometimes the SMR is expressed after multiplying by 100. Thus, a SMR<1.0 (or 100) indicated fewer than expected deaths, an SMR>1.0 (or 100) indicates there were excess deaths. In most analyses, a value of 1.0/100 equals the average mortality. For example, Table 3.8 shows the SMR for coronary heart disease in selected areas of England

Table 3.8 SMR rates due to coronary heart
disease in England, 2012

Area	SMR
Buckinghamshire CC	83.5
Cambridgeshire CC	87.3
Cumbria CC	112.5
Derbyshire CC	110.1
Devon CC	88.9
Dorset CC	80.1
East Sussex CC	81.1
Essex CC	91.8
Gloucestershire CC	95.8
Hampshire CC	84.2
Hertfordshire CC	90.0
Kent CC	96.5
Lancashire CC	113.0
Leicestershire CC	93.2
Lincolnshire CC	99.1
Norfolk CC	94.1
Northamptonshire CC	91.6
North Yorkshire CC	107.6
Nottinghamshire CC	100.1
Oxfordshire CC	78.3
Somerset CC	85.3
Staffordshire CC	101.3
Suffolk CC	95.5
Surrey CC	79.7
Warwickshire CC	84.1
West Sussex CC	86.1
Worcestershire CC	86.3

Table 3.9 Death rates in the home countries, 1981–2001

	Number of deaths			Death rate per 1,000 population			SMR		
	1981	*1991*	*2000*	*1981*	*1991*	*2000*	*Persons*	*Males*	*Females*
Scotland	63.8	61.0	57.8	12.3	12.0	11.3	118	117	117
England	541.0	534.0	501.0	11.6	11.1	10.0	98	98	98
Wales	35.0	34.1	33.3	12.4	11.8	11.3	102	102	102
Northern Ireland	16.3	15.1	14.9	10.6	9.4	8.8	105	105	105
United Kingdom	658.0	646.2	608.4	11.7	11.2	10.2	100	100	100

The data can be used to determine the parts of the country where death rates are highest. Table 3.9 shows that the SMR rates are higher in Lancashire than in Oxfordshire. Similarly, the SMR can be used to compare countries (see Table 3.9). The data show that England has a lower mortality rate than other UK countries, particularly Scotland (General Registrar Office for Scotland, 2012).

Morbidity statistics

Morbidity statistics are often used to determine the prevalence of illness and disease. Again, such data are used to compare morbidity across years and population groups. The databases include a wide range of statistics, from information on the prevalence of specific cancers to individuals who have drug dependency and mental health disorders. In the UK, this information can be found on websites like those of the Office for National Statistics, the Department of Health and the Health Security Agency. Such statistics are only concerned with the population as a whole, not at an individual level.

Individual health measurement tools

At an individual level, health can be measured from several perspectives: by looking at either physical or psychological health or a combination of the two (i.e., health-related quality of life [HRQoL]). There are several measures for assessing the latter, for example, the 36-Item Short Form Survey (Ware & Sherbourne, 1992; Brazier et al., 1992). This generic health survey consists of eight constructs that, when combined, assess the physical and mental health of an individual:

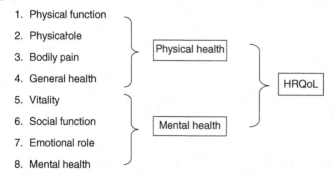

1. Physical function
2. Physical role
3. Bodily pain
4. General health
5. Vitality
6. Social function
7. Emotional role
8. Mental health

Physical health

Mental health

HRQoL

The results of such questionnaires should be interpreted with caution due to the nature of the measures. As the measures rely on self-reports, responses may be biased and socially desirable answers may be received.

Applying this to Dave

Dave could undertake a quality-of-life assessment concerning his angina. This will enable his health care professionals to understand the effect of his illness on him from a social and psychological perspective.

Health promotion

Health promotion is the process of enabling people to increase their control over their health and its determinants, thereby improving their health. It is a core function of public health and contributes to tackling communicable and non-communicable diseases and other threats to health (WHO, 2016).

Broadly, health promotion combines disease prevention and health education to inspire individuals to maintain a healthy lifestyle (see Chapter 2 for more detail).

Approaches to health promotion

Approaches to health promotion vary and will be considered in more detail in the next chapter. However, it is worth briefly outlining the five main approaches and how these can be linked to health inequalities.

Medical model

To ensure individuals remain in good health, the medical model encourages individuals to undertake efforts to ensure good health, such as receiving immunisations. This is done through persuasion. For example, the UK National Health Service (NHS) launched a national immunisation programme in 2008 to protect girls from developing cervical cancer. Girls aged 14–17 are given the human papillomavirus (HPV) vaccine to reduce rates of adult cervical cancer. The NHS has also been following a COVID-19 vaccination programme that is separate from the routine immunisation schedule. The COVID-19 vaccination programme aims to protect the population against the novel coronavirus (SARS-CoV-2), which has caused a global pandemic (NHS, 2022). By addressing specific health issues through targeted vaccination programmes, the NHS is actively working to improve the overall health and wellbeing of the population. This combined approach illustrates the interplay between individual responsibility and public health initiatives, ultimately emphasising the need for a comprehensive strategy to protect and maintain the wellbeing of communities.

Behavioural model

The behavioural model considers the individual's behaviours and attitudes and aims to change these in an attempt to improve health. The government has considered this angle of health promotion in schemes such as the School Fruit and Vegetable Scheme. This programme runs as part of the 5 A Day programme and has been shown to increase children's consumption of fruit and vegetables (Teeman et al., 2010). In using this approach, health promoters take an expert-led, top-down role to influence the individuals' behaviour. Strategies are used to persuade the individual to undertake beneficial health behaviours.

Educational model

The educational model aims to give the individual the required information on healthy lifestyles, such as the benefits of smoking cessation, so they can make an educated decision concerning their health behaviours. Persuasion is not considered in this model; instead, it focuses on providing knowledge to empower the individual to adopt healthy behaviours. Therefore, in this sense, health promotion is purely considered providing information to empower the individual to consider their attitudes towards health behaviours.

Client-led model

The client-led model is predominantly concerned with empowering the individual to understand the health effects of their behaviour. In doing so, the client takes control of their health behaviours in a bottom-up process. The health professional is simply there to guide and advise the client about the behaviour they wish to change. For example, an individual may decide, with the support of their GP, that they want to lose weight. The health professional will simply guide the client and support them in accomplishing their goal. This can be through providing information, support and recourses.

Societal-led model

The societal-led model does not intend to change the individual's behaviour but that of society. In making health behaviours more accessible to all individuals regardless of their socio-economic background, health promotion can tackle health and health inequalities. In doing so, poor health-related behaviours can be made less accessible. For example, the UK Government acknowledges the need to address unhealthy food advertising, particularly aimed at children, and has now banned advertisements for fatty, salty and sugar-laden products on TV and online before 9 pm. This approach represents a top-down process to tackle health issues, such as obesity and cardiovascular disease, by targeting the larger societal structures that influence individual behaviour (Department of Health & Social Care, 2020).

Applying this to Dave

Dave could use the health promotion materials that can be found in local chemists and GP surgeries. He could take a bottom-up approach and start taking control of his health-related behaviours by considering promotional materials on angina and smoking. This may help educate him and motivate him to change. Alternatively, other models could be applied, but these are much more difficult and long term.

Interventions to reduce health inequalities

Interventions aimed at improving the overall health of individuals and reducing health inequalities have been considered an essential part of the UK Government's agenda for many years. According to Ford et al. (2021), the English Health and Social Care Act (2012) legally requires national and local NHS decision-making bodies to address health inequalities. However, the years following the Act saw a reorganisation and fragmentation of services, with little progress on health inequalities. The NHS Long Term Plan (National Health Service England, 2019) aimed to establish a more systematic approach to reducing health inequalities, but it lacked clear guidance on how local and national systems could systematically address the issue. It is clear that the health service cannot tackle this alone—a multidisciplinary approach, involving a combination of local services, will prove the most beneficial.

The UK Department of Health (2012) outlined a move to integrate public health into local government that allowed services to be planned in the context of broader social determinants of health, such as poverty, education, housing and employment. The Public Health Outcomes Framework will be refocused on positive health outcomes and reducing inequalities in health rather than focusing on performance targets. The intended outcomes of the change are to increase healthy life expectancy and reduce differences in healthy life expectancy between communities.

By instigating this change, the Department of Health hopes to remove central control and tailor local health promotion messages that are specific to the target audience. The government proposed to 'reach across and reach out' by being:

- responsive: owned by communities and shaped by their needs
- resourced: with ring-fenced funding and incentives to improve
- rigorous: professionally led, focused on evidence, efficient and effective
- resilient: strengthening protection against current and future threats to health (Department of Health, 2010b, p. 6).

Public Health England's (PHE; now the Office for Health Improvement & Disparities since 2021) strategy for 2020–2025 aimed to address the critical challenges faced by the UK population regarding health and wellbeing, with a strong focus on preventive measures and reducing health disparities. By embracing a multisectoral approach, the department sought to collaborate with local governments, the NHS and other stakeholders to create targeted interventions that considered the wider social determinants of health, such as poverty, education, housing and employment. The strategy emphasised the importance of positive health outcomes, mental health promotion and environmental health, alongside tackling infectious diseases and ensuring workforce development. The ultimate goals of this comprehensive strategy were to extend healthy life expectancy, reduce the differences in healthy life expectancy between communities and create a more resilient and equitable public health system for all.

One of the targeted interventions implemented under PHE's 2020–2025 strategy was the Healthy Minds programme in Manchester, aimed at promoting mental wellbeing and reducing mental health disparities within the community. Manchester was identified as an area with high levels of stress, anxiety and depression, which significantly affected residents' quality of life. The project addressed these concerns by developing a multipronged approach, including public awareness campaigns on mental health;

workshops on stress management and resilience building; and accessible mental health resources, such as peer support groups and digital self-help tools. Additionally, the project collaborated with local schools and employers to create mental health–friendly environments and policies. By employing this multifaceted strategy, the Healthy Minds programme endeavoured to reach a broader audience, raise mental health awareness and ultimately contribute to reducing mental health disparities in the community.

The public health strategy in other UK countries is similarly comprehensive. In Wales, a long-term Public Health Strategy for Wales (2018–2030) was developed to address the country's public health challenges. Although the general health of the Welsh population appears to be improving, as measured by life expectancy, closer inspection of the data reveals a widening gap between the health of the wealthiest and the health of the poorest. These findings indicate that deprivation remains a significant determining factor in people's health status. Objectives within the strategy clearly outline the need to improve health and reduce health inequalities by addressing the wider socio-economic and environmental determinants of health. An updated version outlined the priorities from 2023–2035 (Public Health Wales, 2023):

- influencing the wider determinants of health
- promoting mental and social wellbeing
- promoting healthy behaviours
- delivering excellent public health services
- supporting a sustainable health and care system
- tackling public health effects of climate change

On 31 March 2021, the Welsh Government released its initiative titled *A More Equal Wales: The Socio-economic Duty*. This initiative places equality at the heart of decision-making. The objective is to ensure that decisions made by public bodies consider the effect of socio-economic inequalities and work towards reducing them.

The proposed socio-economic duty would require public bodies in Wales to consider how their decisions and policies could promote greater equality and reduce socio-economic disparities. It intends to address the root causes of inequality, such as poverty and discrimination, and ensure that public resources are used effectively to tackle these issues.

Applying this to Dave

Dave lives in one of the most deprived areas in Wales. The socio-economic duty supports individuals like Dave by promoting equality and progress. Dave can access new education and vocational training opportunities beyond manual labour. Accessible health care and smoking cessation programmes could improve his wellbeing and highlight a positive path for himself and his loved ones. The socio-economic duty drives change, ensuring a fairer society where everyone can thrive.

The public health strategy for Northern Ireland, *Making Life Better – A Whole System Strategic Framework for Public Health 2013–2023*, was published in 2014 as a successor to the 2002 *Investing for Health* strategy. Like other regions in the UK, Northern Ireland has experienced overall population health improvements since the inception of the previous strategy. However, this progress masks persistent health inequalities between the wealthiest and poorest citizens, a pattern observed across the UK. Compared to England, Northern Ireland's population demonstrates poorer health outcomes in certain areas. The *Making Life Better* strategy was developed to address these disparities and adapt to the evolving social, economic and policy landscape.

In response to the persistent health inequalities in Scotland, the Scottish Government and Convention of Scottish Local Authorities jointly introduced the *Public Health Priorities for Scotland* (see Christie, 2018), emphasising the need for a collaborative approach to address health disparities. This initiative acknowledges the strong links between deprivation, inequality and health outcomes by outlining six key priorities to enhance the wellbeing of the entire population, especially the most disadvantaged communities.

Building on these efforts, Public Health Scotland was established in 2020, consolidating resources and expertise to tackle health inequalities effectively and protect the nation's health. This organisation envisions a nation where everybody thrives, despite the country having the lowest life expectancy in Western Europe and a significant gap between the wealthiest and poorest citizens. With a comprehensive 2022–2025 plan, Public Health Scotland focuses on preventing disease, prolonging healthy life and promoting health and wellbeing through various key initiatives, including leading Scotland's vaccination programme, implementing an infectious disease intelligence strategy, utilising health care data to drive performance and improvement, and collaborating with partners to strengthen services and address local public health concerns.

Interventions

Interventions designed to tackle health inequalities can be described as 'upstream' or 'downstream', though, in reality, there is a continuum between the two. Upstream interventions act on the social determinants of health or act to create a healthier environment or culture (e.g., legislation on smoking in public places). Downstream interventions seek to address an existing health problem or risk factor (e.g., smoking cessation services). Another key distinction is whether an intervention is applied at a whole population level (e.g., alcohol minimum unit pricing) or at the individual level (e.g., alcohol brief behavioural interventions). Further information on such interventions is available in other chapters of this book.

Tackling health inequalities at an individual level is important due to the variations within society and individual differences. In attempting to change health inequalities, the government recognised the need to provide individuals with more support when attempting to change lifestyle behaviours, such as smoking. Therefore, implementing various interventions, such as health trainers or (now) health coaches, was considered essential. Health trainers/coaches work in disadvantaged communities with individuals who are engaging in risky behaviours and tailor their support to the needs of the individuals in that specific community. It is recognised that self-efficacy is one of the best predictors of behaviour change in such communities. For example, Cleland et al. (2010) reviewed factors associated with resilience to physical inactivity in women from socio-economically disadvantaged backgrounds. It was found that the strongest factors for achieving the recommended levels of physical activity were factors such as self-efficacy.

However, the social context of the individual and the behaviour should not be overlooked in any training or coaching arena.

Policy-level developments addressing health inequalities

Chapter 2 clearly demonstrates that health promotion must be a central focus for reducing health inequalities. As previously outlined, the public health strategies for England, Wales, Northern Ireland and Scotland recognise that health inequalities must be tackled so that socially disadvantaged groups can enjoy comparable levels of good health to wealthier groups. A recent report by PHE, *Reducing Health Inequalities: System, Scale and Sustainability*, has comprehensively examined the extent of health inequalities in the UK. This document sets out the need for action on health inequalities and an examination of the potential intervention strategies, focusing on implementing effective population-level interventions, reducing health inequalities through service provision and utilising essential tools and resources to reduce health inequalities (PHE, 2017)

Traditional health promotion strategies like the large public health campaigns that raise awareness of health issues are effective, but only, it seems, for the more advantaged groups in society who have greater access to time, resources and finances (Australian Institute of Health and Welfare, 2022; Baah et al., 2019). Consequently, health inequalities are widening because the health of those in higher socio-economic groups is improving faster. Herein the complexity lies. The report (PHE, 2017) explains that the health of disadvantaged groups is not necessarily worsening; it is just not improving at the same rate as their wealthier counterparts. It seems that these socially disadvantaged groups cannot access the same opportunities for good health as the more advantaged groups in society, and this has led to the observed inequalities in health that are apparent in the UK today. Knowing that good health is not equally distributed in society, scarce resources must be targeted to those in greatest need.

Sure start

The UK Government has developed specific health inequality initiatives to close the widening gap between society's wealthiest and poorest. The Sure Start initiative, launched in the UK in 1998, is a good example of how the government has developed and targeted services to families living in deprived areas to tackle inequalities. This government-led initiative identifies that the early years are a crucial stage in the lifespan to address health inequalities through policy development (Cattan et al., 2021). Promoting a healthy start in life is the emphasis of the Sure Start initiative, and this is particularly important because lifestyle factors can have a huge effect on a young child's development and future health. A mother's lifestyle during pregnancy can affect the health of her unborn child and, once born, lifestyle factors (e.g., breastfeeding, diet and parental smoking) can significantly affect a child's health and development (Stephenson et al., 2018). The importance of the early years in governmental policies addressing health inequalities cannot be overstated.

Sure Start programmes are typically designed around objectives related to strengthening families and communities, increasing operations productivity and improving children's social and emotional development, health and ability to learn (Roberts, 2000). The breadth of these objectives acknowledges that health is indeed a multidimensional concept and supports the WHO's definition of health described at the beginning of this chapter.

Preventive work and family support are central components of the programme. The importance of social support for behaviour change is discussed more fully in Chapter 4, but one way social support is believed to improve health is by enhancing healthy lifestyles. In terms of Sure Start, social integration and specific social support for parenting skills and health promotion are ways that social support may operate to enhance behaviour change in harder to reach, disadvantaged families.

The 2021 Institute for Fiscal Studies (IFS) report on the health effects of the Sure Start programme revealed significant benefits for children, particularly those from disadvantaged neighbourhoods (Cattan et al., 2021). The programme led to a notable reduction in hospitalisations by the time children finished primary school, with long-lasting effects that persisted until age 14. Additionally, the IFS report suggested that the reduction in hospitalisations generated long-term savings for the NHS, offsetting around 6% of the programme's cost when children were aged 0–4 and 12% when children were aged 0–11.

Since 2010, one of the most significant changes to the Sure Start programme has been a substantial reduction in funding, leading to the closure of numerous Sure Start Children's Centres across the UK (Cattan et al., 2021). This change primarily resulted from austerity measures introduced in response to the financial crisis in 2008. Local authorities responsible for funding and overseeing Sure Start Children's Centres have faced significant budget cuts, resulting in the reallocation of resources and the prioritisation of other services. Consequently, many centres have been forced to reduce their services, merge with other centres or close altogether. This reduction in funding and the subsequent closure of centres has raised concerns about the accessibility of early years support and intervention services for children and families, particularly those from disadvantaged backgrounds. Critics argue that the closures have disproportionately affected the most vulnerable populations, leading to increased inequality in access to early years support.

Despite these challenges, the Sure Start Children's Centres that have remained open have continued to provide valuable services to their communities, focusing on early intervention and support for children and families.

While the Sure Start model still exists, the concept of family hubs has emerged as a parent-centred approach, taking over as the forefront of family support services. Since its establishment in 1998, Sure Start has primarily focused on early years services, but the transition to family hubs has expanded the scope to encompass a wider age range and placed a strong emphasis on integrated support for families. The family hub concept recognises the vital role of parents and caregivers, treating them as valued partners rather than passive recipients. Thus, under the new family hub model, parents and caregivers are actively involved in the support and decision-making processes (Callan, 2021).

Inequalities and lifestyle

The causes of health inequalities are clearly complex and include lifestyle factors such as smoking, exercise and nutrition. As outlined earlier in this chapter, smoking is considered a significant cause of health inequalities in the UK. Policy-level developments that have reduced these inequalities include the introduction of legislation to ban smoking in public places and vehicles and banning point-of-sale tobacco advertising (Barbry et al., 2015).

Social marketing

Social marketing has also been heralded as a promising new approach to achieve specific behaviour change, particularly in harder to reach or disadvantaged groups. As discussed in Chapter 2, social marketing aims to influence a target audience's behaviour to promote positive behaviour(s) for health or social change. Healthy Families (previously Change4life) is an example of a national social marketing initiative that aims to tackle childhood obesity in the UK (NHS, 2022; see also Department of Health, 2015). A social marketing approach to health promotion can potentially communicate health messages in a more tailored and evidence-based way to influence positive behaviour change, thereby addressing health inequalities in socially disadvantaged groups.

Financial incentives

A recently debated topic and potential intervention that aims to improve medical adherence and participation in vaccination and screening programmes is the use of financial incentives. It is thought that using these schemes could be useful in tackling health inequalities. Incentives can take various forms, such as vouchers for discounts at local retailers or gifts for adherence and attendance. The idea of incentives related to specific behaviours has been previously shown to be effective (Vlaev et al., 2019). Although research has supported the use of incentives for one-off behaviours, such as screening and testing for diseases (Zenner et al., 2012), these behaviours do not require long-term maintenance. More research is needed on using incentives to produce long-term health behaviour changes because the results of studies using incentives have not always been positive (see Mantzari et al., 2015).

In the UK, various incentive programmes and initiatives have encouraged people to switch from smoking to vaping as a harm reduction strategy. PHE has consistently endorsed e-cigarettes as a less harmful alternative to tobacco smoking and has promoted their use as a smoking cessation aid. However, this topic is controversial, as will be discussed in Chapter 8. Nevertheless, the UK Government has introduced a world-first national scheme to provide nearly 20% of smokers in England with a vape starter kit and behavioural support to help them quit smoking. The goal is to reduce smoking rates to 5% or less by 2030. Local authorities are set to participate in the scheme towards the end of 2023, tailoring it to their needs and prioritising specific populations. Additionally, pregnant women will be offered financial incentives and support to stop smoking—a technique with demonstrated, albeit limited, efficacy (Berlin et al., 2021).

Applying this to Dave

Individual-level interventions like those described could help Dave improve his health. For instance, if his local area had health trainers, they could help keep Dave motivated to reduce his smoking habits. Health trainers could also assess and further develop Dave's self-efficacy.

Conclusion

Health inequalities are a key concern to all governments across the UK, and the ill health that results from them is generally preventable. Changing the health behaviour of individuals is challenging, but the systematic changes required to society are even more so. To change behaviour and tackle health inequalities and the social gradient in health, it is necessary to target individuals, cultures and social policy.

Key points

- Health inequalities are the variation in health outcomes and mortality rates between individuals.
- Various factors affect health and health inequalities, such as age, sex, gender identity and sexual orientation, education level, SES and ethnicity.
- The relationship between income and health has produced a social gradient.
- The government has emphasised the importance of reducing the gap in health inequalities.
- Multilayered approaches, such as Dahlgren and Whitehead's (1991) Social Determinants of Health Rainbow, are useful because they acknowledge the complexity of tackling health inequalities.
- The individual's beliefs and reasons behind their health-related and risky behaviours must be considered.
- Measures based on psychological principles can be used to unravel beliefs regarding health-related behaviours.
- Self-efficacy is important when aiming to change health-related behaviour.
- Health promotion and health interventions must reach all individuals in the population if health inequalities are to be successfully reduced.

Points for discussion

- Critically discuss the following statement: 'SES determines health'.
- Consider and discuss the evidence for the various measures of health.
- Describe and evaluate how social factors affect health inequalities.

Further resources

Diemer, M. A., Mistry, R. S., Wadsworth, M. E., López, I. & Reimers, F. (2013). Best practices in conceptualizing and measuring social class in psychological research. Analyses of Social Issues and Public Policy, *13*(1), 77–113. Doi: 10.1111/asap.12001

Marmot, M. (2020). Health equity in England: The Marmot review 10 years on. BMJ, *368*, m693. Doi: 10.1136/bmj.m693

Naidoo, J., & Wills, J. (2010). Developing practice for public health and health promotion (3rd ed.). Edinburgh, Scotland: Bailliere Tindall/Elsevier.

Office for National Statistics. (2022). Health state life expectancies, UK: 2018 to 2020. Newport, South Wales: Author. Retrieved from https://www.ons.gov.uk/peoplepopulationandcommunity/healthandsocialcare/healthandlifeexpectancies/bulletins/healthstatelifeexpectanciesuk/2018to2020

Public Health England. (2019). All Our Health: About the framework. Retrieved from https://www.gov.uk/government/publications/all-our-health-about-the-framework/all-our-health-about-the-framework

World Health Organization. (2021). Health promotion glossary of terms 2021. Geneva, Switzerland: Author.

References

Abel, G. A., Barclay, M. E., & Payne, R. A. (2016). Adjusted indices of multiple deprivation to enable comparisons within and between constituent countries of the UK including an illustration using mortality rates. BMJ Open, 6(11), e012750. Doi: 10.1136/bmjopen–2016-012750

American Psychological Association. (2017). Education and socioeconomic status factsheet. Retrieved from https://www.apa.org/pi/ses/resources/publications/education

Australian Institute of Health and Welfare. (2022). Health across socioeconomic groups. Canberra, ACT: Author. Retrieved from https://www.aihw.gov.au/reports/australias-health/health-across-socioeconomic-groups

Baah, F. O., Teitelman, A. M., & Riegel, B. (2019). Marginalization: Conceptualizing patient vulnerabilities in the framework of social determinants of health—An integrative review. Nursing Inquiry, 26(1), e12268. Doi: 10.1111/nin.12268

Barbry, C., Hartwell-Naguib, S., & Barber, S. (2015). Smoking in public places. Retrieved from https://researchbriefings.files.parliament.uk/documents/SN04414/SN04414.pdf

Berlin, I., Berlin, N., Malecot, M., Breton, M., Jusot, F., & Goldzahl, L. (2021). Financial incentives for smoking cessation in pregnancy: Multicentre randomised controlled trial. BMJ, 375, 1–10.

Brazier, J. E., Harper, R., Jones, N. M., O'Catham, A., Thomas, K. J., Usherwood, T., & Westlake, L. (1992). Validating the SF-36 health survey questionnaire: New outcome measure for primary care. BMJ, 305(6846), 160–164. Doi: 10.1136/bmj.305.6846.160

Callan, S. (2021). Family Hubs: Building on the legacy of Sure Start Children's Centres. Family Hubs Network. Retrieved from https://familyhubsnetwork.com/family-hubs-building-on-sure-start-legacy/

Cattan, S et al. (2021). The health impacts of Sure Start. London: IFS. Available at: https://ifs.org.uk/publications/health-impacts-sure-start (accessed: 25 September 2023).

Christie, B. (2018). Scotland identifies public health priorities. BMJ, 361, 35.

Cleland, V. J., Ball, K., Salmon, J., Timperio, A. F., & Crawford, D. A. (2010). Personal, social and environmental correlates of resilience to physical inactivity among women from socio-economically disadvantaged backgrounds. Health Education Research, 25(2), 268–281. Doi: 10.1093/her/cyn054

Dahlgren, G., & Whitehead, M. (1991). Policies and strategies to promote social equity in health. Stockholm, Sweden: Institute for Future Studies.

Department of Health. (2010b). Healthy lives, healthy people: Our strategy for public health in England [White paper]. London, England: The Stationery Office.

Department of Health. (2010c). Tackling health inequalities in infant and maternal health outcomes: Report of the Infant Mortality National Support Team. London, England: Author.

Department of Health. (2012). Healthy lives, healthy people: Improving outcomes and supporting transparency. London, England: Author.

Department of Health. (2015). Government response to the House of Commons Health Select Committee report on the impact of physical activity and diet on health, sixth report of session 2014–15. Whitehall, England: Her Majesty's Stationery Office. Retrieved from https://assets.publishing.service.gov.uk/government/uploads/system/uploads/attachment_data/file/445984/Cm_9001_accessible.pdf

Department of Health & Social Care. (2020). Tackling obesity: Empowering adults and children to live healthier lives. Retrieved from: https://www.gov.uk/government/publications/tackling-obesity-government-strategy/tackling-obesity-empowering-adults-and-children-to-live-healthier-lives (accessed September 25, 2023)

Dickerson, S. S., & Kemeny, M. E. (2004). Acute stressors and cortisol responses: A theoretical integration and synthesis of laboratory research. Psychological Bulletin, 130(3), 355–391. Doi: 10.1037/0033-2909.130.3.355

Diemer, M. A., Mistry, R. S., Wadsworth, M. E., López, I., & Reimers, F. (2013). Best practices in conceptualizing and measuring social class in psychological research. Analyses of Social Issues and Public Policy, 13(1), 77–113. Doi: 10.1111/asap.12001

Diener, E., Pressman, S. D., Hunter, J., & Delgadillo-Chase, D. (2017). If, why, and when subjective well-being influences health, and future needed research. Applied Psychology: Health and Well-Being, *9*(2), 133–167. doi:10.1111/aphw.12090

Evans, R. G., & Stoddart, G. L. (1990). Producing health, consuming health care. Social Science and Medicine, *31*, 1347–1363.

Ford, J., Sowden, S., Olivera, J., Bambra, C., Gimson, A., Aldridge, R., & Brayne, C. (2021). Transforming health systems to reduce health inequalities. Future Healthcare Journal, *8*(2), 1–6. Doi: 10.7861/fhj.2021-0018

Forster, T., Kentikelenis, A., & Bambra, C. (2018). Health inequalities in Europe. Setting the stage for progressive policy action. Dublin, Ireland: Think-tank for Action on Social Change. Retrieved from https://feps-europe.eu/publication/629-health-inequalities-in-europe-setting-the-stage-for-progressive-policy-action/

Global Health Observatory. (2022). GHE: Life expectancy and healthy life expectancy. Retrieved from https://www.who.int/data/gho/data/themes/mortality-and-global-health-estimates/ghe-life-expectancy-and-healthy-life-expectancy. (accessed September 25, 2023)

Health and Social Care Act. (2012). c. 7. United Kingdom. Retrieved from http://www.legislation.gov.uk/ukpga/2012/7/contents/enacted

Janlert, U., & Hammarström, A. (2009). Which theory is best? Explanatory models of the relationship between unemployment and health. BMC Public Health, *9*, 1–9.

Kontopantelis, E., Buchan, I., Webb, R. T., Ashcroft, D. M., Mamas, M. A., & Doran, T. (2018). Disparities in mortality among 25–44-year-olds in England: A longitudinal, population-based study. Lancet Public Health, *3*(12), E567–E5575. Doi: 10.1016/S2468-2667(18)30177-4

Mackenbach, J. P., Stirbu, I., Roskam, A. J. R., Schaap, M. M., Menvielle, G., Leinsalu, M., & Kunst, A. E. (2008). Socioeconomic inequalities in health in 22 European countries. New England Journal of Medicine, *358*(23), 2468–2481.

Mackenbach, J. P., Valverde, J. R., Artnik, B., Bopp, M., Brønnum-Hansen, H., Deboosere, P., … Nusselder, W. J. (2018). Trends in health inequalities in 27 European countries. Proceedings of the National Academy of Sciences, *115*(25), 6440–6445. Doi: 10.1073/pnas.1800028115

Mantzari, E., Vogt, F., & Marteau, T. M. (2015). Financial incentives for increasing uptake of HPV vaccinations: A randomized controlled trial. Health Psychology, *34*(2), 160

Marmot, M. (2010). Fair society, healthy lives: The Marmot Review. Strategic review of health inequalities in England post-2010. London, England: The Marmot Review. Retrieved from https://www.instituteofhealthequity.org/resources-reports/fair-society-healthy-lives-the-marmot-review

Marmot, M. (2020). Health equity in England: The Marmot review 10 years on. BMJ, *368*, m693. Doi: 10.1136/bmj.m693

Maynou, L., & Saez, M. (2016). Economic crisis and health inequalities: Evidence from the European Union. International Journal for Equity in Health, *15*(1), 135. Doi: 10.1186/s12939-016-0425-6

Ministry of Housing, Communities & Local Government. (2019). The English indices of deprivation 2019 (IoD2019). Statistical release. Retrieved from https://assets.publishing.service.gov.uk/government/uploads/system/uploads/attachment_data/file/835115/IoD2019_Statistical_Release.pdf

National Health Service. (2022). Healthier families. Retrieved from https://www.nhs.uk/healthier-families/

National Health Service. (2019). The NHS long term plan. Retrieved from https://www.longtermplan.nhs.uk/publication/nhs-long-term-plan/

Northern Ireland Statistics and Research Agency. (2017). Northern Ireland multiple deprivation measure 2017 (NIMDM2017). Retrieved from https://www.nisra.gov.uk/statistics/deprivation/northern-ireland-multiple-deprivation-measure-2017-nimdm2017

Notten, G., & Kaplan, J. (2021). Material deprivation: Measuring poverty by counting necessities households cannot afford. Canadian Public Policy, *47*(1), 1–17.

Office for National Statistics. (2022). Ethnic group differences in health, employment, education and housing shown in England and Wales' Census 2021. London, England: Office for National Statistics.

ONS. (2023). SOC2010 volume 3: the National Statistics Socio-economic classification (NS-SEC rebased on SOC2010). Retrieved from https://www.ons.gov.uk/methodology/classificationsandstandards/standardoccupationalclassificationsoc/soc2010/soc2010volume3thenationalstatisticssocioeconomic-classificationnssecrebasedonsoc2010 (accessed September 25, 2023)

ONS. (2023). General health, England and Wales: Census 2021. Retrieved from https://www.ons.gov.uk/peoplepopulationandcommunity/healthandsocialcare/healthandwellbeing/bulletins/generalhealthenglandandwales/census2021 (accessed September 25, 2023)

ONS. (2021). National life tables – Life expectancy in the UK: 2018 to 2020. Retrieved from https://www.ons.gov.uk/peoplepopulationandcommunity/birthsdeathsandmarriages/lifeexpectancies/bulletins/nationallifetablesunitedkingdom/2018to2020#life-expectancy-at-birth-in-uk-countries (accessed October 21, 2023)

Payne, R. A. , & Abel, l. G. A. (2012). UK indices of multiple deprivation-a way to make comparisons across constituent countries easier. Health Stat Q, 53, 2015–2016.

Peçi, B. (2017). Peer influence and adolescent sexual behavior trajectories: Links to sexual initiation. European Journal of Multidisciplinary Studies, 4(3), 96–105. Doi: 10.26417/ejms.v4i3.p96-105

Public Health England. (2017). Reducing health inequalities: System, scale and sustainability. Retrieved from https://assets.publishing.service.gov.uk/government/uploads/system/uploads/attachment_data/file/731682/Reducing_health_inequalities_system_scale_and_sustainability.pdf

Public Health Wales. (2023). Our Long term strategy 2023–2035. Retrieved from https://phw.nhs.wales/about-us/working-together-for-a-healthier-wales/ (accessed September 25, 2023)

Raleigh, V., & Holmes, J. (September 17, 2021). The health of people from ethnic minority groups in England. The King's Fund. https://www.kingsfund.org.uk/publications/health-people-ethnic-minority-groups-england

Roberts, H. (2000). What is sure start? Archives of Disease in Childhood, 82(6), 435–437. doi:10.1136%2Fadc.82.6.435

Rözer, J. J., Hofstra, B., Brashears, M. E., & Volker, B. (2020). Does unemployment lead to isolation? The consequences of unemployment for social networks. Social Networks, 63, 100–111. Doi: 10.1016/j.socnet.2020.06.002

Saracci, R. (May 10, 1997). The World Health Organisation needs to reconsider its definition of health. BMJ, 314(7091), 1409–1410. Doi: 10.1136/bmj.314.7091.1409. PMID: 9161320; PMCID: PMC2126653.

Scottish Government. (2020). Scottish Index of Multiple Deprivation 2020. https://www.gov.scot/collections/scottish-index-of-multiple-deprivation-2020/ (accessed September 25, 2023)

Short, S. E., & Mollborn, S. (2015). Social determinants and health behaviors: Conceptual frames and empirical advances. Current Opinion in Psychology, 5, 78–84. Doi: 10.1016/j.copsyc.2015.05.002

Stephenson, J., Heslehurst, N., Hall, J., Schoenaker, D. A., Hutchinson, J., Cade, J. E., ... & Mishra, G. D. (2018). Before the beginning: Nutrition and lifestyle in the preconception period and its importance for future health. The Lancet, 391(10132), 1830–1841.

Svalastog, A. L., Donev, D., Jahren Kristoffersen, N., & Gajović, S. (2017). Concepts and definitions of health and health-related values in the knowledge landscapes of the digital society. Croatian Medical Journal, 58(6), 431–435. Doi: 10.3325/cmj.2017.58.431. The Institute for Fiscal Studies (2021).

Teeman, D., Lynch, S., White, K., Scott, E., Waldman, J., Benton, T., ...Thomas, J. (2010). The third evaluation of the school fruit and vegetable scheme. London, England: Department of Health.

Townsend, P., & Davidson, N. (1982). Inequalities in health. In Classic and contemporary readings in sociology (pp. 202–209). London: Routledge.

U.S. Department of Health and Human Services. (August 29, 2022). HHS announces over $20 million in awards to implement Biden-Harris administration blueprint for addressing the maternal health crisis; reduce disparities in maternal and infant health [Press release]. Retrieved from https://www.hhs.gov/about/news/2022/08/29/hhs-announces-over-20-million-in-awards-to-implement-biden-harris-administration-blueprint.html

Vlaev, I., King, D., Darzi, A., & Dolan, P. (2019). Changing health behaviors using financial incentives: A review from behavioral economics. BMC Public Health, *19*, 1059. Doi: 10.1186/s12889-019-7407-8

Wardle, J., & Steptoe, A. (2003). Socioeconomic differences in attitudes and beliefs about healthy lifestyles. Journal of Epidemiology & Community Health, *57*(6), 440–443.

Ware Jr, J. E., & Sherbourne, C. D. (1992). The MOS 36-item short-form health survey (SF-36): I. Conceptual framework and item selection. Medical Care, *30*, 473–483.

Welsh Government. (2019). Welsh index of multiple deprivation (WIMD) 2019: Results report. Retrieved from https://www.gov.wales/sites/default/files/statistics-and-research/2019-11/welsh-index-multiple-deprivation-2019-results-report-024.pdf

Widman, L., Choukas-Bradley, S., Helms, S. W., & Prinstein, M. J. (2016). Adolescent susceptibility to peer influence in sexual situations. Journal of Adolescent Health, *58*(3), 323–329. Doi: 10.1016/j.jadohealth.2015.10.253

White, Chris, & Edgar, Grace (2010). Inequalities in healthy life expectancy by social class and area type: England, 2001–03. Health Statistics Quarterly, *45*, 28–56.

World Health Organization. (2016). Shanghai Declaration on promoting health in the 2030 agenda for sustainable development. Retrieved from https://www.who.int/publications/i/item/WHO-NMH-PND-17.5

World Health Organization. (1946). Peng-Keller, S., Winiger, F., & Rauch, R. (2022). The spirit of global health: The World Health Organization and the 'spiritual dimension' of health, 1946–2021 (p. 265). Oxford: Oxford University Press.

Zenner, D., Molinar, D., Nichols, T., Riha, J., Macintosh, M., & Nardone, A. (2012). Should young people be paid for getting tested? A national comparative study to evaluate patient financial incentives for Chlamydia screening. BMC Public Health, *12*(1), 261–267. Doi: 10.1186/1471-2458-12-261

4 Psychology in practice

LEARNING OBJECTIVES

At the end of this chapter you will:

- Have been introduced to the key psychological factors that influence behavioural change.
- Recognise the key barriers to behavioural change.
- Have evaluated how psychological approaches can improve the likelihood of clients following behavioural advice.
- Recognise that getting people to adopt a healthy behaviour is only the start of a process and that people will need continued support to maintain a change.
- Have considered the unique problems involved with attempting to change well-established habits.

Case study

Caroline is a practice nurse in a semi-urban GP practice. Her role at the clinic includes health promotion. When Caroline first joined the practice, she was very enthusiastic about the health promotion aspect of her role. She was convinced of the importance of a healthy lifestyle in preventing chronic disease. Caroline set up a blood pressure clinic and a weight control clinic to support patients who had been advised by the doctor to reduce their blood pressure and/or lose weight. Caroline sees patients shortly after the doctor has told them that their health is at risk; many are worried and anxious. Patients at these clinics are provided with high-quality information and advice about how to change their diet, reduce their drinking and increase their physical activity, and stop smoking if they are smokers. They are directed towards local leisure-centre classes and given suggested meal plans. However, over the 5 years that Caroline has worked at the practice, she has become disillusioned with her health promotion role. Very few people are able to make permanent changes to their eating, drinking or exercise habits and the number of patients diagnosed with Type 2 diabetes and other chronic diseases continues to increase.

DOI: 10.4324/9781003471233-4

At first, Caroline wondered if the quality of the information she was providing was an issue. However, a questionnaire survey amongst the clinic attendees demonstrated that the majority understood the importance of a healthy lifestyle, were aware of the government recommendations for healthy behaviours and knew about the local community leisure facilities. Caroline realises that education is not enough and that patients need support to make and maintain changes and is looking for new approaches to use in her clinic. She has enrolled on a continuing professional development (CPD) module looking at psychological approaches to behavioural change in the hope that it will give her new ideas to improve her practice.

Introduction

A central strategy of health promotion has always been education. Health education involves a combination of risk communication and behavioural advice (Knowledge) as well as developing life skills. As such, it assumes that people may practise unhealthy lifestyle behaviours because they do not understand what is bad or good for their health and that if they had good quality information and appropriate skills, they would make healthy choices (WHO, 2012). Whilst it is clear that educational interventions seldom directly change health behaviour providing information remains an important component of a comprehensive policy approach to health promotion. Individuals have a right to be informed about the known risks and benefits of health behaviours and information and education campaigns can contribute to a holistic package of measures to help communities and people make positive changes. The World Health Organization (WHO) (2018) in their Global Action Plan on Physical Activity recognise the importance of 'systems-based' approaches:

Effective nation action to reverse current trends and reduce disparities in physical activity requires a "systems-based" approach with a strategic combination of "upstream" policy actions aimed at improving the social, cultural, economic and environmental factors that support physical activity combined with "downstream" individually focused (educational and informational) approaches

WHO (2018)

Whole systems approaches are important and within them psychologically informed approaches will play a pivotal role. In line with an educational approach to health promotion psychology has focused on investigating how people understand and respond to the information they receive about health and behaviour. This is often described as a social cognitive approach to behavioural change. Social cognitive approaches assume that behavioural choices reflect the way people see and think about the world. Consequently, if we can understand how people think then we will be able to influence the way they decide to behave. A key aspect of this approach is the recognition that different people may perceive the same thing differently. So, what is unpleasant for one person may be enjoyable for another. In terms of lifestyle choices, one person may find cycling a pleasant way to unwind after work, whilst another cannot face cycling home at the end of a long day.

Decisions about how to behave are postulated to involve some sort of cost-benefit analysis. In its simplest version, any model of behavioural change is a straightforward weighing up of these two factors. Research has then gone on to investigate what other factors are also influential. A number of different theoretical models of health behaviour have been developed to predict people's behavioural choices, expanding on the basic cost-benefit model. It is beyond the remit of this text to provide a description and explanation of the numerous psychological models of behaviour. There are a number of texts where the reader can find a comprehensive review of these models, such as Conner and Norman (2015) or Thirlaway and Upton (2009). However, it is worth acknowledging that health behaviour researchers have recognised that the most effective interventions are 'systems-based' that simultaneously target change mechanisms at different levels (e.g., individual, community and population) and that such complex interventions will probably draw on a range of theories in their design and development.

Michie and Wood (2015) recognised that there is a potentially bewildering array of behavioural change techniques available to health professionals and a clear taxonomy would support practitioners to adopt appropriate techniques for their particular needs and researchers to evaluate and contribute to the continuing development of effective techniques and interventions (Michie & Wood, 2015). The Behavioural Change Wheel is a synthesis of 19 behavioural change frameworks that draw on a wide range of disciplines and approaches. It introduces a systematic method for understanding behaviour and links them to techniques that have been found to be effective (Figure 4.1).

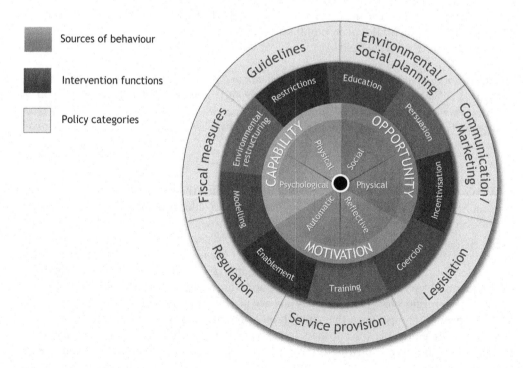

Figure 4.1 The behavioural change wheel. Taken from Michie et al. (2014).

Promoting lifestyle change has traditionally focused on educating people to recognise where a change in behaviour would be good for their health and on motivating people to change. However, more recently the focus has widened to recognise the importance of sustaining health behaviours for the long term (Nigg, 2008; Strobach et al. 2020; Wood & Neal 2016). Lifestyle change needs to be long term to improve health outcomes but unfortunately many people who take up a healthy behaviour soon stop. For example, research has shown that up to 50% of people who start a formal physical activity programme drop out within 6 months (Nigg et al., 2008). Different studies report different levels of attrition ranging from 7–58% but the mechanisms for better adherence are not well established (Linke et al., 2011). Psychological concepts such as self-regulation, habituation and stages of change recognise the long-term issues around behavioural change and the interventions associated with these concepts go some way towards addressing the issue of sustained change (Table 4.1).

Table 4.1 Factors that may influence lifestyle behavioural change

Psychological concept	Associated intervention
Perception of risk	Education, risk communication
Perception of benefits	Education, risk communication
Barriers	Structural change, cognitive behavioural therapy
Social norms	Policy; education; cultural adaptation
Social support	Motivational interviewing; counselling
Self-efficacy	Motivational interviewing; goal setting
Self-regulation	Goal setting; implementation intentions, coping skills
Fear	Risk communication
Habituation	Motivational interviewing; implementation intentions; cognitive behavioural therapy, Mindfulness
Pleasure	Little known, classical conditioning
Stages of change	Various, depending on stage

Applying this to Caroline

Caroline needs a broad toolkit of intervention strategies to deal with the range of factors that could be influencing the lifestyle behaviours in her clients

Psychological concepts

Perception of risk and benefits

A perception of risk is a central factor in the majority of psychological models of behavioural change; it delivers the costs side of the basic behavioural change evaluation. It is based on the assumption that unless people realise a behaviour is risky they will not attempt to alter it.

In 2002, the Cabinet Office Strategy Unit defined risk as:

Uncertainty of outcome, whether positive opportunity or negative threat.

(Cabinet Office Strategy Unit, 2002, p. 7)

However, the Office for Product Safety and Standards (2021) have recently developed a Risk Lexicon in which they define risk as:

an event that can have negative impact (harm)

and opportunity as:

an event that can have a positive impact (benefit).

(Office for Product Safety and Standards, 2021, p. 2)

The Risk Lexicon definition of risk reflects the views of most people that risk is negative and indicates something to worry about (Thirlaway & Heggs, 2005). Indeed, a lot of risk communication is intended to generate fear and anxiety in order to get people to change their behaviour; whether this works will be considered later in the chapter.

A useful definition of risk for health promotion is the one provided by Connolly et al. (2000):

A situation of risk presents some chance of injury, damage or loss, a hazard or dangerous chance.

So the starting point for any health promotion activity has always been to communicate a risk because it is assumed that unless people realise that drinking has the potential to cause harm, they are unlikely to stop. Similarly, people are unlikely to adopt healthy behaviours that they don't enjoy, such as eating fruit, unless they understand that not eating fruit puts their health at risk.

Health professionals collectively decide about what is risky and what is safe. They provide a plethora of information about the 'right' way to behave. In the UK people are advised to drink no more than 14 UK units (8 grams) of alcohol a week. They are advised to eat five portions of fruit and vegetables each day and to do 150 minutes of moderate to vigorous physical activity each week. There is expert advice available on the correct way to brush your teeth, the amount of water to drink, and the speed at which to drive your car. Through risk communication the government informs us both of the *cost* of practising unhealthy behaviours, such as drinking too much, and of the *cost* of avoiding healthy behaviours, such as being physically active. There is an agreed 'correct' risk perception and on the basis of that, an agreed 'correct' decision. However, health promotion has been communicating lifestyle risks for more than two decades with little impact on lifestyle choices. In general the public fail to adhere to the recommendations made by the government (Health Survey for England, 2020; Health Survey (NI), 2021; Scottish Health Survey, 2020; Welsh Health Survey, 2020). Previously it had been assumed that this is because individuals don't understand the risk correctly (Thirlaway & Upton, 2009). Indeed, in 1999 the Department of Health stated that lay risk perceptions must be challenged by more effective risk communications. However, a large body of research has now established that people understand the risks associated with an unhealthy lifestyle but still struggle to make appropriate changes to their behaviour (Blaxter, 2004; Lawton & Conner, 2007).

Applying this to Caroline

Caroline's experience in her clinics has already shown her that providing risk information is only a small aspect of the behavioural change intervention process.

The other main communication that health promotion delivers is behavioural advice and this behavioural advice often informs about the *benefits* of change as well as giving advice about what the change should be. Similarly to risk communications, behavioural advice is generally well understood but it is not generally adhered to (Health Survey for England, 2020; Health Survey (NI), 2021; Scottish Health Survey, 2020; Welsh Health Survey, 2020).

Why don't people respond to risk communications and behavioural advice about their lifestyle by changing their behaviour? Certainly, when asked to evaluate a risk communication people report feeling anxious or worried (Thirlaway & Heggs, 2005). We proposed in 2009 that there are three main reasons risk communications do not result in lifestyle behavioural change (Thirlaway & Upton, 2009). We continue to argue that these are critical to understanding why health behaviour change is so hard.

Firstly, lifestyle behaviours are not practised solely for health reasons. Lifestyle behaviours have other social outcomes that are often more important for people than a future risk to health, so any cost-benefit analysis carried out by individuals may include non-health outcomes that are often not considered by health-focused health professionals.

Secondly, lifestyle health messages are predominantly focused on long-term health outcomes. This requires people to be 'future-orientated' and most people are focused on the present (Thirlaway & Upton, 2009). Health promotion is asking people to make unpalatable changes to their lives now in order to reduce a risk that is a long way in the future. Consequently, people tend to look for other, less difficult ways to reduce the anxiety that a risk communication generates (Thirlaway & Heggs, 2005). It is easier to use strategies such as deciding the source of the message is untrustworthy, or to be unrealistically optimistic about your current behaviour, than it is to actually set about changing.

Thirdly, many established health behaviours have become habitual and are controlled not by cognitive decisions but by automatic responses to the routine situations of our daily lives (Hagger, 2019; Stobach et al., 2020; Verplanken & Melkeviko, 2008). The concept of 'choice architecture' is based on automatic behavioural theory and is defined as trying to change behaviour by altering the presentation of a choice through information or the physical or social micro-environment in which individuals make decisions (Landias et al., 2020). How many of us have decided to give up biscuits with our cup of coffee only to find that we are halfway through one before we remember our decision not to eat them? A simple change such as moving the biscuit tin might help override the automatic behaviour.

Barriers

Barriers refer to those things that are part of our wider social and physical environment that prevent us carrying out behaviours we might otherwise choose to do. Individuals tend to list a set of barriers, such as lack of time, lack of resources, or poor facilities, unsafe environments as the reason for their failure to make positive lifestyle choices. However, what is a barrier for one person, e.g., a three-mile trip to a leisure centre, may not be seen as a barrier at all for another.

The term obesogenic environment has been widely used to refer to the physical, economic, social and cultural barriers in the environment that impede the maintenance of a healthy body weight (Hobbs & Radley, 2020; Lee et al., 2011). Barriers to successful weight maintenance are things like the easy availability of high-fat food and the environmental obstacles to active commuting. However, the government-commissioned Foresight Report on obesity in the UK (Jones et al., 2007) concluded that the influence of the environment on obesity was not straightforward. It is not the environment *per se* that matters but the way individuals perceive it. Jones et al. (2007) have raised concerns that building more cycle paths may only encourage people who already cycle rather than creating more cyclists. Non-cyclists will need support to encourage them to believe that they could use the cycle paths provided in their environment. Recently, the SLOPE study that followed 14,084 children at ages 4–5 and 5,637 at ages 10–11 found mixed results between area characteristics at birth and overweight/obesity at later ages. Relative density of unhealthy food outlets and measures of air pollution were positively associated with overweight/obesity but not in children who moved. Local access to green spaces at time of birth was inversely associated with becoming overweight and obese regardless of migration (Wilding et al., 2020).

Applying this to Caroline

Caroline needs to work at changing her clients' perceptions of the local resources available to them to increase their physical activity. She may be supported in this as active transport policies start to change the cultural norms for cycling and walking. Keeping abreast of community interventions such as perhaps a new Park Run starting and aligning any GP practice promotions may increase uptake.

Social norms

As part of their detailed analysis of obesity in the UK, the Foresight authors (Jones et al., 2007) argue that normative social behaviour, that is, what is acceptable behaviour to the majority of an individual's peer group, is key to understanding and promoting positive lifestyle choices (Jones et al., 2007). Injunctive norms describe the perceived attitudes or approval of behaviours by others and descriptive norms relate to perceptions of peer engagement in behaviours (Dempsey et al., 2018). Descriptive norms appear to be more influential over behaviour than injunctive norms. A clear relationship between what people think their peers are drinking and what they themselves choose to drink has been demonstrated both in adults at work and in students at college (Barrientos-Gutierrez et al., 2007; Mcalaney et al., 2007). Similarly, research has demonstrated that parents influence their adolescent children's consumption of fruit and vegetables through what they do (descriptive norms) rather than what they say (injunctive norms) (Pedersen et al., 2014). Robinson et al. (2013) carried out a systematic review that demonstrated that descriptive social norms, perceptions of what others were eating, influenced choice and quantity of food eaten. Delivering normative feedback about peer behaviour needs to be relevant and specific to the target population to ensure any social norm based intervention is perceived to be realistic and persuasive by participants (Dempsey et al., 2018). In challenging perceptions of peer behaviour, interventions need to recognise that people are generally very optimistic about their own behaviour in comparison to other people (Mcalaney et al., 2007). It is becoming clear that social norms-based strategies are most likely to be effective within a framework of strategies, a whole systems approach, where they may be an important element of a successful behavioural change package (Cislaghi & Heise, 2018; WHO, 2018).

Applying this to Caroline

Caroline could use data from individuals similar to her clients to demonstrate that their behaviour is actually more risky than that of other similar people. She could encourage clients to participate in local activities such as Park Run by sharing data about the number of patients registered at the practice who participate.

Social support

There is considerable evidence that social isolation or lack of social support increases the risk of developing a range of chronic diseases (Cohen & Janicki-Deverts, 2009; Uchino, 2006). Social support clearly matters for health but what is difficult is defining and measuring something so complex. As social support is fundamentally about relationships, a simple way to investigate social support is to count how many relationships an individual has. Other studies have tried to evaluate the quality of social support using questionnaires that ask questions such as:

Do you have someone that you can share your innermost thoughts with and confide in?
(Wang et al., 2005, p. 600)

Another way to think about social support is in terms of emotional support (availability of close emotional support) and social integration (availability of peripheral contacts). Social support is a complex thing; we know that it has health benefits, but it is hard to identify how it is beneficial and therefore develop any strategies to build in what is lacking for the socially isolated. One way that social support is believed to improve health is by enhancing healthy lifestyles. For example, smokers with good social support are more likely to succeed in giving up smoking (Creswell et al., 2015; Pirie et al., 1997). Social network and environmental-based therapies in drinking attempt to use the individual's social environment to help achieve absence through helping clients build social networks supportive of change or by developing engagement in social activities that do not promote alcohol use. The evidence that these approaches work are very much around maintaining change rather than generating change (NICE, 2011).

What is not clear is whether general social support (good emotional support and/or strong social integration) is enough to support individuals attempting to change their behaviour or whether specific support for the attempted activity is necessary. So is it enough to get general emotional support from a partner whilst dieting, or does the partner need to be supportive of the specific dieting behaviour? Similarly, it is not clear whether specific support for changing behaviour, such as that available from personal trainers or support groups, is sufficient to support long-term behavioural change and could provide the social support necessary to facilitate change for the socially isolated. It has been argued that general social support improves health outcomes by acting as a stress buffer (Uchino, 2006). Individuals who have people with whom they can talk through stressful situations and from whom they can receive emotional support may receive direct physiological benefits in terms of lower levels of stress hormones (Uchino, 2006). Equally, they may be less likely to use alcohol, high-fat food or drugs as a stress alleviator (Gruber, 2008; Harvey & Alexander, 2012).

Specific social support such as that provided by weight reduction groups, exercise programme classes or by personal trainers or other health professionals can work at the individual level by providing positive feedback about successful behavioural change and improving self-efficacy (Gruber, 2008) but it can also, over time, provide some of the general emotional support if the relationships persist over time. The therapeutic alliance & therapist competence has long been recognised as a critical factor for success in all types of psychological interventions (NICE, 2011). This is now being recognised as important in early primary care and public health lifestyle change interventions. Make Every Contact Count (MECC) recognises that professionals across a range of settings have the potential to influence health behaviours in every interaction, and perhaps more importantly, recognise that the quality of even the briefest of interactions matters. The strategy recommends that all practitioners delivering behaviour change interventions as suggested by the NHS MECC (2016) policy should be trained in good behavioural change techniques in order to maximise success (NICE, 2019).

Applying this to Caroline

Caroline has recognised that she and her clients will benefit if she develops her skills in behaviour change techniques.

Self-efficacy

Self-efficacy is the belief that you can carry out a specific behaviour in a specific situation (Bandura, 1997). Self-efficacy has been to be a reliable predictor of whether people will change their behaviour across all lifestyle behaviours (Luszczynska & Schwarzer, 2015). University students who reported higher levels of exercise self-efficacy were more likely to be physically active (Williams & French, 2011). Gilles et al. (2006) found that those with low self-efficacy for avoiding heavy drinking in social situations drank more. Higher self-efficacy has been found to predict greater ability to resist peer pressure to have sex (Dilorio et al., 2001) and a better ability to avoid risky sexual behaviour (O'Leary et al., 2008).

Self-efficacy is behaviour specific and is not transferable. So you may have high self-efficacy for taking physical activity but low self-efficacy for practising safe sex. Increasing self-efficacy in one behaviour will not translate into increased self-efficacy in other behaviours. Given the importance of self-efficacy in health behaviours, it is crucial to understand the mechanisms by which self-efficacy can be improved or damaged.

The dieting industry is often detrimental to the self-efficacy of individuals trying to lose weight. There are many diets on the market offering rapid weight loss that is either very difficult to achieve or very difficult to maintain. A series of failed dieting attempts can seriously damage self-efficacy for weight loss. Professionals working with individuals trying to lose weight need to be aware that if they have made multiple failed attempts to lose weight and/or maintain weight loss they are likely to have very little confidence in their ability to succeed. Repeated failure is very damaging to self-efficacy.

Self-efficacy has been argued to be enhanced by personal accomplishment, mastery, vicarious experience or verbal persuasion (Williams & French, 2011). It is important to note that some of the most common behavioural techniques such as persuasion and barrier identification are associated with lower levels of self-efficacy. The strong evidence that self-efficacy is associated with positive health behaviours has generated a number of psychological strategies to develop self-efficacy, including motivational interviewing, coping skills, goal setting and implementation intentions, all of which will be discussed later in the chapter.

Applying this to Caroline

Caroline may want to consider how confident her clinic participants are about making the changes she is suggesting and investigate mechanisms for increasing their self-efficacy for the proposed change.

Self-regulation

Self-regulation in the context of behavioural change refers to efforts by people to alter their responses to situational cues and control their dominant and automatic behaviours. For example, being in a pub and not ordering an alcoholic drink. It is people trying to control the number of calories they consume, the number of units of alcohol they drink, the drugs they take, the cigarettes they consume, the time they spend in sedentary activities or the amount of physical activity they take. It is likely that at any one time a majority of people will be attempting to regulate one or more of their lifestyle behaviours. Self-regulation is closely linked to self-efficacy because if people try and succeed in regulating a behaviour their self-efficacy will increase (Magill et al., 2020). However, if they try and fail to regulate a behaviour, they risk damaging their self-efficacy and are less likely to succeed if they attempt regulation again.

Successful self-regulation involves setting goals for a particular behaviour and sticking to them. So, for instance, many people try to lose weight by going on a calorie-controlled diet where they attempt to limit the amount of calories, they consume each day. Interestingly, people who are dieting are more prone to bouts of disinhibited eating than people who are not attempting to diet (Herman & Polivy, 2004). At first sight this is counterintuitive, in that people who are trying to restrict their calorie intake should be less likely to overeat. However, research consistently shows that if people on a diet are asked to consume food perceived as 'high calorie', such as a rich milkshake, they are more likely than people not dieting to over-consume afterwards (Herman & Polivy, 2004). It would seem that once dieters perceive that they have 'failed' to stick to their daily calorie quota; they feel they might as well eat whatever they like. Herman and Polivy (2004, p. 498) describe this as the 'what-the-hell' effect. This then creates a real problem for health professionals attempting to encourage weight loss because the setting of goals for calorie intake may actually put individuals at greater risk of overeating. In the field of alcohol and drug addiction many treatment programmes aim for total abstinence, which is one response to the problem of disinhibition; however, total abstinence is not an option for weight management.

Fear

When the relationship between behaviour and health was first recognised and health professionals wanted to stop unhealthy behaviours, they used risk communication to try to generate fear.

Fear appeals are based on the fear-drive model which argues that fear is unpleasant, and people want to avoid it. If a communication makes people feel fearful or anxious then the fear-drive model suggests that the recipient will want to reduce this unpleasant state of mind. If the communication also contains advice, then individuals may try to follow this advice in order to escape from the unpleasant feelings of anxiety and fear for their future health. If following the behavioural advice leads to a reduction in fear, then people are likely to continue with their changed behaviour.

Fear is intuitively appealing as a means of promoting behavioural change but the role it plays in initiating behavioural change is not clear-cut or consistent (Simpson, 2017; Thirlaway & Upton, 2009). Often the response to failed fear appeals is to increase the level of fear either by increasing the graphicness of the imagery or by focusing on the worst possible outcome. Gallopel-Morvan et al. (2009) found that graphic images were more effective than text messages alone in changing behavioural intentions, but it is not clear whether this translates into behaviour change. Other research suggests that increasing the level of fear generated by a message does not increase the uptake of behavioural prevention strategies. One reason may be that highly fearful messages are likely to induce denial and therefore fail to have any impact on behavioural choices (Sutton, 1982). Fear appeals may be more effective when combined with self-efficacy messages which can help individuals believe there is an effective action to minimise the risk (Simpson, 2017).

Habituation

Past behaviour is a powerful predictor of future behaviour (Hagger et al., 2002; Conner & Norman, 2015). Consistent patterns of past behaviours are often referred to as habits. Habits are behaviours that may once have been initiated by rational choice but are now under the control of specific situational cues that trigger the behaviour without thinking (Aarts et al., 1997; Landais et al., 2020; Verplanken & Melkeviko, 2008). So, many of the choices we make about what to eat for breakfast, the amount of coffee we consume, whether we walk or drive to work on a day-to-day basis are not conscious choices at all but things we do without thinking. Assumptions that lifestyle choices are always a conscious choice undermine many health promotions (Wood & Neal, 2016).

All lifestyle behaviours have the potential to become habits or even addictions. There is a tendency to assume that behaviours such as smoking and drinking that include a physiological response to the alcohol or the nicotine are harder habits to break because of the combined physiological and psychological reinforcement. However, people struggle to give up smoking long after the physiological addiction is overcome (Thirlaway & Upton, 2009), which implies that psychological addiction can be powerful alone.

Health professionals are faced with a dual problem: they need to help people break unhealthy habits and they need to support the development of healthy habits (Wood & Neal, 2016). Many of the unhealthy habits that older adults struggle with, as the negative consequences of decades of unhealthy living start to materialise, are established in adolescence and early adulthood when health is optimal, and the costs of smoking, drinking, eating badly or not exercising are in the distant future. Important outcomes for young people are identity formation and the establishment of social relationships (Kuther & Timoshin, 2003). Drinking and eating are an integral component of many social events in the UK and alcohol in particular enhances social integration and facilitates the development of relationships. Interventions that attempt to enable young people to set up healthy drinking habits need to focus on the role of alcohol for young people in the present, rather than on the cost of alcohol consumption in the future. On a positive front, sport is often central to socialisation, particularly for young men, and supports the establishment of positive physical activity habits (Thirlaway & Upton, 2009).

Much of early behavioural change work focused on instigating change but more recently the importance of maintaining change for long enough for people to establish habitual behaviour patterns that are easier for them to maintain has been recognised (Gardner et al., 2012; Wood & Neal 2016).

Health starts to become pertinent for individuals as they start to experience ill-health and the costs of unhealthy lifestyles are in the present or the near future rather than in the distant future (Lawton, 2002). Unfortunately, by the time individuals wish to change their unhealthy habits they are likely to be well established and difficult to break. Wood and Neal (2016, p. 73) have argued that *'existing habits are a significant impediment to people adopting and sticking with helping behaviour'*. In the second edition of this text we suggested that research needed to focus on understanding how we can help people change ingrained habits. In 2016, Wood and Neal (2016) reviewed the literature on developing healthy habits and concluded that there are three central habit-forming interventions: behaviour repetition, stable context cues (which can often be supported by implementation plans) and rewards. They also identify three main habit-breaking interventions: cue disruption, environmental re-engineering and vigilant monitoring. It is clear that for habit-breaking context is critical and using transitional changes, such as changing jobs or retiring, as a time to change established behaviours can support success. Similarly environmental re-engineering 'choice architecture' such as building cycle paths, banning smoking or introducing free showers in workplaces can be pivotal to whether a psychological change invention succeeds (Kelly & Barker, 2016; Landais et al., 2020; Wood & Neal, 2016).

Applying this to Caroline

Caroline could work more closely with her local public health team and county council to time interventions with new public health initiatives such as new cycle paths or other local and national lifestyle change initiatives. Setting goals for self-regulation needs to be carefully managed and monitored to ensure that individuals can see success and feel rewarded.

Pleasure

People usually choose to do things that they enjoy. Pleasure can be argued to be the main motivation for lifestyle choices, particularly among the young (Kuntsche & Cooper, 2010). Pleasure can be experienced as a physiological sensation, for instance the response to chocolate in the mouth. Pleasure can also be experienced as a positive emotion, for instance winning a game of sport. Frequently, a pleasurable response includes both physiological and emotive sensations. Some things are innately pleasurable, such as sweet food. Other things we learn to enjoy, such as drinking alcohol. Few young people enjoy their first taste of an alcoholic drink, which is why beverage manufacturers have developed sweetened alcoholic drinks for the teenage market to make the alcohol more palatable and support the initiation of learnt enjoyment of alcohol (Plant & Plant, 2006).

Regardless of whether the pleasure is physiological or psychological, innate, or learnt, if an experience is pleasurable people are more likely to repeat it. Consequently, pleasure is fundamental in the establishment of habitual behaviours. One approach to encouraging healthy lifestyle habits would be to try to elicit pleasurable responses to healthy behaviours. However, we don't understand very well how people learn to enjoy certain behaviours and not others.

Applying this to Caroline

Presumably, most health professionals understand that people do things that they enjoy but they seldom take that into account when offering advice about lifestyle change. Feeling successful is a positive emotion and good goal setting can help individuals start to enjoy activities that they haven't learnt to enjoy previously.

Stages of change

As well as looking at what external factors influence behavioural change, psychologists have also looked at the motivation state of the individual who is trying to change. This approach views change not as a one-off event but as a process and argues that health professionals need to tailor their support for individuals to their stage of change.

According to all stage theories, a person can move through a series of stages in the process of behavioural change. Different models argue for different numbers of stages that last for differing lengths of time. The most well-known stages of change model comes from the trans-theoretical model of change which conceptualises the process of change as having five stages as described in Table 4.2.

Table 4.2 The stages of change, conceptualised using alcohol as the healthy behaviour

Stages of change	Behavioural and motivational characteristics
Pre-contemplation	Individuals are drinking and have no intention of stopping in the next 6 months
Contemplation	Individuals are drinking but they intend to stop in the next 6 months
Preparation	Individuals are drinking less and intend to stop in the next 6 months
Action	Individuals have stopped drinking to excess within the past 6 months. The perceived benefits are greater than the perceived costs. This is the least stable stage
Maintenance	Individuals have been non-drinkers for over 6 months and risk of relapse is small

The model argues that it is important to understand where people are in the process of change before attempting to support them to change, because depending on the stage of change you would use different techniques to encourage a change in behaviour. Whilst it is possible to identify different motivational states in individuals the relationship between these stages and effective interventions has not been clearly established.

Psychological interventions

Making every contact count

Making every contact count (MECC) is an approach to behaviour change that uses the millions of day-to-day interactions that organisations and individuals have with other people to support them in making positive changes to their physical and mental health and wellbeing (Public Health England, 2016). Public Health England recognise that individual behavioural change approaches such as MECC need delivery by people who have been trained in the concepts of effective behavioural change and within an environment that supports behavioural change. They propose that different intensities of behavioural change interventions should be integrated within clinical pathways so many of the psychological interventions that follow could sit in these pathways.

Within Community pharmacies there are now over 3,500 qualified health champions working in over 2,100 'healthy living' pharmacies who are engaging members of the public by using every interaction as an opportunity for a health promoting intervention (Public Health England, 2016) (Figure 4.2).

MECC activity is detailed in the 2 layers at base of the pyramid below

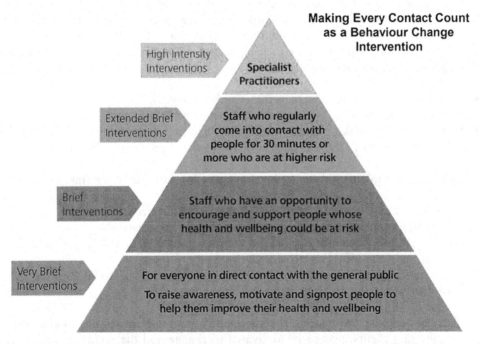

Behaviour change interventions mapped to NICE Behaviour Change: Individual approaches/PH49

Figure 4.2 Making Every Contact Count (MECC) model.

Parchment et al. (2021) demonstrated in their review of 22 studies that '*Healthy Conversations Skills*' had a positive impact on staff competence in supporting behaviour change with some evidence of positive impact on sedentary behaviours and dietary quality of service users. They concluded that '*Healthy Conversations Skills*' was an effective behavioural change intervention for use as a very brief/brief intervention in the MECC framework.

Motivational interviewing

Miller and Rollnick (2002) suggested that motivation is fundamental to change, and they suggest that motivational interviewing is the appropriate approach. Motivational interviewing can be defined as 'a client-centred, directive method for enhancing intrinsic motivation to change by exploring and resolving ambivalence' (Miller & Rollnick, 2002).

Motivational interviewing aims to increase an individual's motivation to consider change rather than showing them how to change. If a person doesn't want to change then it is irrelevant if they know how to do it or not. However, if a person is motivated to change then the interventions aimed at changing behaviour can begin.

Motivational interviewing (MI) is a technique based on cognitive-behavioural therapy which aims to enhance an individual's motivation to change health behaviour. The whole process aims to help the patient understand their thought processes, to identify how their thought processes are helping to produce the inappropriate behaviour and how their thought processes can be changed to develop alternative, health-promoting, behaviours. Motivational interviewing differs from counselling because it is directive; the health care professional elicits and selectively reinforces change talk that resolves ambivalence and moves the client towards change.

Motivational strategies include eight components that are designed to increase the level of motivation the person has towards changing a specific behaviour. It is important to note that the motivation is specific to one behaviour and so being motivated to quit smoking does not simply transfer to being motivated to reduce alcohol consumption. The eight components are as follows:

- Giving advice (about specific behaviours to be changed);
- Removing barriers (often about access to particular help);
- Providing choice (making it clear that if they choose not to change that is their right and it is their choice; the therapist is there to encourage change but not to insist on change);
- Decreasing desirability (of the ambivalence towards change or the status quo);
- Practising empathy;
- Providing feedback (from a variety of perspectives—family, friends, health professionals—in order to give the patient a full picture of their current situation);
- Clarifying goals (feedback should be compared with a standard (an ideal), and clarification of the ideal can provide the pathway to the goal);
- Active helping (such as expressing caring or facilitating a referral, both of which convey a real interest in helping the person to change).

Similarly to cognitive behavioural therapy motivational interviewing has a clear central philosophy that clients need to be motivated to change and that empathy and 'change talk' (Moyers, 2014) mediate change. However, what actually changes behaviours in any particular intervention is not clearly established. There are other mediators that may or may not be included within any motivational interviewing intervention such as goal setting, and feedback that may or may not generate self-regulatory behaviours. This has led to the considerable work on establishing effective behavioural change techniques and mapping to different populations, behaviours & contexts (Kok et al., 2016; Michie et al., 2014) (Table 4.3).

Table 4.3 Key skills for motivational interviewing

Skill	*Comment*
Express empathy	There should be no criticism or blame as acceptance facilitates change
Develop discrepancy	Change is motivated by a perceived discrepancy between present behaviour and personal goal
Roll with resistance	Avoid arguing for change or providing change—see the smoker as the source of information
Support self-efficacy	The smoker's belief in the possibility of change is an important motivator for change
Use open-ended questions	Encourage the client to do most of the talking: 'What are your concerns about smoking?'
Use reflective listening	Reflect back change talk in a statement: 'I had real cravings this morning' to 'You are a little concerned about the cravings in the morning'
Use affirmation	Use to build rapport: 'You are right to be concerned about smoking in front of the children'
Summarise	Link together and reinforce what has been discussed: 'You are concerned that your smoking may cause lung cancer'
Reframe or agree with a twist	Address resistance by reinterpreting: 'My kids nag me about giving up smoking' to 'It sounds like they really care about your health'
Emphasise personal choice	Reinforce that it is the client's choice to change their behaviour
Evocative questions	
Increasing confidence	Use open questions to evoke confidence talk: 'How might you go about making this change?'
Confidence ruler	Use the ruler to ask 'What would it take to score higher?'
Strengths and successes	Review obstacles and how the client has overcome them
Reframing	'I've tried three times to quit and failed' to 'You have had three good attempts already and are learning new skills'
Prompt coping strategies	Ask for potential obstacles and putative coping strategies

Source: Adapted from Miller and Rollnick (2002).

Goal setting

We all set ourselves goals in all areas of life. Some psychologists would argue that goals give meaning to people's lives (Rasmussen et al., 2006). The challenge for health professionals interested in behavioural change is how to utilise goal setting to support change. Goals can vary both in terms of their difficulty (running a marathon is more difficult that running a 10 km race) and in terms of their specificity (Strecher et al., 1995). Someone may have a vague goal 'to eat well' or a more specific goal 'to eat a high-fibre breakfast cereal at least five times a week'.

Evidence suggests that non-specific, vague goals such as wanting to lose weight are less likely to be achieved than more specific goals such as 'I am going to stop eating chocolate biscuits for the next fortnight' (Strecher et al., 1995; Epton et al., 2017; Pearson, 2012). Health professionals therefore can support people in their overarching goals to lose weight, get fitter, control their blood sugar etc. by helping them break down their complex and long-term goals into a set of simpler, short-term sub-goals. SMART goals are a well-established set of criteria to help achieve successful outcomes. Pearson (2012) has proposed an adaptation of SMART goal criteria to START goals (Table 4.4).

Table 4.4 The START criteria for health behaviour goal setting

Criteria	Explanation	Evidence of value
Specificity	Specific, reasonably challenging goals such as 'run 5k 5 times a week' are more effective than vague goals to 'take more exercise'. Specific goals enable effective self-regulation but do risk failure and reduced self-efficacy if too demanding	Locke and Latham (2002)
Timing	Goals that are short-term are directive and serve as an incentive for immediate action, achievement of goals set in the short-term can provide motivation and improve self-efficacy for next goal. Longer-term goals don't provide immediate indicators of progress	Bandara and Simon (1977)
Acquisition	Self-determined and/or collaboratively set goals are more effective than assigned goals.	Ryan and Deci (2000).
Rewards & Feedback	Internal (e.g., pride) & external rewards (e.g., prizes) can both play a motivating role in behaviour change. However, external rewards can be counter-productive if they are not achieved or cannot be maintained. Feedback on progress towards goals, whether personal (from a health professional) or technological (from a fitness device) is critical particularly long-term maintenance and goal adjustment.	Locke and Latham (2002)
Tools	Several tools such as action planning, self-monitoring and coping skills have been identified as important mechanisms in successful behavioural change and progress towards goals.	Pettman et al. (2008).

Source: Adapted from Pearson (2012).

A major benefit of goal-directed behaviour is the possibility of positive feedback. Feedback about goal success can significantly improve subsequent performance, probably by improving self-efficacy. However, for behavioural change, difficult, complex, long-term goals (such as weight loss or fitness) are unlikely to generate immediate positive feedback. This can lead to a reduction in self-efficacy as individuals feel they are not achieving their goal and can lead to individuals giving up and reverting to their original 'bad habits'. Indeed, research suggests that failing to achieve self-regulatory goals can promote a worsening of original bad habits (Herman & Polivy, 2004). Short-term goals are much easier to link to positive feedback and can improve self-efficacy and help people stick to their change. The majority of health behaviours that people wish to change are highly complex and will require careful planning to develop an appropriate goal-setting strategy.

It is generally better to set behavioural goals such as increasing exercise rather than physiological status goals such as increasing VO2 max. Behaviours are more directly under a person's control than are physiological responses. The key strategies for successful goal setting are summarised in Table 4.5.

Table 4.5 Key recommendations for goal-setting behavioural change strategies using weight loss as the example

Strategy	Example
Explore client motivation. This might be done using the stages of change paradigm. Pre-contemplation clients are not ready for goal setting	A client has been referred to you by her GP for weight loss support. The client has been advised to lose 3 stone. Initially, you need to establish the client's personal motivation for weight loss of this magnitude
Break down a complex goal into a series of short-term sub-goals and create an action plan	You might set the client a series of short-term goals such as stop eating biscuits at coffee time for the next fortnight
Attempt where possible to set behavioural goals rather than physiological goals	You may wish to focus on the food an individual chooses to eat or on an activity such as walking rather than pounds lost over a time frame
Evaluate client self-efficacy for the various behaviours involved in goal achievement	Your client may be more confident about restricting food intake than taking exercise and your action plan needs to be tailored to client self-efficacy
Tailor sub-goals to the client to ensure they are challenging but realistic and perceived as such by the client	Your client may wish to set goals that are unrealistic, as rapid weight loss is attractive to most individuals wishing to lose weight. You need to negotiate a goal for which you are likely to be able to deliver positive feedback
Provide regular feedback to the client	Feedback needs to be regular, supportive and reflect behavioural achievements and physiological achievements if appropriate
Goal adaptation	For long-term complex change the short-term sub-goals may need to be reviewed and renegotiated as the client's physiological status and self-efficacy change in response to behavioural adaptation

It is emerging that having an action plan about how to achieve goals that involve particularly ingrained habitual behaviours can be further supported by 'if-then' plans that provide strategies for people to achieve their goals in difficult contexts (see following section on implementation intentions).

Successful goal setting will promote self-efficacy for changing the specified behaviour, giving the client the confidence to believe that having met previous goals, they can meet the next sub-goal and that the overarching goal is possible. Ineffective goal setting, when clients fail to meet their short-term targets, can have the opposite effect and damage self-efficacy, reducing the likelihood that clients will meet their overarching goal.

Effective goal setting needs to be tailored to the individual and supported by regular feedback and encouragement. For long-term goals, such as major weight loss, this will involve considerable and sustained input from a health professional. It is not usual for health professionals to have the resources available to provide this level of individualised support. One avenue that might be worthy of exploration is whether clients can be taught effective goal-setting techniques and could then set and reward their own goals.

Implementation intentions

One of the problems with goal setting and with behavioural change generally is that people may have decided to change, they may want to change very strongly, but because their behaviour is habitual and ingrained they may not be able to overcome the impulse to give in, in situations where they habitually practise an unhealthy behaviour (Wood & Neal, 2016). So people who are trying to give up smoking will have key situational prompts when they find it very hard to overcome the impulse to smoke; perhaps during a coffee break, or in the pub. Gollwitzer and Sheeran (2006) have suggested that people need to develop a set of 'if-then' plans to help them deal with situations where they usually do something they are trying to stop doing. For example, if your goal is to lose weight then you need to identify when you are likely to eat high-fat food and how you will respond differently in that situation. So if you usually have a cup of tea and a biscuit mid-morning you need to formulate an alternative response to replace eating a biscuit, such as eating a low-fat cracker instead.

Building 'if-then' plans into goal-setting action plans increases the involvement and commitment of the health professional. As mentioned under goal setting, it is unlikely that many health professionals currently have the resources to provide this level of support. Encouragingly, Hagger et al. (2012) found that using motivational and implementation interventions delivered using an online format did reduce drinking in participants with high baseline alcohol consumption. Other researchers similarly report that online interventions can be effective (Kypri et al., 2009). Online behavioural change interventions have the potential to provide an efficient way of providing the personalised support that is required.

Cognitive behavioural therapy

Cognitive behavioural therapy (CBT) was originally developed as an intervention for mental health disorders (such as anxiety, depression, panic or agoraphobia) (Westbrook et al., 2007). However, CBT is now well established as an effective intervention for health behaviour change (Conner & Norman, 2015) Indeed, motivational interviewing (described earlier in the chapter) is based on aspects of CBT. However, in some instances, perhaps when the behaviour people are attempting to change is clearly addictive, there may be a place for a more complete cognitive behavioural approach than motivational interviewing. Motivational interviewing is usually a brief therapy (1–4 sessions) for enhancing motivation to change problematic health behaviours (Ismail et al., 2008). Cognitive behavioural therapy is longer (a minimum of six sessions) and aims to help the client identify, challenge, and substitute unhelpful thoughts (cognitions) and behaviours with more constructive ones (Ismail et al., 2008). It is beyond the remit of this book to provide a comprehensive review of CBT and the reader is advised to access one of the many available texts if they wish to explore the subject further (for instance: Kennerley et al., 2016). Ismail et al. (2008) found that CBT improved blood glucose control in patients with diabetes 12 months after the intervention whereas motivational interviewing did not. However, given that motivational interviewing is a brief intervention and CBT is a longer-term intervention, it is possible that it is the length of the intervention that results in the better outcome rather than the type of therapy itself. Longer-term interventions have the potential to provide social support for individuals attempting to change a behaviour, and it may be the social support rather than the therapeutic approach that is important.

Mindfulness

Mindfulness has been defined as the awareness that comes when individuals pay attention to the present non-judgmentally. Mindfulness-based interventions started to emerge for chronic physical and mental conditions in the 2000s and over the last decade, interest and investment into mindfulness interventions for drinking has been considerable (Cavicchioli et al., 2018; Garland & Howard, 2018). Changing habitual behaviours requires paying attention to situation cues, regulating the emotional response to stimuli and self-regulation and it seems intuitive that mindfulness interventions may support individuals trying to change habitual behaviours. However, there is limited evidence about how successful such interventions are for different behaviours and how they could 'fit' in our behavioural change toolkit (Schuman-Oliver et al., 2020).

Working effectively with others

Lifestyle change is a complex challenge which individuals must address outside of health care settings in their daily lives. It is if you like an upstream activity before the descent into primary, secondary or tertiary care and consequently outside of the experience of many traditional health professionals. Few health professionals, even specialists such as dieticians, have time in their workloads to work with individuals to build self-efficacy and or provide the social support that can make lifestyle change more likely. Traditionally, health practitioners in primary care have focused on ensuring that they work effectively with secondary care to identify individuals who have clinical problems that need referral to specialist services such as addiction centres or dieticians. Increasingly, as the complexities of lifestyle change are beginning to be recognised primary care practitioners need to build relationships with a wider range of (health and non-health practitioners) that are community-based and can provide additional support to those embarking on lifestyle change. Understanding how health advice is translated into the normal daily lives of individuals is a different knowledge base to understanding the relationship between health behaviours and disease. If we are to reach individuals who are living in high levels of deprivation and so attempt to tackle the widening health inequalities in society health practitioners will probably need to work with community workers, social workers, probation officers and others who have the experience and expertise in working with individuals most at need of health interventions. Links with non-health practitioners and primary care are beginning to be established. The exercise referral scheme is one established pathway to link primary care to community exercise schemes (see Chapter 6, Being Active). Community pharmacies are increasingly recognised as a local resource where support for lifestyle change could be provided (Parchment et al., 2021; Thirlaway, 2011). There are also private companies such as Weight Watchers, gyms, and personal trainers that can provide valuable support for individuals embarking on change. Any primary care practitioner interested in promoting lifestyle change will need to access resources that can support change on a more regular basis than is possible as an individual practitioner.

Conclusion

The various behaviours implicated in contributing to ill health—eating, drinking, smoking, illicit drug taking and sexual behaviours—are all complex behaviours that have many different roles in individuals' lives. People need to eat to stay alive and hunger is the physiological response that ensures that people do eat and don't starve to death. Viewed in this simplistic way, understanding eating behaviour should be straightforward. People should eat enough to prevent hunger. However, people eat for pleasure, they eat for comfort, they eat because they are bored, they eat because the social situation demands it, and they eat because they have got into the habit of doing so in particular situations or at particular times. Psychological theories of behavioural change have developed to try to understand how these non-biological factors influence the choices people make. Psychological theory to date gives us some clues about the key factors that influence behaviour.

Key points

- Education about the risks and benefits of behaviour is not an effective behavioural change strategy.
- Getting people to change their lifestyle requires them to prioritise their health and change often long-established habits.
- Getting people to change their lifestyle requires them to make unpalatable changes in the 'here and now' for an uncertain benefit in the future.
- Perceptions of barriers to healthy lifestyles are more important than actual barriers; what is insurmountable for one individual will not be a problem for another.
- Self-efficacy is key to successful behavioural change; if you believe you can change you are far more likely to succeed.
- Self-regulation involves the setting of goals but failing to achieve goals can put people at greater risk of excessive consumption. Goal setting requires a delicate balance to arrive at a sufficiently challenging but realistic goal.
- Habitual behaviours need complex 'systems-based' approaches to help individuals break 'negative' habits and establish helpful habits, mindfulness interventions may offer another approach to stopping negative habitual behaviours.
- Social support is complex but indisputably related to health. It is possible, but not yet established, that health professionals and/or support groups could provide useful social support for behavioural change.

Discussion points

- Motivational interviewing requires a client-centred perspective and requires the professional to let the client set their own objectives for change. How can we balance that against a requirement to give professional advice?
- Many people seeking help with weight loss will have tried and failed to lose weight many times before finally seeking professional help. They are likely to have low self-efficacy. How would you go about re-building self-efficacy in such clients?
- Breaking bad habits and establishing new good habits can be a long process. How can health professionals manage to provide sustained support for individuals attempting to change their behaviour?

Further resources

Thirlaway, K.J., & Upton, D. (2009). *The psychology of lifestyle: Promoting healthy behaviour.* London: Routledge.

Conner, M., & Norman, P. (2015). *Predicting and changing health behaviour: Research and practice with social cognition models (3rd Ed.).* Berkshire: Open University Press.

References

Aarts, H., Paulussen, T., & Schaalma, H. (1997). Physical exercise habit: On the conceptualisation and formation of habitual health behaviours. *Health Education Research*, 21, 363–374.

Bandara, A. (1997). *Self Efficacy: The Exercise of Control.* New York: Worth Publishers.

Bandara, A., & Simon, K. P. (1977). The role of proximal intentions in self-regulation of refractory behaviour. *Cognitive Therapy Research*, 1, 177–193.

Barrientos-Gutierrez, T., Gimeno, D., Mangiane, T. W., Harrist, R. B., & Amick, B. C. (2007). Drinking social norms and drinking behaviours. *Occupational and Environmental Medicine*, 64, 602–608.

Blaxter, M. (2004). *Health and lifestyles.* London: Routledge.

Cabinet Office Strategy Unit. (2002). *Risk: Improving government capability to handle risk and uncertainty.* London: Cabinet Office.

Cavicchioli, M., Movalli, M., & Maffei, C. (2018). The clinical efficacy of mindfulness-based treatments for alcohol and drug use disorders: A meta-analytic review of randomised and nonrandomised controlled trials. *European Addiction Research*, 24137–24162. Doi 10.1159/000490762

Cislaghi, B., & Heise, L. (2018). Using social norms theory for health promotion in low-income countries. *Health Promotion International*, 34, 616–623. Doi 10.1093/heapro/day017

Cohen, S., & Janicki-Deverts, D. (2009). Can we improve our physical health by altering our social networks? *Perspectives on Psychological Science*, 4(4), 375–378.

Conner, M., & Norman, P. (2015). *Predicting and changing health behaviour: Research and practice with social cognition models (3rd Ed.).* Berkshire: Open University Press.

Connolly, T., Arkes, H. R., & Hammond, K. R. (2000). *Judgement and decision making: An interdisciplinary reader.* Cambridge: Cambridge University Press.

Creswell, K. G., Cheng, Y., & Levine, M. D. (2015). A test of the stress-buffering model of social support in smoking cessation: is the relationship between social support and time to relapse mediated by reduced withdrawal symptoms? *Nicotine and Tobacco Research*, 556–571. Doi 10.1093/ntr/ntu192

Dempsey, R. C., McAlaney, J., & Bewick, B. M. (2018). A critical appraisal of the social norms approach as an intervention strategy for health-related behaviour and attitude change. *Frontiers in Psychology*, 9, 2180. Doi 10.3389/fpsyg2018.02180

Dilorio, C., Dudley, W. N., Kelly, M., Soet, J., Mbwara, J., & Sharpe Potter, J. (2001). Social cognitive correlates of sexual experience and condom use among 13 though 15 year old adolescents. *Journal of Adolescent Health*, 29, 208–216.

Epton, T., Currie, S., & Armitage, C. J. (2017). *Journal of Consulting and Clinical Psychology*, 85(12), 1182–1198. Doi 10.1037/ccp0000260

Gallopel-Morvan, K., Gabriel, P., Le Gall-Ely, M., Rieunier, S., & Urien, B. (2011). The use of visual warnings in social marketing: The case of tobacco. *Journal of Business Research*.

Garland, E. L., & Howard, M. O. (2018). Mindfulness-based treatment of addiction: current state of the field and envisioning the next wave of research. *Addiction Science & Clinical Practice*, 13, 14. Doi 10.1186/s13722-018-0115-3.

Gardner, B., Lally, P., & Wardle, J. (2012). Making health habitual: The psychology of 'habit-formation' and general practice. *British Journal of General Practice*. Doi 10.3399/bjgp12X659466

Gilles, D. M., Turk, C. L., & Fresco, D. M. (2006). Social anxiety, alcohol expectancies, and self-efficacy as predictors of heavy drinking in college students. *Addictive Behaviors, 31,* 388–398.

Gollwitzer, P. M., & Sheeran, P. (2006). Implementation intentions and goal achievement: A meta-analysis of effects and processes. *Advances in Experimental Social Psychology, 38,* 69–119.

Gruber, K. J. (2008). Social support for exercise and dietary habits among college students. *Adolescence, 43*(171), 557–575.

Hagger, M. (2019). Habit and physical activity: Theoretical advances, practical implications and agenda for future research. *Psychology of Sport and Exercise, 42,* 118–129.

Hagger, M. S., Lonsdale, A. J., & Chatzisarantis, N. L. D. (2012). A theory-based intervention to reduce alcohol drinking in excess of guideline limits among undergraduate students. *British Journal of Health Psychology, 17,* 18–43.

Hagger, M. S., Chatzisarantis, N. L. D., & Biddle, S. J. H. (2002). A meta-analytic review of the theories of reasoned action and planned behaviour in physical activity: Predictive validity and the contribution of additional variables. *Journal of Sport and Exercise Psychology, 24,* 3–32.

Harvey, I. S., & Alexander, K. (2012). Perceived social support and preventative health behavioural outcomes among older women. *Journal of Cross Cultural Gerontology, 27*(3), 275–290. Doi 10.1007/s10823-012-9172-3.

Health Survey for England. (2020). *Health survey for England 2019: Adults' health-related behaviours.* London: NHS Digital, www.digital.nhs.uk

Health Survey (NI). (2021). *Health survey (NI) first results 2020/21.* Belfast: Information Analysis Directorate. www.health-ni.gov.uk/topics/doh-statistics& research/health-survey-northern Ireland.

Herman, C. P., & Polivy, J. (2004). The self-regulation of eating: Theoretical and practical problems. In R. F. Baumeister & K. D. Vohs (Eds.), *Handbook of Self Regulation: Research, Theory and Applications.* London: The Guilford Press.

Hobbs, M., & Radley, D. (2020). Obesogenic environments and obesity: A comment on 'are environmental area characteristics at birth associated with overweight and obesity in school-aged children? Findings from the SLOPE (studying life-course obesity predictors) population-based cohort in the south of England. *BMC Medicine, 18,* 59. Doi 10.1186/s12916-020-0153 8-5.

Ismail, K., Thomas, S. M., Maissi, E., Chalder, T., Schmidt, U., Barlett, J., Patel, A., Dickens, C. M., Creed, F., & Treasure, J. (2008). Motivational enhancement therapy with and without cognitive behaviour therapy to treat type 1 diabetes. *Annals of Internal Medicine, 149,* 708–719.

Jones, A., Bentham, G., Foster, C., Hillsdon, M., & Panter, J. (2007). *Tackling obesities: Future choices – Obesogenic environments – Evidence review.* London: United Kingdom Government Foreign Programmes Office of Science and Innovation. Crown Copyright.

Kelly, M. P., & Barker, M. (2016). Why is changing health-related behaviour so difficult? *Public Health, 136,* 109–116. Doi 10.1016/j.puhe.2016.03.030

Kennerley, H., Kirk, J., & Westbrook, D. (2016). *An introduction to cognitive behavioural therapy: Skills and applications.* London: Sage.

Kok, G., Gottlieb, N. H., Peters, G. Y., Mullen, D. P., Parcel, G. S., Ruiter, R. A. C., Fernandez, M. E., Markham, C., & Bartholomew, K. L. (2016). A taxonomy of behavioural change methods: An intervention mapping approach. *Health Psychology Review, 10*(3), 297–312. Doi 10.1080/17437199.2015.1077155

Kuntsche, E., & Cooper, M. L. (2010). Drinking to have fun and to get drunk: Motives as predictors of weekend drinking over and above usual drinking habits. *Drug and Alcohol Dependency, 110*(3), 259–262. Doi 10.1016/j.drugalcdep.2010.02021

Kuther, T. L., & Timoshin, A. (2003). A comparison of social cognitive and psychosocial predictors of alcohol use by college students. *Journal of College Student Development, 44,* 143–154.

Kypri, K., Hallett, J., Howat, P., McManus, A., Maycock, B., Bowe, S. J., & Horton, N. J. (2009). Randomized controlled trial of proactive web-based alcohol screening and brief intervention for university students. *Archives of Internal Medicine, 169,* 1508–1514.

Landais, L. L., Damman, O. C., Schoonmade, L. J., Timmermans, D. R. M., Verhagen, E. A. L. M., & Jelsma, J. G. M. (2020). Choice architecture interventions to change physical activity and sedentary behaviour: A systematic review of effects on intention, behavior and health outcomes during and after intervention. *International Journal of Behavioral Nutrition and Physical Activity*, 17(47). Doi 10.1186/s12966-020-00942-7.

Lawton, J. (2002). Colonising the future: Temporal perceptions and health-relevant behaviors across the adult life-course. *Sociology of Health and Illness*, 24, 714–733.

Lawton, R., & Conner, M. (2007). Beyond cognition: Predicting health risk behaviours from instrumental and affective beliefs. *Health Psychology*, 26, 259–267.

Lee, R. E., McAlexander, K. M., & Banda, J. A. (2011). *Reversing the obesogenic environment.* USA: Human Kinetics.

Linke, S. E., Gallo, L. C., & Norman, G. J. (2011). Attrition and adherence rates of sustained vs. intermittent exercise interventions. *Annals of Behavioral Medicine*, 42(2), 197–209.

Locke, E. A., & Latham, G. P. (2002). Building a practically useful theory of goal setting and task motivation. *American Psychologist*, 57, 705–717.

Luszczynska, A., & Schwarzer, R. (2015). Chapter 7 social cognitive theory. In M. Conner & P. Norman (Eds.), *Predicting and changing health behaviour: Research and practice with social cognition models* (3rd Ed.). New York: Open University Press.

Magill, M., Scott Tonigan, J., Kiluk, B., Ray, L., Walters, J., & Carroll, K. (2020). The search for mechanisms of cognitive behavioural therapy for alcohol or other drug use disorders: A systematic review. *Behaviour Research and Therapy*, 131, 103648.

Mcalaney, J., & McMahon, J. (2007). Normative beliefs, misperceptions and heavy episodic drinking in a British student sample. *Journal of Studies on Alcohol and Drugs*, 68(3), 385–392.

Michie, S., Atkins, L., & West, R. (2014). *The behaviour change wheel.* Surrey: Silverback Publishing.

Michie, S., & Wood, C. E. (2015). Chapter 11. Health behaviour change techniques. In M. Conner & P. Norman (Eds.), *Predicting and changing health behaviour: Research and practice with social cognition models* (3rd Ed.). New York: Open University Press.

Miller, W. R., & Rollnick, S. (2002). *Motivational interviewing: Preparing people for change* (2nd Ed.). New York: Guilford Press.

Moyers, T. B. (2014). The relationship in motivational interviewing. *Psychotherapy*, 51(3), 358–363. Doi 10.1037/a0036910

NICE. (2011). Alcohol-use disorders. *Diagnosis, assessment and management of harmful drinking and alcohol dependence. National clinical practice guideline 115.* The British Psychological Society & The Royal College of Psychiatrists.

NICE. (2019). *Alcohol Interventions in secondary and further education.* Public Health England. Doi www.nice.org.uk/guideline/ng135

Nigg, C. R., Borrelli, B., Maddock, J., & Dishman, R. K. (2008). A theory of physical activity maintenance. *Applied Psychology: An International Review*, 57(4), 544–560.

Office for Product Safety and Standards. (2021). *OPSS risk lexicon.* London: Uk Government. www.gov.uk

O'Leary, A., Jemmott, L. T., & Jemmott, J. B. (2008). Mediation analysis of an effective sexual risk-reduction intervention for women: The importance of self-efficacy. *Health Psychology*, 27(2), 180–184.

Parchment, A., Lawrence, W., Perry, R., Rahman, E., Townsend, N., Wainwright, E., & Wainwright, D. (2021). Making every contact count and healthy conversations skills as very brief or brief behaviour change interventions: A scoping review. *Journal of Public Health.* Doi 10.1007/s10389-0210-01653-4

Pedersen, S., Gronhoj, A., & Thogersen, J. (2014). Following family or friends. Social norms in adolescent healthy eating. *Appetite*, 86, 54–60. Doi 10.1016/j.appet2014.07.030.

Pearson, E. S. (2012). Goal setting as a health behavior change strategy in overweight and obese adults: A systematic literature review examining intervention components. *Patient Education and Counselling*, 87, 32–42. Doi 10.1016/j.pec.2011.07.018

Pirie, P., Rooney, B., Pechacek, T., Lando, H., & Schmid, L. (1997). Incorporating social support into a community-wide smoking cessation contest. *Addictive Behaviour*, 22(1), 131–137.

Plant, M., & Plant, M. (2006). *Binge Britain*. Oxford: Oxford University Press.

Pettman, T. L., Misan, G. M. H., Owen, K., Warren, K., Coates, A. M., & Buckley, J. D. et al. (2008). Self management for obesity and cardio-metabolic fitness: Description and evaluation of the lifestyle modification program of a randomised clinical controlled trial. *International Journal of Behaviour, Nutrition & Physiology Action*, 5, 1–15.

Public Health England. (2016). *Making every contact count (MECC): Consensus statement*. London: Public Health England

Rasmussen, H. N., Wrosch, C., Scheier, M. F., & Carver, C. S. (2006). Self-regulation processes and health: The importance of optimism and goal adjustment. *Journal of Personality*, 74(6), 1721–1747.

Robinson, E., Thomas, J., Aveyard, P., & Higgs, S. (2013). What everyone else is eating: A systematic review and meta-analysis of the effect of informational eating norms on eating behaviour. *Journal of Academic Nutrition and Diet*, 114, 414–429. Doi 10.1016/j.jand.2013.11.009.

Ryan, R. M., & Deci, E. L. (2000). Self-determination theory and the facilitation of intrinsic motivation, social development and well-being. *American Psychologist*, 55, 68–78.

Schuman-Olivier, Z., Trombka, M., Lovas, D. A., Brewer, J. A., Vago, D. R., Gawande, R., Dunne, J. P., Lazar, S. W., Loucks, E. B., & Fulwiler, C. (2020). Mindfulness and behavior change. *Harvard Review of Psychiatry*, 28(6), 371–394. Doi 10.1097/HRP0000000000000277

Scottish Health Survey (2020). *The Scottish health survey 2019 edition volume 1 main report*. Belfast: Scottish Government. www.gov.scot

Simpson, K. J. (2017). Appeal to fear in health care: Appropriate or inappropriate? *Chiropractic & Manual Therapies*, 25, 27. Doi 10.1186/s12998-017-0157-8

Strecher, V. J., Seijts, G. H., Kok, G. J., Latham, G. P., Glasgow, R., DeVellis, B., Meertens, R. M., & Bulger, D. W. (1995). Goal setting as a strategy for health behaviour change. *Health Education Quarterly*, 22(2), 190–200.

Strobach, T., Englert, C., Jekauc, D., & Pfeffer, I. (2020). Predicting adoption and maintenance of physical activity in the context of dual-process theories. *Performance Enhancement and Health*, 8. Doi 10.1016/j.peh2020.100162.

Sutton, S. (1982). Fear-arousing communications: A critical examination of theory and research. In J. R. Eiser (Ed.), *Social psychology and behavioural medicine*. London: Wiley, pp. 303–337.

Thirlaway, K. J., & Heggs, D. (2005). Interpreting risk messages: Women's responses to a health story. *Health, Risk and Society*, 7, 107–121.

Thirlaway, K. J., & Upton, D. (2009). *The psychology of lifestyle: Promoting healthy behaviour*. London: Routledge.

Thirlaway, K. (2011). Lifestyle change. *Welsh Chemist Review*. Winter 2011: 18–19.

Uchino, B. N. (2006). Social support and health: A review of physiological processes potentially underlying links to disease outcomes. *Journal of Behavioral Medicine*, 29(4), 377–387.

Verplanken, B., & Melkeviko, O. (2008). Predicting habit: The case of physical activity. *Psychology of Sport and Exercise*, 9(1), 15–26.

Wang, H. X., Mittleman, M. A., & Orth-Gomer, K. (2005). Influence of social support on progression of coronary heart disease in women. *Social Science and Medicine*, 60, 599–607.

Welsh Health Survey. (2020). *National survey for Wales 2019/20*. Welsh Government.

Westbrook, D., Kennerley, H., & Kirk, J. (2007). *An Introduction to Cognitive Behaviour Therapy: Skills and Applications*. London: Sage.

Wilding, S., Ziauddeen, N., Smith, D., Roderisk, P., Chase, D., & Alwan, N. A. (2020). Are environmental area characteristics at birth associated with overweight and obesity in school-aged children? Findings from the SLOPE (studying life-course obesity predictors) population-based cohort in the south of England. *BMC Medicine*, 18, 43. Doi 10.1186/s12916-020-01513-0.

Williams, & French (2011). What are the most effective intervention techniques for changing physical activity self-efficacy and physical activity behavior- and are they the same? *Health Education Research*, 26(2), 308–322.

WHO. (2012). *Health education: Theoretical concepts, effective strategies and core competencies.* Geneva: World Health Organisation.

WHO. (2018). *Global action plan on physical activity 2018–2030. More active people for a healthier world.* Geneva: World Health Organisation. 2018: CC BY-NC-SA 3.0 IGO.

Wood, W., & Neal, D. T. (2016). Healthy through habit: Interventions for initiating and maintaining health behaviour change. *Behavioural Science & Policy*, 2(1), 71–83.

5 Eating well

Case Study

Michael is a 28-year-old man who works in the finance office of a large supermarket chain. Mike, as he likes to be called, has worked in an office since completing his accountancy degree a few years ago. Mike has always had a problem with his weight, but since his son was born 5 years ago, his weight has ballooned, and he now tips the scales at 23 stone (or 146 kilos). He has found that a regular wage packet, limited exercise, regular nights out and access to a plentiful food supply (he has a staff discount) mean he has put on considerable weight.

Mike is married and has a five-year-old son, Jacob, although he and his wife are trying for another child. His wife is also obese, and they fear that their weight is getting in the way of them having another child. Jacob is rather chubby and takes great delight in eating fish fingers and chips to the exclusion of most other food!

Mike now finds that his regular diet of takeaways and pre-packaged meals with limited fruit and vegetables is creating a downward spiral. He used to play five-a-side football with 'the lads' but given his weight and because he becomes out of

DOI: 10.4324/9781003471233-5

breath easily, he has stopped playing, merely turning up for the post-match drinking session.

Mike has recently had a health scare; he had a pain in the centre of his chest and was rushed to hospital, where he was admitted overnight for observation. This caused great family concern, and they all started to worry about their lifestyle. Although the hospital tests revealed no significant problems, his blood pressure was high (160/100 mmHg), and his Body Mass Index (BMI) (44) placed him in the morbidly obese category. He was referred to you to reduce his weight and improve his overall weight control.

Applying this to Mike In order to help Mike and work with him and his family to reduce his weight and improve his lifestyle, it is important to consider three main things: improving his diet, reducing his weight and installing an exercise regime.

Introduction

Unlike many of the other behaviours discussed in this text (e.g., smoking or drinking alcohol), we all eat, and we all have to eat. Eating can have a protective benefit; for example, a healthy diet protects from a third of all cancers, diabetes, osteoporosis, heart disease, strokes and tooth decay. In contrast, having an unhealthy diet can lead to considerable health damage, such as osteoporosis, heart disease and cancer. According to the Global BMI Mortality Collaboration, it is estimated that obesity, on average, is associated with a 14% increased mortality rate in Europe, thus indicating that BMI can predict mortality (The Global BMI Mortality Collaboration, 2016). Forecast estimates suggest that improving diet could result in significant reduction in mortality rates—more than 11 million deaths worldwide—from a variety of causes (see Table 5.1, Wang et al., 2019).

Government recommendations

The UK national guidelines suggest that a healthy diet is a balanced diet based on five major food groups: breads, other cereals and potatoes; fruit and vegetables; milk and dairy foods; meat, fish and alternatives; and foods containing fats and sugars (see Photograph 5.1). The UK Department of Health (DOH, 1999) defines good nutrition in the *Saving Lives: Our Healthier Nation* document as 'plenty of fruit and vegetables, cereals, and not too much fatty and salty food'. The NHS advice has developed over time

Table 5.1 Numbers of preventable deaths from attributable to poor diet in 190 countries/ territories in 2017 (adapted from Wang et al., 2019)

Cause	Preventable deaths
Total deaths	6,978,411 (5,768,476–8,100,019)
Cancer	1,210,648 (548,606–1,795,445)
Coronary heart disease	1,878,810 (1,261,245–2,425,734)
Stroke	304,520 (-435,230 to 911,193)
Respiratory disease	964,393 (544,924–1,289,152)
Neurodegenerative disease	446,211 (247,771–604,154)
Kidney disease	258,156 (-21,509–434,609)
Diabetes	206,265 (126,597–275,809)
Digestive system disease	806,709 (448,812–1,048,322)

and now provides information for some commonly adopted special diets (such as vegan and vegetarian), although the basic eating well advice remains centred around the five basic food groups:

> Starchy foods such as rice and pasta should make up just over a third of our diet; with plenty of fruit and vegetables; some protein-rich foods such as meat, fish and lentils; some milk and dairy foods or dairy alternatives; and small amounts of unsaturated fats in the form of oils or spreads. It is advised that saturated fat, salt, sugar or processed foods should be limited and eaten in small amounts only, since they are not needed in our diet. (NHS, 2012)

The Eatwell guide applies to all people except children under 2, who have specific nutritional needs (Figure 5.1).

In addition to this general 'eat well' guidance, there are more specific government recommendations as suggested by the government initiative Healthy Families (previously called Change4Life). These evidence-based guidelines appear relatively simple but can be confusing and difficult to implement for certain sections of society. The recommendations are many. First, eat at least five portions of fruit and vegetables per day. Each portion is around 80 g (e.g., one medium apple or three heaped tablespoons of peas). That being said, potatoes do not count as part of the five a day; more than one serving of

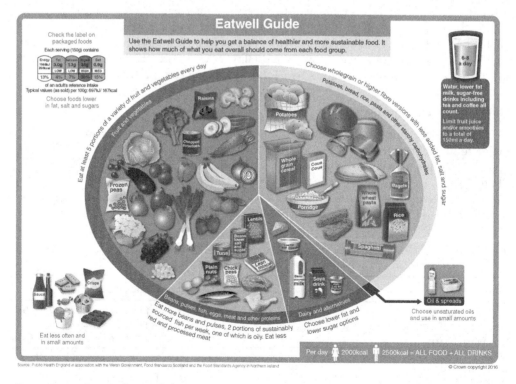

Figure 5.1 Balance of a good diet.

Source: UK gov, https://www.gov.uk/government/publications/the-eatwell-guide, © Crown copyright 2012. Crown copyright material is reproduced with permission under the terms of the Click-Use Licence.

beans and pulses is fine but only counts as one of the five a day; and while fruit juice and smoothies also count for a serving, the limit is 150 ml per day. Salt should be consumed at a maximum quantity of 3 g per day for 4–6 year-olds, 5 g per day for 7–10 year-olds and 6 g per day for those 11 years and older. For sugar, the maximum consumption should be 19 g per day for 4–6-year-olds, 24 g per day for 7–10-year-olds and 30 g per day for those 11 years and older. For saturated fat, the maximum consumption is advised to be 18 g per day for 4–6-year-olds, 22 g per day for 7–10-year-olds and 28 g per day for those 11 years and older. The recommendation that has been the focus of most marketing and advertising is that at least five portions of fruit and vegetables are consumed daily (NHS, 2012; World Health Organization [WHO], 2020). The consensus appears to be that most people are not eating enough fruits and vegetables (FVs).

Applying this to Mike

Mike eats a limited amount of fruit and vegetables, in addition to consuming a lot of processed and takeaway convenience foods that can contain high levels of salt. Therefore, Mike should reduce the amount of convenience foods he eats alongside increasing the amounts of fruit and vegetables consumed to ensure he stays within recommended government guidelines. Abiding by this will positively impact his health.

Evidence from the *National Diet and Nutrition Survey: Diet, nutrition and physical activity in 2020: A follow up study during COVID-19* found that consumption of fruit and vegetables was 2.8 portions per day for children. In addition, only 8% of children and 27% of adults (19–64 years) ate the recommended 'five a day' (PHE, 2020).

The overall rates of daily fruit and vegetable consumption per government guidelines for adults aged 16 years and above varied considerably by country according to various national surveys: *Sport England Active Survey, Scottish Health Survey* (2016–2019), *Welsh Health Survey* (2018–2020) and *Health Survey Northern Ireland* (2019–2020). England observed the highest overall rate of adults (55%) meeting the recommended daily intake of at least five portions of fruit and vegetable, followed by Northern Ireland (44%), Wales (25%) and Scotland, which had the lowest (22%). The percentage of adults meeting these guidelines has increased since 2003, except for in Wales, where there has been a decline in the rate of adults consuming the recommended five a day. Gender differences exist within the data. Across all four home countries, proportionately more women than men meet government guidelines to consume at least five portions of fruit and vegetables daily (see Table 5.2).

Social class differences are also apparent (see Chapter 3 for more information), with those in the working class consuming up to 50% fewer FVs than those in professional groups. Research suggests that food distribution and total food expenditure are two important factors driving the limited consumption of fruit and vegetables in lower socio-economic groups. That is, affordable FVs may not always be accessible. Conversely, unhealthy sugar- and fat-laden alternatives tend to be cheap and accessible. As a result, children's diets have become a particular area of concern and a national and international focus. For example, the latest release from the Australian Bureau of Statistics report on

Table 5.2 The percentage of men and women living in the UK achieving the government guidelines for daily fruit and vegetable consumption (based on guidelines set out in '5-a-day' DoH)

Source of Data	% of adults achieving 5 or more portions of fruit and vegetables daily	% of men achieving 5 or more portions of fruit and vegetables daily	% of women achieving 5 or more portions of fruit and vegetables daily	% of adults not consuming any fruit and vegetables daily
Health Survey for England (2008)	27%	25%	29%	Not reported
Health Survey for Scotland 2010 (Bromley and Given, 2011)	22%	20%	23%	10%
Welsh Health Survey (Welsh Assembly Government, 2011)	35%	33%	36%	8%
Health Survey Northern Ireland 2010/ 2011(Department of Health, Social Services and Public Safety, 2011)	33%	27%	36%	Not reported

dietary behaviour (2020–2021) states that 5.3% of children aged 2–17 did not eat fruit, and 4.1% did not eat vegetables.

Despite considerable effort, increased marketing commitment and expenditures towards increasing the consumption of fruit and vegetables, there has been little success (Rekhy & McConchie, 2014). From a socio-economic perspective, people may know which foods they should eat to stay healthy, but many cannot afford to buy them.

Health consequences of a poor diet

A poor diet can contribute to a range of illnesses, including both coronary heart disease (CHD) and cancer (see Table 5.3). A poor diet can also result in increased falls and fractures in older people, low birth weight, increased childhood morbidity and mortality and increased dental cavities in children (see Table 5.4 for links between specific nutrient deficits and poor health). There is also evidence to support the link between poor diet and antisocial behaviour, not to mention growing concern over the economic implications of the population's weight gain.

Table 5.3 Diseases associated with obesity

Cardiovascular disease
Cancer
Diabetes
Stroke
Hypertension
Angina
Dental decay

Table 5.4 Health risks associated with lack of dietary elements

	Found in	Health risk
Vitamin A	Liver, cheese, eggs and oily fish	Weakening of immune system
Vitamin B6	Poultry, whole cereals and peanuts	Depression and irritability
Vitamin B12	Meat, salmon, cheese and eggs	Anaemia
Vitamin C	Oranges, peppers, broccoli, cabbage	Bleeding gums, aching joints
Vitamin D	Oily fish, eggs	Muscle weakness and aching bones
Calcium	Milk, cheese, broccoli and cabbage	Bone and tooth decay
Folic acid	Broccoli, Brussel sprouts, peas, brown rice	Anaemia
Iron	Meat, bones, whole grains and watercress	Anaemia
Magnesium	Spinach, nuts, bread	Tiredness and bone and tooth decay
Vitamin B3	Beef, pork, eggs and milk	Skin problems, dizziness, swelling of tongue
Potassium	Bananas, vegetables, nuts	Irregular heartbeat, irritability and nausea
Vitamin B2	Mushrooms, rice, eggs and milk	Skin problems, difficulty sleeping
Vitamin B1	Peas and other vegetables, pork, milk and cheese	Headaches and tiredness
Zinc	Meat, shellfish, milk and cheese	Hair loss, skin problems, diarrhoea

Several public health documents and government policies highlight the benefits of an improved diet. For example:

- High cholesterol levels are one of eight risk factors that account for many cardiovascular-related deaths. For instance, high non-HDL cholesterol was found to cause approximately 3.9 million deaths worldwide (Taddei et al., 2020). Reducing the intake of saturated fat could reduce these numbers (WHO, 2020).
- The incidence of strokes could be decreased by increasing consumption of FVs.
- Hypertension could be reduced by reducing salt intake and, therefore, positively affect the incidence of cardiovascular diseases such as CHD/stroke (Cheema et al., 2022). In fact, modelled projections suggest that reducing salt intake to a maximum of 5 mg per day (per WHO guidelines; see WHO, 2013) could result in 1.4 million fewer instances of hypertension by 2035.
- Approximately 40% of endometrial cancer and 10% of breast and colon cancers would be avoided by maintaining a healthy weight (i.e., a BMI of 25 or less).
- Increased dietary fibre is associated with a decreased risk of colorectal and pancreatic cancer.

Obesity may be a risk factor in several chronic diseases such as heart disease, stroke, some cancers and Type 2 diabetes (Keaver et al., 2020). Figures from The Health and Social Care Information Centre, NHS (2017) suggest that in 2015, 43% of men and 37% of women who were classified as obese suffered from high blood pressure compared to 21% of men and 19% of women who were not classified as obese. Greater awareness of the disease burden associated with obesity has led to concern over the economic implications of the population's weight gain. The Department of Health and Social Care (2021) estimates that overweight and obesity currently cost the NHS £6 bn per year, with more spent each year on treating obesity and diabetes than the police, fire service and judicial system combined. According to Frontier Economics, the latest estimates of total costs (health care costs coupled with indirect costs such as loss of earnings) suggest that obesity costs the UK upwards of £58 bn annually (Palmer, 2022).

The consequences of a poor diet are more than just obesity. A strong connection exists between being overweight or obese and an increased risk of cancer. Research conducted by the American Cancer Society indicates that excessive body weight is believed to contribute to approximately 11% of cancer cases in women and 5% in men in the United States. Further, overweight and obesity are estimated to contribute to around 7% of all cancer-related deaths in the United States (American Cancer Society, 2019) and an estimated 3.9% of all cancer-related deaths globally (Feletto et al., 2022). A diet involving significant intake of high-fat foods, high salt and low fibre levels appears to be particularly implicated (World Cancer Research Fund, 2018). In addition to cancer, excessive fat intake has been implicated in disease and death from several serious illnesses, including CHD. According to recent research, cardiovascular-related deaths and others are related to the type and quality of our food. A study by Zheng et al. (2019) showed that a decrease in red meat consumption and an increase in whole grains, vegetables and alternative protein sources were associated with a reduced risk of death in both women and men. Replacing red meat with nuts, fish, whole grains, poultry without skin, vegetables without legumes, dairy, eggs or legumes led to a substantial decrease in mortality risk, with the most significant risk reductions observed for nuts and fish. Conversely, increasing processed meat intake by one serving per day over 8 years was linked to a 19% higher risk of death from cardiovascular disease and a 57% higher risk of death from neurodegenerative diseases in the subsequent 8 years. These findings highlight the importance of healthier dietary choices to promote longevity and reduce the risk of specific diseases. Losing as little weight as 5% has been proven to reduce health risks significantly (Ryan & Yockey, 2017). Obesity is an important issue in the poverty–poor diet–poor health cycle. A systematic analysis of the Global Burden of Disease study reports that 11 million deaths reported that food-related ill health was responsible for about 11 million premature deaths worldwide in 2017 (GBD, 2017 Diet Collaborators, 2019). According to a recent Australian Institute of Health and Welfare study, unhealthy eating is the new smoking. The most recent data suggests the cost associated with overweight and obesity amounts to $4.3 billion, surpassing the $3.3 billion cost attributed to smoking, a story replicated in most Western nations. It should be emphasised that this chapter will explore the obesity 'epidemic' and this side of the diet equation rather than the malnutrition side of a poor diet (although the latter has been suggested to cost the NHS some £13 billion a year, i.e., higher than the cost of obesity; Eliaand & Russell, 2009).

Applying this to Mike

Mike is at an increased risk of developing cancer, heart disease, diabetes and other chronic diseases due to his poor diet. Also, his poor intake of FVs could leave him with low levels of potassium, folic acid and vitamin C.

Obviously, eating the right foods can prevent illness and promote health. For example, eating FVs may offer protection against some forms of cancer (e.g.,

Schwingshackl et al., 2018). Block et al. (1992) suggested that, based on 132 of 170 studies, there is evidence to suggest that FVs offer significant protection against cancer. However, other reports (e.g., Key, 2011) suggest that Block et al. (1992) study was less convincing than initially considered, given that, along with many others, it failed to take into account confounding variables such as smoking (World Cancer Research Fund, 2018) and that the relationship between fruit and vegetable intake and cancer is somewhat dubious. However, specific phytonutrients (certain plant chemicals) may protect against certain cancers; cruciferous vegetables—such as broccoli, cabbage and cauliflower—and carotenoids—such as lycopene, found in tomatoes and β-Carotene, in orange and yellow FVs—have demonstrated unique anticarcinogenic properties (Pilátová et al., 2011; Tanaka et al., 2012). Key (2011) disputed that FVs offer specific 'broad spectrum' cancer protection amongst otherwise well-nourished individuals but does draw a link between their role in decreasing nutrient deficiencies and consequentially reducing cancer risk in those with a poor diet. Other studies have indicated that fruit and vegetable intake also benefits stroke and heart disease (Aune et al., 2017).

Assessment of diet

There are many ways of assessing diet, but a food diary is the most easily employed within a clinical setting (see Table 5.5). In this case, the patient or client would be asked to record their daily intake of various foodstuffs (based on the categories in the eat well plate).

The other method of assessing diet consequences is to infer it from body measurements. The most common form of body measurement is the BMI. BMI is calculated using the equation weight (kg)/height (m^2) or can be read from a graph (see Figure 5.2). Although BMI is a good way of assessing body fat levels for the average person, there are problems when using this method to assess muscular people (overestimates are possible) and older people (for whom true BMI may be underestimated). For example, athletes and well-trained bodybuilders have a very low percentage of body fat, but their BMI may be in the overweight range. This is because BMI does not distinguish between fat mass and lean mass. Similarly, others have argued that it is overestimated in tall people and underestimated in shorter people, with the need for a new, revised formula (see: http://people.maths.ox.ac.uk/trefethen/bmi.html). However, this suggestion has not been widely accepted, and the simple formula for BMI calculation is certainly easy to calculate and understand.

Table 5.5 How to get waist and hip measurements

Use a measuring tape to take the waist and hip measurement:
Waist: This measurement should be taken at the smaller section of the natural waist, usually located just above the belly button.
Hips: Hip measurement should be taken at the hips on the widest part of your buttocks.
Healthy waist-to-hip ratios
A healthy waist-to-hip ratio for women is **0.8** or lower.
A healthy ratio for men is **1.0** or lower.
Ratios above **0.8** for women and **1.0** for men are associated with obesity and are linked to greater risk of health complications and diseases.

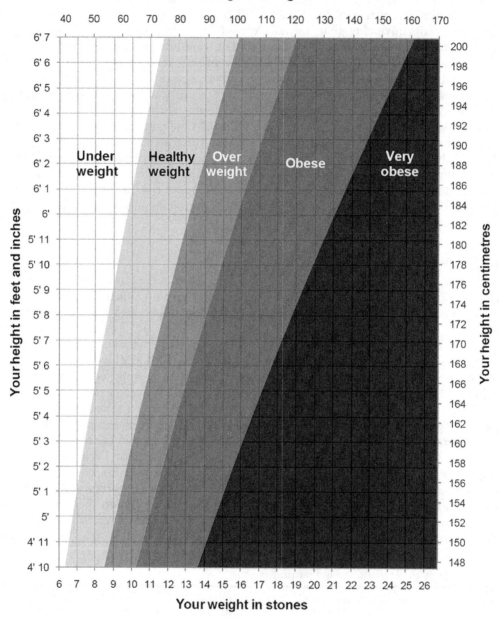

Figure 5.2 BMI measurements.

BMI provides a simple guide to whether weight matches height appropriately for adults. However, BMI is more complex for children because weight varies with height as children grow. It is calculated the same way as for adults but then compared to typical values for other children of the same age and biological sex.

Applying this to Mike

Mike weighs 23 stone (146 kilos), and his BMI is 44. This places him in the morbidly obese category on the BMI measurement graph and at a high risk of developing weight-related health problems.

Using the UK National BMI percentile classification system for children aged 2–15, overweight and obesity are categorised as follows:

Description	BMI centile for child's exact age
Not overweight	91st centile or below
Overweight	Over 91st to 98th centile
Obese	98th centile or over

Although it is rather crude and imprecise, BMI is a useful measure of adiposity and correlates well with the risk of obesity-related diseases (Khanna et al., 2022). In many studies, BMI is calculated using self-reported height and weight. However, a recent systematic review has demonstrated that this self-reported BMI may be lower than a measured BMI; that is, some obese individuals are being misclassified as non-obese based on self-reported BMI (Robinson, 2017). Importantly, this self-report misclassification is not random: moderately obese individuals are more likely to side with non-obese than severely obese, the latter having a BMI further away from the obese/non-obese cut-off value. Consequently, you should always take recordings of height and weight rather than relying on self-reporting, as this may be an underestimate. Another issue may be the time of day measurements are taken. Certain diurnal variations in weight may result in over or underestimation of BMI (Routen et al., 2011). Again, care should be taken to ensure consistent recordings.

An alternative method for assessing body size is to measure waist circumference. Although most people can measure their waist size, they usually do so at the smallest point rather than the appropriate place (see Table 5.6). The waist-to-hip ratio is the final method for assessing body shape (see Table 5.6). The waist-to-hip ratio is a simple measure of where fat is stored in the body. Most people store their body fat in two places: around their waist and around their hips. Storing extra weight around your waist

Table 5.6 Risk of associated disease according to BMI and waist size

BMI		Waist less than or equal to 40 in. (men) or 35 in. (women)	Waist greater than 40 in. (men) or 35 in. (women)
18.5 or less	Underweight		N/A
18.5–24.9	Normal	–	N/A
25.0–29.9	Overweight	Increased	High
30.0–34.9	Obese	High	Very high
35.0–39.9	Obese	Very high	Very high
40 or greater	Extremely obese	Extremely high	Extremely high

Table 5.7 Decisional balance sheet

	Benefits/Pros	Costs/Cons
Making a change		
Not changing		

Applying this to Mike

On the basis of the case study presented at the start of the chapter, Mike's decision balance sheet could look like this:-

	Benefits/Pros	Costs/Cons
Making a change	Reduce weight, BMI and blood pressure.	Extra financial costs e.g., joining a gym.
	Improve general fitness—in time he will be able to return to his five-a-side football team.	Cost implications of buying fresh produce for the whole family
	Reduce risks of developing conditions such as cancer and diabetes.	
	Increase the chances of conception (as Mike and his wife want another child).	
	Saving money—having regular takeaways will be more expensive than eating home-prepared meals.	
Not changing	Mike can eat all the foods he likes.	Health implications.
	Mike can still partake in his post-match drinking sessions.	Reduced life expectancy.
		Reduced healthy life expectancy.

(apple-shaped) creates a higher health risk than someone carrying extra weight around their hips and thighs (pear-shaped). The waist-to-hip ratio is calculated by dividing the waist measurement by the hip measurement. Both BMI and waist sizes come with cut-offs that suggest whether the individual has a problem with their size or not (see Table 5.7).

Why do people eat unhealthily?

There have been several explanations for why people eat what they do, ranging from the genetic to the social-environmental and including media and cognitive factors along the way. Although it is impossible in this brief review to cover all these different proposals, it is worth exploring how some of them translate into interventions.

The media

The media is often cited as one of the major reasons for the increase in diet problems in the developed world (Tudor, 2022). Several studies have linked TV viewing and childhood obesity and concluded that television viewing is associated with obesity (Rosiek et al., 2015). There are several potential explanations for this link, but two predominate. On the one hand, it may be that watching TV encourages a sedentary lifestyle. Alternatively, it may be that media advertising promotes unhealthy consumption, and research has confirmed that this may be the case (Delfino et al., 2020;

Harris et al., 2009). The WHO (2000) has identified food marketing for junk food as detrimental to health and wellbeing. Based on this advice, many countries have regulations to restrict this type of advertising to younger children. Crucially, however, such regulation does not typically cover food marketing on the internet/social media. Research is now expanding on this and revealing the potentially harmful effects of social media consumption and technology on exercise and eating habits (Kucharczuk et al., 2022). Interestingly, the detrimental effects of technology use (i.e., screen time) on health go beyond the direct influence of junk food advertising and/or lack of physical activity. Rosen et al. (2014), for example, identified an association between technology and ill health independent of the factors of diet and exercise.

Obesogenic environments

The term 'obesogenic environment' was coined by Swinburn et al. (1999), who argued that the physical, economic, social and cultural environments of the developed world promote positive energy balance (i.e., calorie intake exceeding calorie output) and consequently weight gain and obesity. According to Park et al. (2020), the prevalence of sedentary activities, such as long hours of screen time, computer work and reduced physical activity, contributes to decreased energy expenditure, making it easier to gain weight. Indeed, urbanisation and a lack of green spaces can contribute to the obesogenic environment (Dempsey et al., 2018). While many studies have investigated the relationship between the environment and weight status, the evidence is complex and often inconclusive. The SLOPE study by Wilding et al. (2020) contributed valuable longitudinal data, examining environmental characteristics' associations with over-weight and obesity in school-aged children. The study found that the relative density of unhealthy food outlets and air pollutants were positively associated with overweight/obesity in children who did not move homes. However, greenspace coverage was negatively associated with the risk of overweight/obesity in all children, regardless of residential mobility. The study suggests that increased access to green space may contribute to preventing childhood obesity. The findings emphasise the importance of considering environmental factors in addressing obesity and promoting future research to understand their impact on health behaviours and outcomes further.

However, to focus on eating, examples of environmental influences that may encourage us to eat more than we need include the marketing of energy-dense drinks and snacks—for example, through television advertising and vending machines in schools—and increased portion sizes where an average meal may provide up to 2,000 kcal, almost the entire recommended daily intake for most adults. According to the Food and Agriculture Organization of the United Nations (2017), time constraints on workers have increased demand for convenience food, pre-packaged foods with short preparation times and food consumption away from the home. These have decreased structured meals and increased snacking, which is often (although not always) densely calorific, and caused the emergence of fast-food restaurants, which are associated with a high-fat diet. Modern lifestyles and work demands can lead to increased stress, which may trigger emotional eating and overconsumption of comfort foods high in calories, sugar and unhealthy fats (Schnepper et al., 2020; Singh, 2014). In some areas, access to fresh and healthy foods is limited, leading to increased reliance on highly processed and calorie-dense foods, which can lead to weight gain (Carvajal-Aldaz et al., 2022). Government policies and agricultural subsidies can influence food prices, making unhealthy foods more affordable than healthier options. The food industry's focus on profit can lead to the production and promotion of foods with high profit margins but low nutritional value.

Applying this to Mike

Mike works in an office and spends a lot of time sitting down each day. Alongside this, his work in the supermarket gives him a discount on the food he purchases. His sedentary behaviour and his motivation to purchase food are both environmental contributors to his poor diet and weight gain.

Psychosocial factors

Some key social factors associated with a poor diet include:

Low income and debt: Healthier foods are generally more expensive than the less healthy alternatives. Fresh fruit and vegetables are less affordable.

Poor accessibility to affordable healthy foods: Many local shops are closing and being replaced with larger, out-of-town stores. This is particularly an issue in deprived areas where such developments mean increased costs within the local shops, poor-quality foodstuffs and less local choice. The out-of-town public stores may have poor transport links and, consequently, not be as easily accessible as the local shops with poor-quality and expensive food.

Factors involved in food production and the food chain: The cheap nutrient level of easily available foodstuffs such as TV dinners may contain high fat, sugar or salt.

Poor literacy and numeracy skills: These are barriers to maintaining a healthy diet, household budget, management and employment.

Food labelling: The recently introduced food labelling agreement means more information is available to the consumer. However, there is still some disagreement about the nature of the information provided and the value derived by the consumer from the information.

Food marketing: Adverts to children usually focus on food that is high in fat or sugar. Consequently, the UK government is introducing new restrictions on what can be advertised and marketed to young children (Department of Health and Social Care, 2021).

Developmental approach

Eating is typically a social event for infants and children. Hence, from a social learning perspective, it could be suggested that children's preferences for and consumption of disliked vegetables are enhanced when children observe peers selecting and eating foods that the observing child dislikes. Parental behaviour and attitudes are central to the process of social learning; however, this association is not straightforward, as parents often differentiate between themselves and their children in terms of food-related motivations and food choice, and it has been suggested that food preferences in children are influenced more by genetic than acquired factors (Persky & Yaremych, 2020). The promise of a reward is a time-honoured parental tactic for promoting the consumption of healthy food. Nevertheless, it has been argued that treating food consumption in this way may decrease liking for that food (Birch, 1999, p. 53). This is a debated topic. It has been acknowledged that the relationship between eating behaviour and rewards is not simple, and different rewarding techniques are beneficial when considering differing outcomes, that is, consumption v. liking (Cooke et al., 2011).

The developmental model emphasises the importance of learning and focuses on developing childhood food preferences. From this perspective, eating behaviour is influenced by exposure, social learning and associative learning.

Applying this to Mike

Jacob will develop eating behaviours partly through social learning from Mike. Therefore, if Mike can change his dietary habits and eat a healthier diet, this should influence Jacob.

Cognitive approach

Cognitive models of eating behaviour explore the extent to which cognitions predict and explain behaviour. Most research from a cognitive perspective has drawn on social cognition models, and several models have been developed (see Chapter 7 for details on some of these models): the Health Belief Model (Becker & Rosenstock, 1984), Protection Motivation Theory (Rogers, 1985), Health Action Process Approach (Schwarzer, 1992), Theory of Reasoned Action (Fishbein & Ajzen, 1975) and its descendant the Theory of Planned Behaviour (Ajzen, 1985). All five models assume that attitudes and beliefs are major determinants of eating behaviour; however, they vary in terms of the cognitions they include and whether they use behavioural intentions or actual behaviour as their outcome measure.

These cognitive models of eating behaviour explore the extent to which cognitions predict and explain behaviour. Cognitive models are informative concerning their ability to predict behaviour and provide helpful insight into ways of influencing this behaviour (Ogden, 2019).

Improving diet

The National Institute for Health and Clinical Excellence (NICE, 2007) published a set of generic principles that can be used as the basis for planning and delivering interventions to change health-related behaviours. The guidance is for health care professionals with direct or indirect responsibility for helping people to change their health behaviour. NICE recommended that practitioners working with individuals should select interventions that motivate and support people to:

- understand the short-, medium- and long-term consequences of their health-related behaviours for themselves and others
- feel positive about the benefits of health-enhancing behaviours and changing their behaviour
- plan changes as easy steps over time

- recognise how their social contexts and relationships may affect their behaviour and identify and plan for situations that might undermine the changes they are trying to make
- plan explicit 'if–then' coping strategies to prevent relapse
- make a personal commitment to adopt health-enhancing behaviours by setting (and recording) goals to undertake clearly defined behaviours in particular contexts over a specified time
- share their behaviour change goals with others.

This guidance should be read in conjunction with other health guidance issued by NICE. For example, NICE (2014) published specific recommendations on increasing interventions' ability to improve diet and reduce energy intake. In this case, NICE recommended that dietary interventions should:

- be multicomponent (i.e., including dietary modification, targeted advice, family involvement and goal setting)
- be tailored to the individual
- provide ongoing support
- include behaviour change strategies
- include awareness-raising promotional activities as part of a long-term, multi-component intervention rather than a one-off activity.

Hence, the health care professional needs to be aware of the available interventions—whether they are structural, psychological or medical. Several interventions have been developed and implemented to improve diet and eating behaviours. These have been at both individual and community levels. Those that are most relevant to the practising health care professional are presented here. How they can be implemented with individuals will be described so that essential tips can be appreciated.

Applying this to Mike

If Mike had a wider selection of foods available from which Jacob could choose, and choosing healthy food was positively reinforced by Mike and his wife, this might lead to improved eating habits for Jacob.

Applying Research in Practice

Access With Education Improves Fruit and Vegetable Intake in Preschool Children (Smith et al., 2020). This study investigated the effects of a multi-component intervention on fruit and vegetable consumption among preschool-aged children (3–5 years) enrolled in the Head Start programme in a rural county in Ohio. The study employed a pre–post group (classroom) randomised control trial design.

During the 8-week intervention, 61 children were assigned to Treatment A and 82 children to Treatment B. Both groups received high-carotenoid FVs during this period. In addition to the FVs, children in Treatment B also received weekly FV education, and their caregivers were provided with FV information and recipes. In contrast, the comparison group, consisting of 66 children, did not receive any FVs or education during the study. Baseline measurements were completed before randomisation, and postintervention carotenoid scans were conducted approximately 8 weeks later.

The access-only treatment group also showed improved carotenoid scores by 16%, highlighting the benefits of providing FVs to children's homes.

Further, adding nutrition education to FV access led to further improvements in carotenoid scores, demonstrating the incremental effect of education.

The study's findings demonstrate that ensuring access to FVs and providing nutrition education may play important roles in promoting healthier eating habits in preschool-aged children.

Individual-level interventions

Individual-level interventions provide strategies for the target population. Medical practitioners, alongside health professionals, can advise individuals on strategies that impact and result in behaviour change.

Prescriptions for fruit and vegetables

At the level of the health practitioner, Buyuktuncer et al. (2014) report on a brief preventative intervention deployed in primary care consultations in a deprived area in North West England. At the centre of the scheme is a prescription for FVs, which GPs, nurses, health visitors and midwives issue to patients opportunistically. Each prescription contains four vouchers offering a £1 discount when £3 or more is spent on fruit and vegetables. As the health professionals issue the prescription, they link it explicitly to key five-a-day messages. Researchers found that the FVs prescription scheme effectively engages participants and improves awareness of key diet-related health messages, but further intervention is required to produce significant, lasting change.

Primary care remains the public's preferred source of food and health information. It provides a natural setting for health promotion, which is usually long term and characterised by trust. Hence, all primary care consultations should be accompanied by some health promotion message, whether concerning diet, weight, smoking or alcohol.

Although such food prescriptions can be useful and encourage a more focused approach to dietary selection, there are psychological principles that help explain why a person succeeds in changing their diet and why they ask for assistance in the first place. One important concept that has been highlighted throughout this text is self-efficacy.

Self-efficacy

One of the most important concepts when examining the success of psychological interventions is self-efficacy (Dennis & Goldberg, 1996; French et al., 1996). Self-efficacy regarding weight loss (Rodin et al., 1988), the ability to handle emotions, life situations (Jeffery et al., 1984) and exercise have been related to later weight loss maintenance. It is thought that developing and changing an individual's self-efficacy during an intervention phase could be crucial to weight loss (Byrne et al., 2012). More information on self-efficacy is presented in Chapter 4.

Decisional balance

One way to prompt individuals to change is to encourage them to consider the *pros* and *cons* of changing their behaviour. Pros and cons were originally derived from Janis and Mann's (1977) model of decision-making and have become critical constructs in the transtheoretical, or stages of change, model. The balance between the pros and cons varies depending on which stage of change the individual is in. However, change is unlikely until the reasons for change outweigh the reasons for staying the same.

When considering change, most of us do not really consider all 'sides' in a logical way. Instead, we often do what we think we 'should' do, avoid doing things we do not feel like doing or feel confused or overwhelmed and give up thinking about it. Thinking through the pros and cons of changing or not changing is one way to help us ensure we have fully considered the consequences of our behaviour. This can help us to 'hang on' to our plan in times of stress or temptation.

The material in Table 5.8 can be used to make a list of the pros and cons associated with changing diet or eating behaviour. For most people, 'making a change' will probably mean eating healthily, but it is important to state the *specific* changes that individuals might want to make, for example, cutting down on saturated fat and sugar, eating five portions of fruit and vegetables a day or trying to eat less salt (no more than 6 g a day).

Table 5.8 The 10 processes of change

Process of change	What this means	Related to diet
Consciousness raising	Increasing information about self and problem: observations, confrontations, interpretations, bibliotherapy	Look for information on improving diet. Leaflets and information guidance
Self-re-evaluation	Assessing how one feels and thinks about oneself with respect to a problem: value clarification, imagery, corrective emotional experience	Feel disappointed with self when eating something unhealthy
Self-liberation	Choosing and commitment to act or belief in ability to change: decision-making therapy, New Year's resolutions, commitment-enhancing techniques	Making a decision to quit, and making a commitment to it
Counter-conditioning	Substituting alternatives for problem behaviours: relaxation, desensitisation, assertion, positive self-statements	Rather than grabbing a chocolate biscuit, have an apple or replace eating with a form of relaxation

(Continued)

Table 5.8 (Continued)

Process of change	What this means	Related to diet
Stimulus control	Avoiding or countering stimuli that elicit problem behaviours: restructuring one's environment (e.g., removing alcohol or fattening foods), avoiding high-risk cues, fading techniques	Remove fattening foods from the home. Replace with healthy foods
Reinforcement management	Rewarding oneself or being rewarded by others for making changes: contingency contracts, overt and covert reinforcement, self-reward	Make sure that friends and other members of the family provide reinforcement.
Helping relationships	Being open and trusting about problems with someone who cares: therapeutic alliance, social support, self-help groups	Weight watchers groups: social support from others
Dramatic relief	Experiencing and expressing feelings about one's problems and solutions: psychodrama, grieving losses, role playing	Emotional link between health and diet—worry and concern about their weight, or a recent health threat
Environmental re-evaluation	Assessing how one's problem affects the physical environment: empathy training, documentaries	How can the physical environment be improved by changing behaviour?
Social liberation	Increasing alternatives for non-problem behaviours available in society: advocating for rights of repressed, empowering, policy interventions	Wider adverts for healthy eating in society

Source: Based on Prochaska et al. (1988).

Goal setting

Once the individual has decided to change their behaviour and start eating healthily, they must be given specific goals. It is of limited value to suggest that the individual 'loses weight' or 'eats more healthily'; the guidance must be specific—'lose two kilos' or 'start to eat five portions of fruit and vegetables per day'. In this way, the goals need to be specific, measurable, achievable, realistic and timed (SMART):

Specific: Specific goals are essential to diet improvement programmes. They represent the difference in focus and motivation between 'I should lose some weight' and 'I'm going to lose a kilo a week for the next 7 weeks—this means in 7 weeks' time I'll be 7 kilos lighter'.

Measurable: The starting point, the weight goal and milestones along the way are all required so that progress can be checked at regular intervals to maintain confidence and ensure the plan is on track.

Achievable: It must be possible to achieve the goal; this is the key to success. If the goals are large—losing two or more stones—they should be broken down into smaller steps, an initial goal of half a stone, for example. Once you have achieved your first goal, a new milestone goal can then be set.

Realistic: There is no point attempting to be half a stone lighter by the end of next week. Even if it were possible, it would be setting the client up for failure in the long term.

Timed: Setting a time frame for the goal gives the client a clear target to work towards. Remember, the time frame must be measurable, achievable and realistic!

Applying this to Mike

The case study presented at the start of the chapter can be used to set SMART targets for both Mike and Jacob. This will help to keep them both motivated and on target.

Mike's SMART targets:

I will increase my fitness and reduce my blood pressure by walking for 45 minutes from 6.00 pm–6.45 pm, 3 days a week (Tuesday, Thursday and Saturday). I will do this in the park and I will take my sports clothes with me to work so I can go on my way home. On a Saturday, I can take Jacob with me so we both get some exercise. In 2 months, I will aim to reduce my blood pressure and my weight.

Jacob's SMART targets:

I will reduce the number of fish fingers and chips that I eat. Each week for 4 weeks, I will reduce the fish finger and chip portions I eat by one. In 1 month, I will have reduced the number of fish fingers and chips portions I eat to one portion a week, which I will have on a Saturday.

You need to develop these goals in conjunction with the client, and the client should be asked:

What are you going to do?
How are you going to do it?
Where are you going to do it?
When are you going to do it?
With whom are you going to do it?
Once the goals are set, the process outlined in Figure 5.3 can be followed.

Changing diet through motivational interviewing

The technique described in Figure 5.3 is based on the stages of change model and using a motivational interviewing technique. Motivational interviewing is a directive, client-centred counselling technique for enhancing intrinsic motivation. Motivational interviewing works by helping the patient articulate why they need to change and increasing their self-efficacy to have the confidence to do so. It is usually used alongside the transtheoretical model (TTM) (Prochaska & DiClemente, 1983), which is discussed in detail throughout this text. In short, the model suggests that change proceeds through a series of stages. The model (see Figure 5.4) is important as it allows the practitioner to

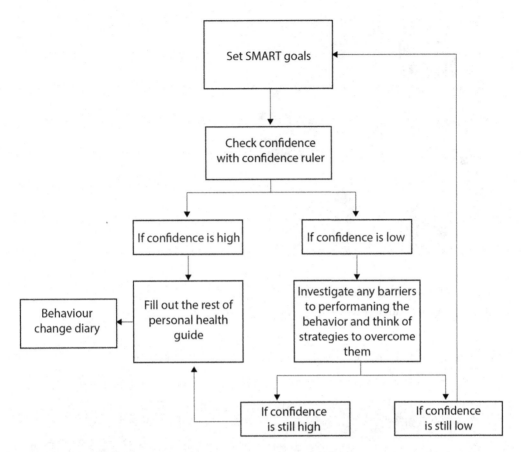

Figure 5.3 Process for encouraging weight loss.

identify where individuals are in their behaviour; with this in mind, appropriate interventions can be developed and implemented. The five stages of change are:

1 *Pre-contemplation:* the patient has no intention of making any changes.
2 *Contemplation:* the patient is considering making some changes.
3 *Preparation:* the patient is making small changes, has developed a plan of action and intends to initiate it soon.
4 *Action:* the patient is actively participating in the new behaviour.
5 *Maintenance:* the patient has continued the new behaviour over an extended period.

Applying this to Mike

Mike is currently in the contemplation stage of change. He has acknowledged that he needs to change his lifestyle, and with help and support, changes can be made.

Jacob is currently in the pre-contemplation stage. He doesn't realise that changes to his lifestyle would be beneficial.

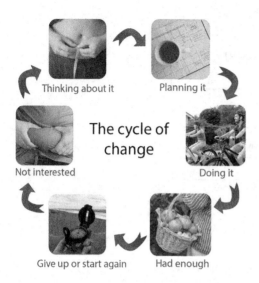

Figure 5.4 The transtheoretical stages of change model.

Source: Adapted from Prochaska, DiClemente and Norcross (1992).

On a scale of 1 to 10, how certain are you that you want to change this behaviour?

1	2	3	4	5	6	7	8	9	10
Not certain at all					Very certain				
Pre-contemplation			Contemplation		Preparation			Action	

Figure 5.5 Readiness ruler: Improving diet.

Any intervention will require the patient to adapt their behaviour in one way or another, be it taking time to attend a hospital appointment, adapting their diet or incorporating new exercise into their daily lives. Adhering to such advice requires the person to be ready and prepared to accept this change. One way to assess a patient's 'readiness' to change is by using the readiness ruler (see Figure 5.5). The readiness ruler can be used at the beginning of an intervention to help target the appropriate stage of change. Alternatively, it can be used during the intervention to encourage the patient to talk about reasons for change.

Thinking that change is important is not always enough for a person to move into the action phase. Sometimes, a person is ready to change but not confident they can. For this reason, both readiness and confidence are addressed in motivation-based interventions.

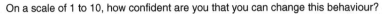

On a scale of 1 to 10, how confident are you that you can change this behaviour?

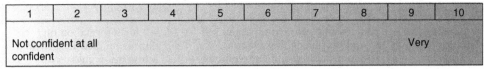

Figure 5.6 Confidence ruler.

The confidence ruler (see Figure 5.6) can be used to assess how confident patients are that they can adapt their behaviour, or it can be used as a hypothetical question to encourage patients to talk about how they would make a change. It is not necessary to show the patient a ruler, but it may be helpful, especially for young children or patients with low literacy and numeracy skills.

Based on the patient's confidence score, the health care professional might ask:

- You said your confidence was a 4, why not a 1 or a 2?
- Why not an 8 or a 9?
- What would it take to make it a 10?

The client's answers to these questions will tell you how resourceful they feel and what potential barriers they have to conquer along the way. The final question will encourage the client to develop their own solutions, tactics and ways to remove obstacles to change. It may also prove helpful to encourage the client to remember previous successes and to review obstacles and how they overcame them.

A person's belief in their ability to change is an important motivator (i.e., their self-efficacy). The health care professional can enhance a person's motivation to change by using open questions to elicit 'confidence talk'. Using negotiation and confidence building to persuade patients that they can change their behaviour is an important part of motivational interviewing.

Applying this to Mike

Mike could use the readiness and confidence rulers to assess his motivation to change his lifestyle and diet. For example, he could consider how important it is for him to eat more fruit and vegetables, to start doing exercise and to cut down his consumption of fatty foods.

Processes of change

While stages of change represent dimensions that allow an understanding of *when* changes occur, the processes of change (Prochaska et al., 1988), outlined in Table 5.9, allow an understanding of *how* changes occur. Ten processes of change have been identified, and specific processes are associated with particular stages of preparation for change. There is integration between the processes of change and the stages of change.

Table 5.9 The 10 processes of change

Process of change	What this means	Related to diet
Consciousness raising	Increasing information about self and problem: observations, confrontations, interpretations, bibliotherapy	Look for information on improving diet. Leaflets and information guidance
Self-re-evaluation	Assessing how one feels and thinks about oneself with respect to a problem: value clarification, imagery, corrective emotional experience	Feel disappointed with self when eating something unhealthy
Self-liberation	Choosing and commitment to act or belief in ability to change: decision-making therapy, New Year's resolutions, commitment-enhancing techniques	Making a decision to quit, and making a commitment to it
Counter-conditioning	Substituting alternatives for problem behaviours: relaxation, desensitisation, assertion, positive self-statements	Rather than grabbing a chocolate biscuit, have an apple or replace eating with a form of relaxation
Stimulus control	Avoiding or countering stimuli that elicit problem behaviours: restructuring one's environment (e.g., removing alcohol or fattening foods), avoiding high-risk cues, fading techniques	Remove fattening foods from the home. Replace with healthy foods
Reinforcement management	Rewarding oneself or being rewarded by others for making changes: contingency contracts, overt and covert reinforcement, self-reward	Make sure that friends and other members of the family provide reinforcement.
Helping relationships	Being open and trusting about problems with someone who cares: therapeutic alliance, social support, self-help groups	Weight watchers groups: social support from others
Dramatic relief	Experiencing and expressing feelings about one's problems and solutions: psychodrama, grieving losses, role playing	Emotional link between health and diet—worry and concern about their weight, or a recent health threat
Environmental re-evaluation	Assessing how one's problem affects the physical environment: empathy training, documentaries	How can the physical environment be improved by changing behaviour?
Social liberation	Increasing alternatives for non-problem behaviours available in society: advocating for rights of repressed, empowering, policy interventions	Wider adverts for healthy eating in society

Source: Based on Prochaska et al. (1988).

Effective self-change depends on doing the right things (processes) at the right time (stages). A successful behavioural change is unlikely to occur with a mismatch in stages and processes. Figure 5.7 highlights how these can be integrated when attempting to change an individual's diet.

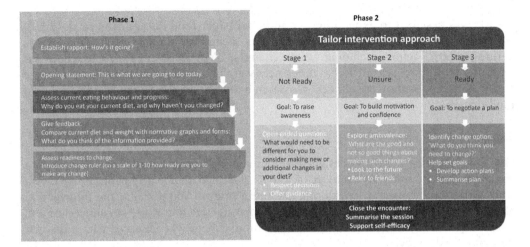

Figure 5.7 Changing diet through motivational interviewing.

Applying this to Mike

Different processes of change will be useful for Mike in order to change his behaviour.

Stimulus control would be a starting point. He could remove any high-fat foods and takeaway menus he has at home. Consciousness-raising would also help him learn about dietary composition and healthy eating. In addition, Mike could also go to Weight Watchers, which would provide some social support. Combining these processes of change would improve Mike's chances of losing and then maintaining his weight.

Efficacy of mobile applications for weight management

Mobile apps have shown promising results in aiding weight loss, either on par with or superior to traditional paper-and-pencil interventions and often outperforming minimal intervention control groups (see Ufholz & Werner, 2023 for a review). Some of the weight loss apps that have been empirically investigated are included below.

Noom

Noom, a commercially available app, features health coaches trained to deliver the CDC's Diabetes Prevention Programme. The app includes daily messaging with a health coach, social support and self-monitoring. In a randomised control trial by Toro-Ramos et al. (2020), participants receiving the Noom intervention lost significant weight and reduced their BMI, highlighting the app's efficacy in weight loss, with reductions lasting up to 1 year.

Well-D

Well-D was designed to expand upon traditional paper food diaries. Ahn et al. (2020) compared Well-D to traditional paper diaries, achieving similar results for various anthropometric factors, including weight changes, BMI, waist circumference, body fat mass and skeletal muscle mass. No differences were observed in terms of nutrient intake either. Both groups showed significant losses in body fat, suggesting the efficacy of digital food diaries.

Oviva

Oviva is a mobile phone app designed to remotely deliver personalised support from a dietician. A pilot study by Haas et al. (2019) revealed that participants using Oviva showed significant weight loss during the intervention. Additionally, the intervention also resulted in improvements in other health parameters like waist circumference and body fat percentage. However, much of this improvement was observed within the first 3 months of delivery.

AKTDIET

According to Apiñaniz et al. (2019), The AKTDIET physical activity and diet tracking mobile app was minimally effective in supporting weight loss when participants engaged with it. There were no statistically significant differences observed in weight, blood cholesterol, blood pressure, adherence to diet recommendations or physical activity between the control and intervention groups. The authors note that patients in the contemplation stage of change may require further behavioural support before weight loss. Thus, in the face of limited evidence of efficacy, the authors do not recommend the AKTDIET app for weight loss.

Fitbit App with push notifications

A randomised control trial by Hernández-Reyes et al. (2020) found that the Fitbit app with additional push notifications for personalised motivational messages led to more significant reductions in body fat and maintenance of muscle mass in overweight women. The push notification group also showed greater weight loss, although this difference was not statistically significant.

Another study, by Bender et al. (2017), found that the PilAm Go4Health intervention, which included a Fitbit and mobile app, was feasible and showed potential efficacy in reducing diabetes risks in overweight Filipino Americans with those with Type 2 diabetes. Both intervention and waitlist groups achieved significant weight loss, supporting mobile-based health interventions for addressing obesity and diabetes risks in this population. These studies combined indicate the potential for increased participant engagement and weight management in participants using Fitbit.

MyFitnessPal

MyFitnessPal is a popular app for tracking diet and weight. In a study by Patel et al. (2019), a standalone weight loss intervention using the MyFitnessPal app, with tailored goals and automated reminders, led to clinically significant weight loss in adults who were overweight or obese. The order in which participants tracked their weight and diet did not significantly impact the outcomes, indicating that both sequential and simultaneous self-monitoring approaches were effective. The results suggest that digital health treatments using mobile apps can be a viable and lower-intensity option for weight management.

Mobile apps taken together promote various strategies, including self-monitoring of diet, exercise and weight, along with social support and educational content. However, the effectiveness of different app types remains inconclusive. The level of user engagement with the app appears to impact the success of these types of interventions significantly. The lack of apps and app-based studies catering to older adults, individuals with limited tech-savviness, ethnic/racial minorities and those with a low income should be noted. Additionally, there is a scarcity of longer-term studies investigating the sustained impact of these apps.

Community-level interventions

Food in Schools Programme: This will promote a 'whole school approach' and encourage greater access to healthier choices within schools.

Work with the food industry: This will address the amount of fat, salt and added sugar in the diet (with the Food Standards Agency).

New GP contract: Practices will be required to offer relevant health promotion advice to patients.

National Food Strategy: Launched in July 2021. It is an independent review for the government, which has a strong focus on making food environments healthier. The government is expected to respond to this in the coming months.

Restricting 'junk food' advertising: This is a recent initiative by the Department of Health and Social Care has now placed restrictions on when foods high in fat, salt and sugar (HFSS foods) can be advertised on television—'The watershed will apply from 9 pm to 5.30 am, meaning HFSS adverts can only be shown during these times' (GOV.UK, 2019). However, there is still doubt about the finer details of this approach, and given its recent introduction, its success has yet to be assessed. However, projections suggest that these restrictions could prevent around 7.2 billion calories from being consumed by children per year. Hopefully, this would prevent more than 20,000 children from becoming obese.

Tackling Obesity Strategy: Launched in July 2020. It includes a suite of new policies to change the food consumption environment in the UK and supports people to make healthier choices. The strategy includes banning all adverts for high fat, salt or sugar products on TV and online before 9 pm; calorie labelling in large restaurants/takeaways; and a new health promotion campaign from Public Health England (PHE), 'Better health—let's do this!'

5-a-day programme

Devised by the Department of Health, the campaign aimed to increase the public's awareness of the government's recommendations for the daily consumption of FVs. An evaluation of the scheme, underpinned by the incentive to prevent illness and health inequalities, indicates promising results. Improvements in the awareness of portion sizes, alongside the recommended daily consumption of FVs, have been seen from the latest evaluation of the scheme (Bremner et al., 2006).

The 5-a-day programme also incorporates the school fruit and vegetable scheme. The scheme entitles children between 4 and 6 years old to receive a free piece of fruit or a vegetable at school to increase consumption alongside increasing awareness of healthy eating. Combined fruit and vegetable consumption was seen to increase due to the programme. However, the effects were not seen to translate to the home setting (Teeman et al., 2010). Thus, dietary changes must translate between environments to ensure a long-lasting dietary impact.

Traffic light system

To guide individuals to make healthy choices, the Food Standards Agency devised the traffic light system that gives the public an indication of the nutritional values of food. Food products are labelled with green-, red- or amber-coloured labels, which represent low, high or medium amounts of fat, saturated fat, salt and sugar. The labels provide a quick and easy guide for individuals to make healthier dietary choices. However, it is thought that only one in four shoppers look at this information (The European Food Information Council, 2008). Evidence has shown a consistent link between the use of nutrition labels and healthier diets, but that may result from healthier eaters seeking out and using the information rather than the labels promoting better diets (Campos et al., 2011). With government efforts being made to address the poor diets of the nation, it is also important to understand the gap between the individuals' understanding of such healthy eating government campaigns and their implementation.

Applying this to Mike

Mike could use all the resources from the government campaigns to help him change his dietary habits. The Change4Life website provides information and advice on healthy eating and exercise, including recipe and exercise ideas. In addition, Mike could start to use the traffic light system and start looking at the labels on the foods that he purchases in an attempt to eat a more balanced diet.

Working effectively with others

In attempting to tackle obesity, various professions, such as psychologists and health professionals, can help and support individuals aiming to tackle obesity. Outlined below are examples of such professionals.

Dieticians

A dietician is a professional who advises on dietary intake and its impact on health. They offer advice to individuals to help them make health-conscious decisions. Using the science behind nutrition, they work with an individual to draw up a dietary plan according to specific goals (weight loss) or requirements (allergies). Dieticians can also treat dietary-related problems and educate individuals who require specific diets as part of a medical regime (e.g., diabetes and kidney disease).

Physiologists

Physiologists are concerned with the impact of our modern lifestyle and how this affects health and wellbeing. They consider external influences and the impact of those influences on science within the human body. Physiologists are trained to assess individuals' health and work with clients to develop behaviour change strategies.

Physical training instructors

Physical training instructors work in many settings, including gyms, health clubs and the NHS. Working with their client, physical training instructors devise personal training and diet plans and give general advice regarding fitness. In addition, they can work with the client to set goals so the client reaches their target weight. The advice and input from physical training instructors can provide individuals with much-needed motivation when considering weight loss.

Applying this to Mike

To help Mike address his health and weight concerns, he could seek the advice of many professionals who will provide him with support in many areas. In addition, while helping him understand the impact of his diet on his health, it will also advise him on ways to change his dietary behaviour. For instance, he could join a gym and devise an exercise regime with the help of a physical training instructor. In turn, the physical training instructor could help keep Mike motivated and on target to lose weight.

Conclusion

The consequences of a poor diet are more than just obesity. A poor diet can contribute to various illnesses, including CHD, cancer and Type 2 diabetes. Conversely, eating the 'right' foods can prevent illness and promote health. Despite the wealth of evidence endorsing diet's positive and negative impact on health, research suggests that many people do not eat a sufficiently healthy diet.

Several explanations have been offered for why people eat what they do, ranging from the media to the social-environmental and psychosocial. This chapter also explored two key psychological models of eating behaviour: the developmental approach, which emphasises the importance of learning and the development of food preferences, and the cognitive approach, which explores the extent to which cognitions explain and predict behaviour.

Numerous interventions have been introduced to tackle the nation's poor diet; however, the effectiveness of such interventions remains poor. Future attempts to improve the nation's diet should be multicomponent, include behaviour change strategies and provide ongoing support and, most importantly, be tailored to the needs of the individual; after all, one size does not fit all.

Key points

- Diet can affect health through an individual's weight but also plays a role in developing diseases such as CHD, cancer and diabetes.
- Food-related ill health is estimated to be responsible for about 10% of morbidity and mortality in the UK.
- Healthy eating can be understood in terms of five major food groups and is important for promoting health and treating ill health.
- Eating behaviour has been shown to be influenced by the media, the environment and social barriers such as availability, cost and time.
- The developmental approach emphasises the importance of learning and focuses on developing food preferences in childhood. From this perspective, eating behaviour is influenced by exposure, social learning and associative learning.
- Research has demonstrated that self-efficacy, that is, the belief in one's ability to exercise control over challenging demands, plays an important role in weight loss and maintenance.
- Decisional balance, or the individual's evaluation of the pros and cons, is a crucial component in modifying dietary behaviours, as change is unlikely to occur until the reasons for change outweigh the reasons for staying the same.
- SMART goals are essential to diet improvement; that is, goals need to be specific, measurable, achievable, realistic and timed.
- Motivational interviewing is a client-centred approach for eliciting behaviour change. It works by helping the patient articulate why it is important for them to change while increasing their confidence that they can do so.
- According to the TTM, behaviour change can be thought of as a progression through a series of stages: pre-contemplation, contemplation, preparation, action and maintenance.
- Ten processes have been identified that explain how progression through the stages of change can occur. Effective self-change depends on doing the right things (processes) at the right time (stages).
- Community-level interventions have been outlined and can be used in a combined effort as a long-term prevention strategy for the current obesity concern. However, the effectiveness of these is questionable.
- Health professionals such as dieticians, physiologists and physical training instructors can be useful in guiding and motivating the client to make behaviour changes.

Points for discussion

- Imagine that you wanted to decrease your intake of high-fat foods and maintain your level of intake in the long term. How would you do this, and what interventions would be useful?
- Critically discuss the developmental model of eating behaviour.
- Compare and contrast two cognitive models of eating behaviour.
- Consider Mike's son Jacob. How would you improve his diet using psychological principles?
- Also consider:
  o how you would assess Jacob's diet
  o how Jacob's environment might influence his eating behaviour.

Further resources

Conner, M., & Norman, P. (2007). Predicting and changing health behaviour (3rd ed.) Berkshire, UK: Open University Press.

Ogden, J. (2010). The psychology of eating: From healthy to disordered behaviour (2nd ed.) Oxford, UK: Blackwell.

Thirlaway, K., & Upton, D. (2009). The psychology of lifestyle: Promoting healthy behaviour. London, UK: Routledge.

Upton, D., & Thirlaway, K. (2014). Promoting healthy behaviour: A practical guide (2nd ed.). Camebridge: Routledge. 10.4324/9781315819105

Useful web links

An online calculator for working out and interpreting a child's BMI is available at www.healthforallchildren.co.uk on the parent's page.

Food Dudes healthy eating program; http://www.fooddudes.co.uk/

Eat well, be well—the Food Standards Agency website for consumer advice on healthy eating. It is packed with information and tips on eating a healthy, balanced diet http://www.eatwell.gov.uk/

Cancer Prevention Research Centre provides a detailed overview of TTM, including the stages of change, processes of change, decisional balance and self-efficacy http://www.uri.edu/research/cprc/transtheoretical.htm

Motivational interviewing: resources for clinicians, researchers and trainers—provides background information on the practice of motivational interviewing http://www.motivationalinterview.org/

The Food Standards Agency—Traffic Light System: http://tna.europarchive.org/20100910172942/http://www.eatwell.gov.uk/foodlabels/trafficlights/

References

Ahn, J. S., Lee, H., Kim, J., Park, H., Kim, D. W., & Lee, J. E. (2020). Use of a smartphone app for weight loss versus a paper-based dietary diary in overweight adults: Randomized controlled trial. JMIR MHealth UHealth, *8*, e14013. 10.2196/14013

Ajzen, I. (1985). From intention to actions: A theory of planned behaviour. In J. Kuhl and J. Beckman (Eds.), Action control: From cognition to behaviour (pp. 11–89). Heidelberg, Germany: Springer. Retrieved from http://www.people.umass.edu/aizen/publications.html

American Cancer Society. (2019). Cancer prevention & early detection facts & figures 2019–2020. Atlanta, Georgia: American Cancer Society.

Apiñaniz, A., Cobos-Campos, R., Sáez de Lafuente-Moríñigo, A., Parraza, N., Aizpuru, F., Pérez, I., ...García, L. (2019). Effectiveness of randomized controlled trial of a mobile app to promote healthy lifestyle in obese and overweight patients. Family Practice. *36*, 699–705. 10.1093/fampra/cmz020

Aune, D., Giovannucci, E., Boffetta, P., Fadnes, L. T., Keum, N., Norat, T., Greenwood, D. C., Riboli, E., Vatten, L. J., & Tonstad, S. (2017). Fruit and vegetable intake and the risk of cardiovascular disease, total cancer and all-cause mortality—a systematic review and dose-response meta-analysis of prospective studies. International Journal of Epidemiology, *46*, 1029–1056.

Becker, M. H., & Rosenstock, I. M. (1984). Compliance with medical advice. In A. Steptoe and A. Mathews (Eds.), Health care and human behaviour. London, United Kingdom: Academic Press.

Bender, M. S., Cooper, B. A., Park, L. G., Padash, S., & Arai, S. (2017). A feasible and efficacious mobile-phone based lifestyle intervention for Filipino Americans with Type 2 diabetes: Randomized controlled trial. JMIR Diabetes, *2*, e30. 10.2196/diabetes.8156

Birch, L. (1999). Development of food preferences. Annual Review of Nutrition, *19*, 41–62.

Block, G., Patterson, B., & Subar, A. (1992). Fruit, vegetables and cancer prevention: A review of the epidemiological evidence. Nutrition and Cancer, *18*, 1–29.

Bremner, P., Dalziel, D., & Evans. (2006). Evaluation of the 5 a Day programme, final report. Surrey, United Kingdom: TNS Social.

Bromley, C., & Given, L. (2011). The Scottish health survey 2010, volume 1: Main report. Edinburgh, United Kingdom: The Scottish Government. Retrieved from http://www.scotland.gov.uk/Publications/2011/09/27084018/914

Buyuktuncer, Z., Kearney, M., Ryan, C. L., Thurston, M., & Ellahi, B. (2014). Fruit and vegetables on prescription: A brief intervention in primary care. Journal of Human Nutrition and Dietetics, *27*(s2), 186–193. 10.1111/jhn.12109

Byrne, S., Barry, D., & Petry, N. M. (2012). Predictors of weight loss success. Exercise vs. dietary self-efficacy and treatment attendance. Appetite, *58*(2), 695–698.

Campos, S., Doxey, J., & Hammond, D. (2011). Nutrition labels on pre-packaged foods: A systematic review. Public Health Nutrition, *14*, 1496–1506.

Carvajal-Aldaz, D., Cucalon, G., & Ordonez, C. (2022). Food insecurity as a risk factor for obesity: A review. Frontiers in Nutrition, *9*, 1012734. 10.3389/fnut.2022.1012734

Cheema, K. M., Dicks, E., Pearson, J., & Samani, N. J. (2022). Long-term trends in the epidemiology of cardiovascular diseases in the UK: insights from the British Heart Foundation statistical compendium. Cardiovascular Research, *118*(10), 2267–2280.

Cooke, L. J., Chambers, L. C., Añez, E. V., & Wardle, J. (2011). Facilitating or undermining? The effect of reward on food acceptance. A narrative review. Appetite, *57*(2), 493–497.

Delfino, L. D., Tebar, W. R., Silva, D. A. S., Gil, F. C. S., Mota, J., & Christofaro, D. G. D. (2020). Food advertisements on television and eating habits in adolescents: A school-based study. Revista de Saúde Pública, *54*, 55. 10.11606/s1518-8787.2020054001558

Dempsey, S., Lyons, S., & Nolan, A. (2018). Urban green space and obesity in older adults: Evidence from Ireland. SSM—Population Health, *4*, 206–215. https://doi.org/10.1016/j.ssmph.2018.01.002

Dennis, K. E., & Goldberg, A. P. (1996). Weight control self-efficacy types and transitions affect weight-loss outcomes in obese women. Addictive Behaviour, *21*, 103–116.

Department of Health, Social Services and Public Safety. (2011). Health Survey Northern Ireland: First results from the 2010/11 survey. Belfast, United Kingdom. Available at: http://www.dhsspsni.gov.uk/index/stats_research/stats-public-health.htm

Department of Health and Social Care (2021). New advertising rules to help tackle childhood obesity. London, United Kingdom: UK Government. Retrieved from https://www.gov.uk/government/news/new-advertising-rules-to-help-tackle-childhood-obesity

Elia, M., & Russell, C. (2009). Combating malnutrition: Recommendations for action. Redditch, United Kingdom: British Association for Parenteral and Enteral Nutrition. Retrieved from http://www.bapen.org.uk/pdfs/reports/advisory_group_report.pdf

The European Food Information Council. (2008, 25 September). EUFIC Press Release from 25/09/2008: One in four UK consumers look for nutrition information on food labels. Retrieved from http://www.eufic.org/jpage/en/page/PRESS/fftid/Consumer-InsightsUK-results/

Feletto, E., Kohar, A., Mizrahi, D., Grogan, P., Steinberg, J., Hughes, C., ...Yu, X. Q. (2022). An ecological study of obesity-related cancer incidence trends in Australia from 1983 to 2017. The Lancet Regional Health—Western Pacific, *29*, 100575. 10.1016/j.lanwpc.2022.100575

Fishbein, M., & Ajzen, I. (1975). Belief, attitude, intention and behaviour. An introduction to theory and research. Reading, MA: Addison-Wesley. Retrieved from http://www.people.umass.edu/aizen/publications.html

Food and Agriculture Organization of the United Nations. (2017). The future of food and agriculture. Retrieved from https://www.fao.org/3/i6583e/I6583E.pdf

Food Standards Agency. (2008). The eatwell plate. Retrieved from http://www.eatwell.gov.uk/healthydiet/eighttipssection/8tips

French, S. A., Perry, C. L., Leon, G. R., & Faulkerson, J. A. (1996). Self-esteem and change in body mass index over 3 years in a cohort of adolescents. Obesity Research, 4(1), 27–33.

GBD 2017 Diet Collaborators. (2019). Health effects of dietary risks in 195 countries, 1990–2017: A systematic analysis for the Global Burden of Disease Study 2017. The Lancet, 393(10184), 1958–1972. Retrieved from 10.1016/s0140-6736(19)30041-8

GOV.UK. (2019). Introducing further advertising restrictions on TV and online for products high in fat, salt and sugar: Government response. Retrieved from https://www.gov.uk/government/consultations/further-advertising-restrictions-for-products-high-in-fat-salt-and-sugar/outcome/introducing-further-advertising-restrictions-on-tv-and-online-for-products-high-in-fat-salt-and-sugar-government-response

Haas, K., Hayoz, S., & Maurer-Wiesner, S. (2019). Effectiveness and feasibility of a remote lifestyle intervention by dietitians for overweight and obese adults: Pilot study. JMIR MHealth UHealth, 7, e12289. 10.2196/12289

Harris, J. L., Bargh, J. A., & Brownell, K. D. (2009). Priming effects of television food advertising on eating behavior. Health Psychology, 28(4), 404–413. 10.1037/a0014399

Hernández-Reyes, A., Cámara-Martos, F., Molina Recio, G., Molina-Luque, R., Romero-Saldaña, M., & Moreno Rojas, R. (2020). Push notifications from a mobile app to improve the body composition of overweight or obese women: Randomized controlled trial. JMIR MHealth UHealth, 8, e13747. 10.2196/13747

Horne, P. J., Tapper, K., Lowe, C. F., Hardman, C. A., Jackson, M. C., & Woolner, J. (2004). Increasing children's fruit and vegetable consumption: A peer modelling rewards-based intervention. European Journal of Clinical Nutrition, 58, 1649–1660.

Janis, I. L., & Mann, L. (1977). Decision making: A psychological analysis of conflict, choice and commitment. New York, New York: Free Press.

Jeffery, R. W., Bjornson-Benson, W. M., Rosenthal, B. S., Lindquist, R. A., Kurth, C. L., & Johnson, S. L. (1984). Correlates of weight loss and its maintenance over two years of follow-up among middle aged men. Preventive Medicine, 13, 155–168.

Kearney, M., Bradbury, C., Ellahi, B., Hodgson, M., & Thurston, M. (2005). Mainstreaming prevention: Prescribing fruit and vegetables as a brief intervention in primary care. Journal of the Royal Institute of Public Health, 119, 981–986.

Keaver, L., Xu, B., Jaccard, A., & Webber, L. (2020). Morbid obesity in the UK: A modelling projection study to 2035. Scandinavian Journal of Public Health, 48(4), 422–427. 10.1177/1403494818794814

Key, T. J. (2011). Fruit and vegetables and cancer risk. British Journal of Cancer, 104(1), 6–11.

Khanna, D., Peltzer, C., Kahar, P., & Parmar, M. S. (2022). Body mass index (BMI): a screening tool analysis. Cureus, 14(2).

Kucharczuk, A. J., Oliver, T. L., & Dowdell, E. B. (2022). Social media's influence on adolescents' food choices: A mixed studies systematic literature review. Appetite, 168, 105765. 10.1016/j.appet.2021.105765

NICE. (2007). Behaviour change at population, community and individual levels. Retrieved from http://www.nice.org.uk/nicemedia/pdf/PH006guidance.pdf

NICE. (2014). Obesity: Identification, assessment and management. Retrieved from https://www.nice.org.uk/guidance/cg189/resources/obesity-identification-assessment-and-management-pdf-35109821097925

NHS. (2012). Live Well. http://www.nhs.uk/Livewell/Goodfood/Pages/Healthyeating.aspx

Office of Communications. (2006). Annex 7—Impact assessment consultation on television advertising of food and drink to children (Joint FSA/DoH Analysis; no. 2). London, UK: Office of Communications.

Ogden, J. (2019). Health psychology: A textbook (64th ed.). Milton Keynes: Open University Press.

Palmer, D. (2022). Estimating the full costs of obesity—A report for Novo Nordisk. Frontier Economics. Retrieved from https://policycommons.net/artifacts/3350310/estimating-the-full-costs-of-obesity/4149181/

Park, J. H., Moon, J. H., Kim, H. J., Kong, M. H., & Oh, Y. H. (2020). Sedentary lifestyle: Overview of updated evidence of potential health risks. Korean Journal of Family Medicine, *41*(6), 365–373. 10.4082/kjfm.20.0165

Patel, M. L., Hopkins, C. M., Brooks, T. L., & Bennett, G. G. (2019). Comparing self-monitoring strategies for weight loss in a smartphone app: Randomized controlled trial. JMIR MHealth UHealth, 7, e12209. 10.2196/12209

Persky, S., & Yaremych, H. E. (2020). Parents' genetic attributions for children's eating behaviors: Relationships with beliefs, emotions, and food choice behavior. Appetite, *155*, 104824. 10.1016/j.appet.2020.104824

Pilátová, M., Chripková, M., & Mojžiš, J. (2011). Cruciferous vegetables in cancer prevention. Acta Facultatis Pharmaceuticae Universitatis Comenianae, *53*(1), 62–71.

Prochaska, J. O., & DiClemente, C. C. (1983). Stages and processes of self-change smoking: Towards and integrative model of change. Journal of Consulting and Clinical Psychology, *51*, 390–395.

Prochaska, J. O., DiClemente, C. C., & Norcross, J. C. (1992). In search of how people change: Application to addictive behaviors. American Psychologist, *47*(9), 1102–1114.

Prochaska, J. O., Velicer, W. F., DiClemente, C. C., & Fava, J. (1988). Measuring processes of change: Applications to the cessation of smoking. Journal of Consulting and Clinical Psychology, *56*, 520–528.

PHE. (2020). National diet and nutrition survey: Diet, nutrition and physical activity in 2020. A follow up study during COVID-19. Retrieved from https://assets.publishing.service.gov.uk/government/uploads/system/uploads/attachment_data/file/1019663/Follow_up_stud_2020_main_report.pdf

Rekhy, R., & McConchie, R. (2014). Promoting consumption of fruit and vegetables for better health. Have campaigns delivered on the goals? Appetite, *79*, 113–123. 10.1016/j.appet.2014.04.012

Robinson, E. (2017). Overweight but unseen: A review of the underestimation of weight status and a visual normalization theory. Obesity Reviews, *18*(10), 1200–1209. 10.1111/obr.12570

Rodin, J., Elias, M., Silberstein, L. R., & Wagner, A. (1988). Combined behavioural and pharmacologic treatment for obesity: Predictors of successful weight maintenance. Journal of Consulting and Clinical Psychology, *56*, 399–404.

Rogers, R. W. (1985). Attitude change and information integration in fear appeals. Psychological Reports, *56*, 179–182.

Rosen, L. D., Lim, A. F., Felt, J., Carrier, L. M., Cheever, N. A., Lara-Ruiz, J. M., Mendoza, J. S., & Rokkum, J. (2014). Media and technology use predicts ill-being among children, preteens and teenagers independent of the negative health impacts of exercise and eating habits. Computers in Human Behavior, *35*, 364–375. 10.1016/j.chb.2014.01.036

Rosiek, A., Frąckowiak Maciejewska, N., Leksowski, K., Rosiek-Kryszewska, A., & Leksowski, Ł. (2015). Effect of television on obesity and excess of weight and consequences of health. International Journal of Environmental Research and Public Health, *12*(8), 9408–9426. 10.3390/ijerph120809408

Routen, A., Edwards, M., Upton, D., & Peters, D. (2011). The impact of school-day variation in weight and height on national child measurement BMI determined weight category in Year 6 children. Child Care Health Development, *37*(3), 360–367.

Ryan, D. H., & Yockey, S. R. (2017). Weight loss and improvement in comorbidity: Differences at 5%, 10%, 15%, and over. Current Obesity Reports, *6*(2), 187–194. 10.1007/s13679-017-0262-y

Scarborough, P., Morgan, R., Webster, P., & Rayner, M. (2011). Differences in coronary heart disease, stroke and cancer mortality rates between England, Wales, Scotland and Northern Ireland: The role of diet and nutrition. BMJ Open, *1*(1), e000263.

Schwarzer, R. (1992). Self-efficacy in the adoption and maintenance of health behaviours: Theoretical approaches and a new model. In R. Schwarzer (Ed.), Self-efficacy: Thought Control of Action. Washington, DC: Hemisphere.

Schwingshackl, L., Schwedhelm, C., Hoffmann, G., Knüppel, S., Laure Preterre, A., Iqbal, K., Bechthold, A., De Henauw, S., Michels, N., Devleesschauwer, B., Boeing, H., & Schlesinger, S. (2018). Food groups and risk of colorectal cancer. International Journal of Cancer, *142*(9), 1748–1758. 10.1002/ijc.31198

Singh, M. (2014). Mood, food, and obesity. Frontiers in Psychology, *5*, 925. 10.3389/fpsyg.2014.00925

Smith, E., Sutarso, T., & Kaye, G. L. (2020). Access with education improves fruit and vegetable intake in preschool children. Journal of Nutrition Education and Behaviour, *52*, 145–151. 10.1016/j.jneb.2019.07.016

Schnepper, R., Georgii, C., Eichin, K., Arend, A.-K., Wilhelm, F. H., Vögele, C., ...Blechert, J. (2020). Fight, flight,—or grab a bite! Trait emotional and restrained eating style predicts food cue responding under negative emotions. Frontiers in Behavioral Neuroscience, *14*, 91. 10.3389/fnbeh.2020.00091

Swinburn, B. A., Egger, G. J., & Raza, F. (1999). Dissecting obesogenic environments: The development and application of a framework for identifying and prioritising environmental interventions for obesity. Preventative Medicine, *29*, 563–570.

Taddei, C., Zhou, B., Bixby, H., Carrillo-Larco, R. M., Danaei, G., Jackson, R. T., ...NCD Risk Factor Collaboration. (2020). Repositioning of the global epicentre of non-optimal cholesterol. Nature, *582*(7810), Article 7810. 10.1038/s41586-020-2338-1

Tanaka, T., Shnimizu, M., & Moriwaki, H. (2012). Cancer chemoprevention by carotenoids. Molecules, *17*(3), 3202–3242.

Teeman, D., Lynch, S., White, K., Scott, E., Waldman, J., Benton, T. ...Thomas, J. (2010). The third evaluation of the school fruit and vegetable scheme. London, United Kingdom: Department of Health.

The Global BMI Mortality Collaboration. (2016). Body-mass index and all-cause mortality: Individual-participant-data meta-analysis of 239 prospective studies in four continents. The Lancet, *388*(10046), 776–786. Retrieved from 10.1016/s0140-6736(16)30175-1

The Health and Social Care Information Centre, NHS. (2017). Statistics on obesity, physical activity and diet: England. Retrieved from https://assets.publishing.service.gov.uk/government/uploads/system/uploads/attachment_data/file/613532/obes-phys-acti-diet-eng-2017-rep.pdf

Toro-Ramos, T., Michaelides, A., Anton, M., Karim, Z., Kang-Oh, L., Argyrou, C. ...Miller, J. D. (2020). Mobile delivery of the diabetes prevention program in people with prediabetes: Randomized controlled trial. JMIR MHealth UHealth, *8*, e17842. 10.2196/17842

Tudor, C. (2022). The nexus between pollution and obesity and the magnifying role of media consumption: International evidence from GMM systems estimates. International Journal of Environmental Research and Public Health, *19*(16), 10260. 10.3390/ijerph191610260

Ufholz, K., & Werner, J. (2023). The efficacy of mobile applications for weight loss. Current Cardiovascular Risk Reports, *17*, 83–90. 10.1007/s12170-023-00717-2

UK Department of Health. (2009). Change4Life marketing strategy. London, United Kingdom: UK Department of Health.

UK Department of Health. (1999). Saving lives: Our healthier nation. London, United Kingdom: The Stationery Office.

UK Department of Health. (2011b). Healthy lives, healthy people: A call to action on obesity in England. Retrieved from http://www.dh.gov.uk/prod_consum_dh/groups/dh_digitalassets/documents/digitalasset/dh_130487.pdf

Wang, D. D., Li, Y., Afshin, A., Springmann, M., Mozaffarian, D., Stampfer, M. J., Hu, F. B., Murray, C. J. L., & Willett, W. C. (2019). Global improvement in dietary quality could lead to substantial reduction in premature death. The Journal of Nutrition, *149*(6), 1065–1074. 10.1093/jn/nxz010

Welsh Government. (2011). Welsh Health Survey 2010. Retrieved from http://www.wales.gov.uk/statistics

Wilding, S., Ziauddeen, N., Smith, D., Roderick, P., Chase, D., & Alwan, N. A. (2020). Are environmental area characteristics at birth associated with overweight and obesity in school-aged children? Findings from the SLOPE (Studying Lifecourse Obesity PrEdictors) population-based cohort in the south of England. BMC Medicine, *18*, 43. 10.1186/s12916-020-01513-0

World Cancer Research Fund. (2018). Diet, nutrition, physical activity and cancer: A global perspective. Washington, DC: American Institute for Cancer Research.

WHO. (2020). Healthy diet [Fact sheet]. Retrieved from https://www.who.int/news-room/fact-sheets/detail/healthy-diet

WHO. (2013). *Prevention and control of noncommunicable diseases: Formal meeting of Member States to conclude the work on the comprehensive global monitoring framework*, including indicators, and a set of voluntary global targets for the prevention and control of noncommunicable diseases: Report by the director-general. Retrieved from https://apps.who.int/iris/handle/10665/78617

Zheng, Y., Li, Y., Satija, A., Pan, A., Sotos-Prieto, M., Rimm, E., Willett, W. C., & Hu, F. B. (2019). Association of changes in red meat consumption with total and cause specific mortality among US women and men: Two prospective cohort studies. BMJ (Clinical Research ed.), *365*, l2110. 10.1136/bmj.l2110

6 Being physically active

LEARNING OBJECTIVES

At the end of this chapter you will:

- Understand what being physically active means.
- Recognise how much physical activity is recommended to maximise health.
- Understand physical activity patterns in the UK and the wider world.
- Appreciate why some people do not achieve the recommended level of physical activity to remain healthy.
- Have explored available interventions to help people increase their levels of physical activity.
- Recognise the role of 'systems-based' approaches in supporting the physical activity of individuals.

Case Study

Dafydd is a 40-year-old manager of an estate agent based in Cardiff. He is responsible for the performance of his team. He works long hours since money is tight and commutes by car about 5 miles to and from work every day, this can take him up to 40 minutes each way in rush hour. Dafydd is married with three young children all in primary school. His partner also works full-time but works locally to their home. They find caring for three young children and working very tiring and limits available time for themselves as a couple and also for themselves, individually. The family have one car and it is needed in the evenings to take the children to their various leisure activities. Whilst he enjoyed playing football at school, Dafydd stopped playing in his 20's due to a persistent knee injury. He has taken no exercise since, other than occasionally going swimming with the children. Over the past decade his weight has crept up and he is now over the recommended weight for his height, and therefore overweight, although not yet in the obese range.

Recently, Dafydd has been under a lot of pressure at work. He went to the GP reporting difficulty in sleeping and heart palpitations. After ensuring that Dafydd had no underlying severe physiological condition that was responsible for his symptoms, Dafydd's doctor diagnosed stress and depression and suggested he could try and

DOI: 10.4324/9781003471233-6

manage his symptoms by changing his lifestyle but if that was not successful, he would be prescribed an anti-depressant together with beta blockers to control the heart palpitations. Dafydd and the doctor agreed that he would return in 3 months to see if the symptoms had improved through lifestyle adjustments.

Dafydd does not want to take either of the medications prescribed by the doctor. He comes to the GP practice wellbeing clinic to discuss alternative strategies to manage his symptoms. When he realises that being physically active can be an effective treatment for stress and depression, he is initially very enthusiastic about it but soon becomes despondent when he realises that it may not be possible with all his family commitments. He is struggling to see how he could incorporate an appropriate level of physical activity into his already busy day, sufficient enough to meet national recommendations and to enable him to manage his stress and depression. He fears his partner will not be supportive of him being away from home any longer than he already is.

Introduction

There can be many opportunities for people to be physically active during the day because physical activity in its broadest sense includes any bodily movement. Formally, physical activity is defined by the World Health Organisation (WHO) as:

Any bodily movement produced by skeletal muscles that requires energy expenditure. Physical activity refers to all movement including during leisure time, for transport to get to and from places, or as part of a person's work.

World Health Organisation (WHO) 2020

For many people across the world in middle and high income countries normal daily occupations no longer require even moderate levels of physical activity and this trajectory of work and domestic tasks becoming less active and more sedentary shows no sign of stabilising or reversing over the next decade. Countries such as China and Brazil, are seeing rapid reductions in occupational physical activity causing high rates of decline in overall physical activity and are forecast to reach US and UK total physical activity levels by 2030 (Guthold et al., 2018; Ng & Popkin, 2012). India has proven more resistant to declining physical activity particularly in rural areas. In the US and the UK distance walked per year has been declining and vehicle miles travelled increasing but there is some evidence that UK governments promotion of active transport is supporting uptake of walking and cycling (Department of Transport, 2020). A useful review of international levels of physical inactivity and the impact of income on these levels identifies the importance of physical activity at a national and international level (Guthold et al., 2018). This has led to global calls for addressing the factors affecting population and individual physical activity levels by the WHO in 2018 and later updated in 2022 (WHO, 2018; 2022). There is increasing recognition that a systems-based approach is required that strategically links 'upstream' policy actions to improve social, cultural, economic, and environmental factors with 'downstream' local, community and individual interventions (WHO, 2018).

At an individual level, health professionals tend to focus on encouraging clients to increase their physical activity in their leisure-time through exercise, physical activity, or active transport. Another approach to increasing physical activity is through workplace physical activity interventions that can range from campaigns and information, behavioural and social through to environmental and policy approaches. There is some evidence that workplace led interventions, particularly when developed as part of the workplace system, can be effective (Mulchandani et al., 2019).

Applying this to Dafydd

Dafydd's occupation and mode of transport is predominantly sedentary. So unless his workplace introduces work-based physical activity opportunities any increase in his current physical activity will be either leisure-based or through changing his commute to active transport. Given his family commitments, active transport may be the best option for him and to support this he could explore with his workplace any schemes to purchase a bicycle. He will be influenced by the safety of the route to work, his competence and confidence to ride 10 miles a day, and the opportunities available to store a bike safely, wash and change before work, plus the time it takes for him to do this.

Exercise can be conceptualised as a deliberate act to improve or maintain physical or mental health. Khan et al. (2012) define exercise as:

'planned, structured and repetitive bodily movement, the objective of which is to improve or maintain physical fitness'.

Sport includes an element of competition that is not present in exercise activities. Rejeskis and Brawley 1998, cited in Biddle and Mutrie (2008, p. 10) define sport as:

'Rule-governed, structured and competitive and involves gross motor movement characterised by physical strategy, prowess and chance'.

The relationship between physical activity, exercise and sport can be conceptualised as a range of overlapping activities as illustrated in Figure 6.1.

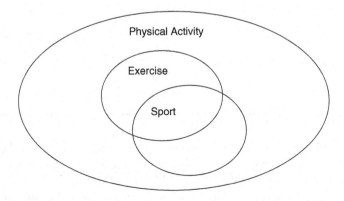

Figure 6.1 The relationship between physical activity, exercise and sport.

At the start of the twenty-first century, government strategies to increase physical activity in the population focused on encouraging more people to take up sport as a leisure-time activity: 'Sport for all' (www.olympic.org, accessed July 2009). Then the focus moved away from sport towards exercise and then away from exercise towards physical activity, active transport, and active recreation because significant uptake of sport or exercise had not been achieved. Consequently, the emphasis of public health initiatives in the twenty-first century have been on encouraging non-sporting physical activity such as walking, cycling, gardening or housework, and more recently active transport, partly in response to the climate change agenda (Department of Health, 2011; Department of Health, Physical Activity, Health Improvement and Protection, 2011; Scottish Government, 2011; Welsh Government, 2011; National Institute for Health and Clinical Excellence NICE, 2007; 2008a; 2008b; 2010; 2011). The most recent UK Chief Medical Officers' Physical Activity Guidelines (UK Chief Medical Officers, 2019) retains this focus, and in fact, partly due to the concerns about inactivity levels, the climate change agenda, and increasing demands on health service from non-communicable diseases, the emphasis continues to grow compared to previous years.

In the second edition of this book published in 2011 it was reported that after many years of policy and interventions to encourage the population to meet the 30 minutes of exercise five times a week recommended by the Department of Health (1999) only a 40% or less of the populations of England, Wales, Scotland, and Northern Ireland were meeting these criteria (Table 6.1). Scottish men were the most likely to meet the weekly target but still less than half were physically active.

Table 6.1 The percentages of men and women living in the UK achieving the government guidelines for weekly physical activity as set out in Start Active, Stay Active (Department of Health, Physical Activity, Health Improvement and Protection, 2011)

Source of data	% of people achieving government activity guidelines	% of men achieving government activity guidelines	% of women achieving government activity guidelines
Health Survey for England 2008 (Department of Health 2011)	34%	39%	29%
Health Survey for Scotland 2010 (Scottish Governmentm 2011)	39%	45%	33%
Welsh Health Survey 2010 (Welsh Government, 2011)	30%	37%	24%
Health Survey Northern Ireland 2010/11 (Department of Health, Social Services and Public Safety 2011)	38%	44%	35%

At first sight physical activity levels seem to have improved over the last decade. The WHO (2018) report that across all four nations of the UK more than 50% of adults aged between were meeting their guidelines for sufficient physical activity during 2012, 2013 & 2014 (Table 6.2). More recent surveys confirm that 61% of adults in England in

Table 6.2 Percentage of adults meeting World Health Organization physical activity recommendations of 150 minutes of moderate or vigorous physical activity per week across the four nations of the UK

Nation	% Adults meeting weekly MVPA guidelines 2012, 2013 & 2014	Age	Source	% Adults meeting weekly MVPA guidelines 2019, 2020 & 2021	Age	Sex Male Female		Source
England	67%(Male)44% (Female)	19-64 / over 65	UK PA Fact sheet 2018 (WHO)	61.4%	Over 16	63%	60%	Active Lives Adult Survey 2020–21 (Sport England 2022).
Northern Ireland	55%	Over 19	UK PA Fact sheet 2018 (WHO)	Question not asked in 2020/21 survey	NA	NA	NA	Health Survey (NI) 2020/21 Information Analysis Directorate (2021)
Scotland	63%	Over 16	UK PA Fact sheet 2018 (WHO)	66%	Over 16	71%	61%	Scottish Health Survey 2019 The Scottish Government (2020)
Wales	59%	Over 19	UK PA Fact sheet 2018 (WHO)	53%	Over 16	58%	49%	National Survey for Wales 2019/20 Welsh Government (2020).

2020/21, 66% of adults in Scotland in 2019 and 53% of adults in Wales in 2019/20 were achieving at least 150 minutes of Moderate to Vigorous Physical Activity (MVPA) a week. However, these increases should be interpreted with caution as the move from a daily recommendation to a weekly recommendation is undoubtedly influencing the outcomes. Previously, people may have been categorised as not achieving the daily guidelines but still have been accumulating 150 minutes a week. Whilst the move to a weekly total may be easier to measure and achieve it does create challenges in evaluating the population changes in response to government policy on physical activity.

Despite the increase in adults meeting the revised weekly physical activity guidelines it remains a serious concern that 34% of adults in Scotland and fewer in England, Wales and Northern Ireland are meeting the minimum levels of physical activity for health. It is likely far fewer reach the 300 minutes at the top end of the recommendations. Furthermore, evaluations of self-report measures of moderate to vigorous activity suggest that many people significantly over-estimate effort (Fukuoka et al., 2016). The impact of decades of interventions to increase physical activity are disappointing. In 2013, the WHO set a target to reduce physical inactivity to 10% by 2025 (WHO, 2013). A large-scale pooled analysis of 358 surveys of physical activity including 1.9 million people concludes that currently member states are not on track. It indicated that 27.5% of adults were not meeting the recommended guidelines. Physical activity levels fluctuate considerably between different countries with lowest levels of physical inactivity in low-income countries (16.2%). Prevalence of inactivity was much greater in high-income countries, such as the UK, where prevalence was 36.8% (Guthold et al., 2018).

The majority of adults do some walking, 71% of adults in England walk once a week (Hirst, 2020). The Department for Transport (2020) reported after increases in miles walked a year between 2015 and 2019 the annual miles walked fell in 2019 to 205 miles. Cycling miles also dropped in 2019 after gradually increasing since 2002. However, despite some gains in cycling distances since 2002, only 11% of people in the UK cycle and whilst walking is common for short journeys rates drop off when the journey is longer than a mile (Hirst, 2020). The UK continues to report some of the lowest levels of walking and cycling in Europe, ranking 11th (out of 28) in 2013.

It has been consistently argued that active transport could be a key factor in the achievement of healthy levels of physical activity (Department of Transport, 2020; Jones et al., 2007). In 2020 a parliamentary briefing paper once again presented the benefits of active travel for increasing population physical activity levels, improving air quality, tackling climate change, reducing congestion, and supporting the local economy (Hirst, 2020). Despite somewhat disappointing success of previous strategies all four nations have recently renewed their commitment to active travel introducing a range of interventions aimed at increasing levels of cycling and walking and these will be considered later in the chapter (Department for Infrastructure, 2022; Department for Transport, 2020; Transport Scotland, 2020; Welsh Parliament, 2022).

Physical activity is currently the only lifestyle behaviour where men are more likely to achieve government guidelines than women (Tables 6.1 and 6.2). Sport is often seen as a male dominated activity, which may contribute to this finding. The Scottish Health Survey 2010 (The Scottish Government, 2011) reported far more men engaged in team sports than women who are more likely to participate in exercise classes such as aerobics.

Applying this to Dafydd

Dafydd is similar to many people who were physically active through sport participation in his youth but has not maintained his physical activity through the life course.

As both men and women get older their activity levels decline (Sport England, 2022; Scottish Government, 2020; Welsh Government, 2020; WHO, 2018). The age-related decline in activity is more marked in men than women, but fewer women are active initially so by the time men and women are in their 60's their activity levels are similar. This supports the notion that men are achieving higher physical activity levels because they play more sport. Sporting participation decreases with age more markedly than any other physical activity (Scottish Government, 2011).

Physical activity declines in relationship to social class, as measured by the National Statistics Socio-Economic Classification (NS-SEC) with those who are long-term unemployed or have never worked (NS-SEC 6–8), the least likely to be active (Sport England, 2022; Welsh Government, 2020). What is of particular concern is that the gap between the most (NS-SEC1-2) and the least (NS0SEC 6-8) affluent groups has increased from 16.2% in 2015/16 to 18.9%. The widening gap is due to levels of physical activity declining in the least affluent from 54.8% to 52.3% (Sport England, 2022). This inequality in physical activity is mirrored in globally. Chastin (2020) reported that economic inequalities, particularly in high- and middle-income countries were contributing to physical inactivity. In the UK only Sport England (2022) reported on physical activity in different ethnic minority groups. Compared to the whole population, Chinese, Black and Asian adults were less likely to participate in physical activity of any kind. Asian adults were the most inactive with only 50% meeting the 150 minutes a week MVPA guidelines (Sport England, 2022). Activity levels in Chinese, Black and Asian adults dropped during the COVID pandemic but unlike the population as a whole their physical activity has not increased to pre-pandemic levels and so the gap in physical activity between these groups and the whole population has widened from 14% pre-pandemic to 18% in 2020/21 (Sport England, 2022).

Government recommendations for physical activity

In the 1999 Department of Health document 'Saving Lives: Our Healthier Nation', the government recommended that adults took:

30 minutes of moderate exercise 5 times a week.

Department of Health (1999)

In 2019 the Chief Medical Officers of England, Wales, Scotland, and Northern Ireland launched their latest UK-wide physical activity guidelines. (UK Chief Medical Officers, 2019). Whilst remaining broadly the same in terms of amount of activity it is now a weekly guideline instead of a daily guideline (Table 6.3).

Table 6.3 The UK physical activity recommendations for adults (UK Chief Medical Officers 2019)

Physical activity guidelines for adults
Adults (19–64 years)
1 For good physical and mental health, adults should aim to be physically active every day. Any activity is better than none, more is better still.
2 Adults should do activities to develop or maintain strength in the major muscle groups. These could include heavy gardening, carrying heavy shopping, or resistance exercise. Muscle strengthening activities should be done on at least 2 days a week, but any strengthening activity is better than none.
3 Each week, adults should accumulate at least 150 minutes (2 ½ hours) of moderate intensity activity (such as brisk walking or cycling); or 75 minutes of vigorous intensity activity (such as running); or even shorter durations of very vigorous intensity activity (such as printing or stair climbing); or a combination of moderate, vigorous and very vigorous intensity activity.
4 Adults should aim to minimise the amount of time spent being sedentary, and when physically possible should break up long periods of inactivity with at least light physical activity.

Older Adults (65+ years)
1 Older adults should participate in daily physical activity to gain health benefits, including maintenance of good physical and mental health, wellbeing, and social functioning. Some physical activity is better than none: even light activity brings some health benefits compared to being sedentary, while more daily physical activity provides greater health and social benefits.
2 Older adults should maintain or improve their physical function by undertaking activities aimed at improving or maintaining muscle strength, balance and flexibility on at least 2 days a week. These could be combined with sessions involving moderate aerobic activity or could be additional sessions aimed specifically at these components of fitness.
3 Each week older adults should aim to accumulate 150 minutes (2 ½ hours) of moderate intensity aerobic activity, building up gradually from current levels. Those who are already regularly active can achieve these benefits through 75 minutes of vigorous intensity activity, or a combination of moderate and vigorous activity, to achieve greater benefits. Weight-bearing activities which create an impact through the body help to maintain bone health.
4 Older adults should break up prolonged periods of being sedentary with light activity when physically possible, or at least with standing, as this has distinct health benefits for older people.

The UK guidelines are fully aligned with the WHO (2020) physical activity guidelines for adults (Figure 6.2). The new guidelines increase the emphasis on strengthening activities to delay age-related declines in bone density and muscle mass. The value of high-intensity interval exercise (HIIT) is mentioned for the first time (Table 6.3).

The importance of sedentary time in relationship to health was acknowledged by the Department of Health in 2010 and continues to be emphasised in the 2019 UK guidelines. Over the last decade the evidence of negative health impacts from long periods of inactivity has increased and is demonstrably independent of levels of moderate-to-vigorous physical activity (MVPA). Prolonged sitting is harmful even in people who achieve physical activity guidelines (WHO, 2020). The WHO (2020) has also recognised the independent impact of sedentary behaviours on health and their latest guidelines are for both physical activity and sedentary behaviour. They describe Sedentary Behaviours as:

Any waking behaviour characterized by an energy expenditure of 1.5 METS or lower while sitting, reclining, or lying. Most desk-based office work, driving a car and watching television are examples of sedentary behaviours; these can also apply to those unable to stand, such as wheelchair users

WHO (2020)

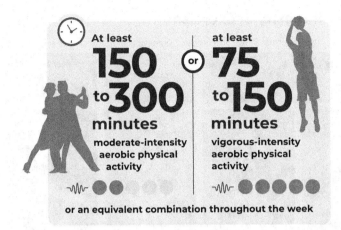

Figure 6.2 The WHO (2020) physical activity guidelines for adults aged 18 to 24.

Encouraging activities such as gardening, walking, and cycling, even if they are not meeting the criteria for moderate physical activity still have the potential to reduce time spent sedentary and so improve health outcomes. Despite the accumulating evidence of the dangers of long periods of sedentary time neither the WHO (2020) nor the UK chief medical officers felt able to provide evidence-based guidance on minimum sedentary time (UK Chief Medical Officers, 2019; WHO, 2020). Private companies have been less reticent in offering advice. Apple Watch reminds wearers to move hourly (Toppa, 2015).

An important issue in all these recommendations is the use of the words 'light, moderate and vigorous'. What is perceived as moderate by one person may be considered vigorous or light for the next. The 2019 guidelines provide some useful guidance about what constitutes sedentary, light, moderate, vigorous and very vigorous activity (Figure 6.3).

The 2019 guidelines (UK Chief Medical Officers, 2019; WHO, 2020) recommends higher levels of physical activity for children than adults (Figures 6.4 and 6.5).

Applying this to Dafydd

It is important when communicating with Dafydd about his plans to increase his physical activity that what is meant by light, moderate and vigorous is clearly explained and agreed by both parties.

All policy documents acknowledge that the appropriate level of physical activity for good health is not definitive. For weight loss and prevention of weight regain after weight loss there is evidence that higher levels of physical activity are required (UK Chief Medical Officers, 2019; WHO, 2020; Saris et al., 2003). Furthermore, there is clear evidence, particularly for coronary heart disease and type 2 diabetes that greater participation brings greater benefits (McKinney, 2016). In the past there have been strong calls in the UK for the advice to change from 'moderate' to 'vigorous', perhaps in recognition that a practitioner understanding of the term 'moderate' may be more

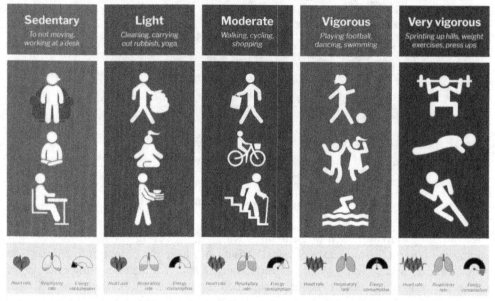

Figure 6.3 UK Chief Medical Officers Exercise Intensity Guidelines.

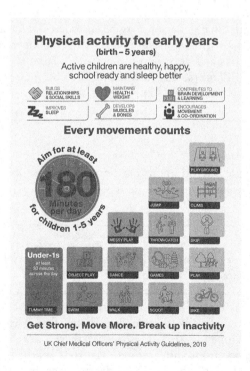

Figure 6.4 Physical activity for early years (birth–5 years).

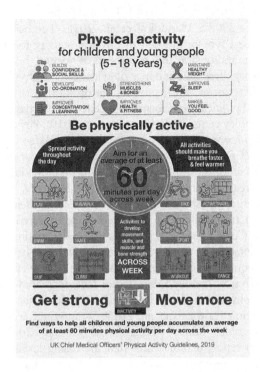

Figure 6.5 Physical activity for children and young people (5–18 years).

demanding than a lay understanding of it (BBC News, 2007). The counterargument is that even small increases in physical activity can improve health (Wen et al., 2011) and setting more challenging targets may deter sedentary individuals from attempting to take up physical activity. As discussed in later in the chapter, and in Chapter 4, setting achievable goals is a cornerstone of effective behavioural change (Ajzen, 1998). From a public health perspective the greatest benefits are perceived to be achieved from moving the sedentary to light or moderate activity levels (Department of Health, 2009; McKinney, 2016; UK Chief Medical Officers, 2019; WHO, 2020).

Applying this to Dafydd

Any increases in physical activity that Dafydd can make are likely to bring some health benefits regardless of whether he reaches the government recommended 150 minutes per week.

Mental health

The 2011 physical activity guidelines were aimed at improving physical health with an acknowledgement of the additional benefits to mental health. In 2019 physical activity is positioned as valuable for physical and mental health but also for building strong communities and supporting the economy. The value of physical activity for psychological well-being is firmly established both to help maintain general well-being and to treat mental health problems (Crone et al., 2009; NICE, 2008c; Mandolesi et al., 2018; Teychenne, 2020). It is still not established what is the best type or amount of physical activity for an improvement or maintenance of well-being and/or for the treatment of mental health conditions. However, despite this lack of clarity there is abundance of evidence that physical activity is beneficial for a number of holistic reasons. For example, the promotion of the concept of 'physical literacy' has gained global political prominence in recent years across the public health, sport and education sectors (Dudley et al., 2017; Cairney et al., 2019). Physical literacy is defined as *'the motivation, confidence, physical competence, knowledge and understanding to value and take responsibility for engagement in physical activities for life'* (Whitehead, 2013; Edwards et al., 2017). It is a holistic approach considering an individual's physical, psychological, social, and cognitive reasons for engaging with physical activity. The premise of physical literacy is that person-centred positive experiences will lead to lifelong engagement with physical activity, which in turn will allow for a multitude of physical, psychological, social, and cognitive benefits. Current evidence suggests that participating in even low levels of physical activity may be effective in improving psychological well-being, irrespective of the levels recommended and required to improve physical health (Crone et al., 2009; Teychenne et al., 2020). Successful physical literacy programmes have increased the competence, motivation, confidence, and physical activity levels of individuals in the community (Morgan et al., 2022), in education (Edwards et al., 2019; Wainwright et al., 2018) and in health-based settings with older adults (Roetert and Ortega, 2019). Furthermore, a recent Sport England (2022) report demonstrates that increasing levels of physical activity are associated with increasing feelings of happiness and life satisfaction, suggesting more physical activity can lead to greater improvements in wellbeing (Sport England, 2022). In 2020 Teychenne et al. reviewed the literature to see if physical activity guidelines for mental health were needed. They concluded that although the benefits of physical activity for mental health are clear even at low doses the impact is domain specific. They propose that if individuals are encouraged to participate in small amounts of enjoyable physical activity the likelihood of achieving mental health benefits would increase.

Applying this to Dafydd

Dafydd is sedentary and looking to reduce his stress and depression. He is not currently obese. Setting him a goal of moderate physical activity that he will enjoy should deliver the mental health benefits that he requires and may offer additional protective benefits against further weight gain. Setting too hard a target or exercise he doesn't like may be unrealistic and potentially detrimental to his self-efficacy. Consideration for Dafydd's physical, psychological, social, and cognitive reasons for engaging in physical activity is crucial for his lifelong engagement,

---

Health consequences of low levels of physical activity

If you are physically active you are likely to live longer than your sedentary colleagues regardless of whether you are young or old, male, or female and regardless of ethnicity or social class (US Department of Health and Human Services, 2008; Department of Health, 2009; Department of Health, Physical Activity, Health Improvement and Protection, 2011; Wen et al. 2011; Zhao et al. 2020; WHO, 2022). Indeed, it has been suggested that adults who keep physically fit through activity are 50% less likely to die prematurely than sedentary adults (Warburton et al., 2006). Others are more conservative in their estimates of benefits. The WHO (2022) suggest that physical activity is the 4th leading risk factor for mortality and people who are insufficiently active have a 20% to 30% increased risk of all-cause mortality compared to those meeting recommended guidelines.

Physical activity influences a wide range of health conditions. For example, people who are physically active can achieve up to a 40% reduced risk of developing coronary heart disease, stroke, diabetes, and some cancers (Department of Health, Physical activity, Health Improvement and Health Protection, 2011; Booth, 2012). Physical activity can also play a role in reducing mental health problems such as depression, stress, and anxiety (Crone et al., 2009; NICE, 2008c, 2009; Mandolesi, 2018; Teychenne, 2020). Newly diagnosed individuals with such chronic diseases face not only a reduction in life expectancy but also a potential reduction in quality of life for the remainder of their lives. Whilst the relationship of physical activity to each disease is valuable, what makes physical activity particularly important is that it can prevent so many different diseases. Physical activity has an important role in treatment, but it is its potential to prevent or delay disease onset that is so impressive.

Applying this to Dafydd

Dafydd has a number of health and lifestyle concerns including stress, depression, physical inactivity, sedentary lifestyle, and weight gain. One benefit of utilising physical activity as an intervention is that he can tackle all of his current concerns simultaneously, whereas the medical option involves two different types of medication, and only address his stress and depression. Furthermore, stress and depression, if untreated, are both related to weight gain, cardiovascular problems and ultimately reduced mortality. Consequently, being more physical activity to help manage and relieve stress and depression will also serve a preventative function for Dafydd, reducing his risk of obesity, cardiovascular disease, Type 2 diabetes and increase his mortality.

Weight maintenance

Levels of obesity are rising throughout the Western world and the UK has one of the highest prevalence of overweight and obesity in Europe (Cancer Intelligence Team, 2022). In 2011 the Department of Health in England described overweight and obesity as:

'Probably the most widespread threat to health and wellbeing in this country'
(Department of Health, 2011, p. 5)

Across all four home countries there was a threefold increase in obesity from 1980 to 2011 (Department of Health, 2011; Department of Health, Physical Activity, Health Improvement and Protection, 2011; Scottish Government, 2011; Welsh Government, 2011a; Department of Health, Social Services and Public Safety, 2011).

Since 2011, a decade of weight management interventions have reduced the rate of increase but the proportion of people who are overweight or obese still increased slightly and in 2019 68% of men and 60% of women in the UK were overweight or obese. The significant risk to health and wellbeing to nearly two-thirds of the UK population from being overweight or obese remains (Cancer Intelligence Team, 2022). The Cancer Intelligence Team (2022) have concluded that if current overweight and obesity prevalence trends continue average adult overweight and obesity will increase to 71% by 2040, that equates to 42.2 million people (20.6 million overweight and 21.6 million obese).

Obesity is often associated with physical inactivity leading the Department of Health in 2004 to conclude that:

Obesity is the main visible sign of inactivity.

Department of Health (2004, pg. 20)

However, it is important to recognise that it is possible to be obese and still achieve high levels of physical activity that will have benefits for health regardless of whether recommended body weight is maintained.

Maintaining a healthy body weight should be straightforward. At its simplest, energy input simply has to equal energy output and weight will remain constant. If your energy intake exceeds your energy output, you will gain weight. Physical activity increases energy output and so decreases the likelihood that an individual will gain weight. However, moderate physical activity is unlikely to make a major contribution to weight loss. Physical activity, at the level suggested by the government, by itself can result in modest weight loss of between 1% and 3% (Pate et al., 2010). Higher levels of physical activity can have more dramatic effects on body weight but suggesting that obese individuals take even higher levels of physical activity than those recommended by the government is potentially dangerous and probably too challenging for currently sedentary individuals to achieve. Nevertheless, many health professionals and academics have called for new guidelines for weight-loss physical activity to be established. However, the UK Chief Medical Officers' Physical Activity Guidelines (2019) do not make separate activity recommendations for the overweight and simply comment that in combination with dietary change, physical activity can support weight loss. Previously, the Chief Medical Officer for England did make additional recommendations in his 2004 report, saying:

45–60 minutes of moderate activity per day may be needed to prevent the development of obesity ... and people who have been obese and have managed to lose weight may need to do as much as 60–90 minutes activity a day in order to avoid regaining weight.

Department of Health (2004, p. 5)

The decision not to recommending increasing exercise to prevent weight re-gain concurs with recent evidence by Chin et al. (2016) who concluded that although diet +

exercise interventions were more effective than diet only interventions for inducing weight loss the evidence to support the value of exercise for maintaining lost weight is sparse.

Applying this to Dafydd

If Dafydd were to achieve an increase in his physical activity levels on its own it is unlikely to result in weight loss but were he to add some changes to his diet, through eating more healthily and reducing his portion size, he may see a reduction in his weight.

Assessment of physical activity

It is beyond the scope of this text to provide a comprehensive review of all the available tools to measure physical activity—over 30 different measures have been reported—but there are a number of good textbooks where this can be obtained (e.g., Stensel et al., 2021; Thompson et al., 2009). To report the physical activity levels of different groups in the population you will need a measure that is quick and easy to administer to a large number of people. To measure physical activity as part of an individualised fitness programme, you might want a very detailed and accurate measure.

When you are thinking about measuring physical activity you need to consider whether you simply want to know the total time spent physically active in a given period or whether you wish to explore the physical activity in more depth. You may wish to know the time spent at different intensities of physical activity. You may wish to understand the impact that the physical activity is having on the physical state of an individual. You may wish to know the amount of energy a person is using, which might be particularly useful if you are interested in weight control or weight loss. You can measure levels of physical activity in one of four ways, described in Table 6.4.

The first three methods are objective assessments of activity whereas observation is a more subjective assessment (Table 6.4). Objective measures of energy expenditure are

Table 6.4 Categories of physical activity measurement

Method of measurement	Assessment	Information available
Measuring a physiological response to physical activity	Objective	Duration Intensity
Calculating the energy expenditure of physical activity	Objective	Duration Intensity
Assessing physiological adaptations to physical activity	Objective	Duration Intensity
Observing (either directly or indirectly) physical activity	Subjective	Duration Intensity Type Frequency

Measures of physical activity can provide information about how often people exercise (frequency), how long they exercise (duration), how hard they work (intensity) and what type of activity (type) they choose to do (Table 6.5).

more precise, giving reliable information about the duration and intensity of activity, but they can be costly and often not practical for large-scale studies. Furthermore, objective measures cannot tell you much about the type of activity undertaken. The most usual form of observation is to use a questionnaire. The more complex questionnaires can provide detailed information about the type of activities undertaken and good information about duration and frequency but only imprecise information about the intensity of the activity (Table 6.4).

If you are going to use a questionnaire-based assessment of physical activity it is very important to use an established questionnaire that has been tested for reliability and validity. The best questionnaires will have been validated by an objective measure of physiological response to physical activity (such as heart-rate monitoring) or an objective measure of energy expenditure, such as doubly labelled water (Shepard, 2003). Shepard (2003) draws attention to the limited reliability and validity of physical activity questionnaires in general and advises that questionnaires can only be use for simple classification of activity levels and not to estimate individual overall energy expenditure.

Why are people physically inactive?

The government guidelines for physical activity are not daunting and indeed many health professionals would like them to be more challenging, yet more between 34% and 47% of the population of the UK remain largely sedentary (UK Chief Medical Officers, 2019). The reasons why are undoubtedly complex and not simply down to individual choices. In physical activity the role of the physical environment is recognised as pivotal to the choices individuals have (Hirst, 2020; Jones et al., 2007; Department for Transport, 2020; WHO, 2018). Environmental, social, demographic, psychological and biological factors have all been implicated in physical activity and the relationship between these factors has been usefully conceptualised by Jones *et al.* in 2007 as shown in Figure 6.6. The WHO (2018) have tasked all nations with taking a 'systems-based' approach that strategically links policies for social, cultural, economic and environment developments to support physical activity that with local, community and individualised interventions (WHO, 2018).

Obesogenic environments

Health promotion and education are often focused on the individual and persuading the individual to change, but the unsupportive nature of the modern environment is recognised to play a role in the low levels of physical activity in Western societies (NICE, 2008a; Department for Transport, 2020; Department of Health, Physical Activity, Health Improvement and Protection, 2011; Jones et al., 2007; WHO, 2018). The term obesogenic has been adopted by policy makers and refers to an environment that is both supportive of high-calorie intake and unsupportive of physical activity (Foster et al., 2006; Jones et al., 2007; Townsend & Lake, 2017).

So what is an obesogenic environment? It has not been clearly characterised, but certainly includes cultural, social, economic, and physical characteristics. A robust evidence-base evaluating the impact of the environment on physical activity is starting to accrue. A 2006 review of interventions that used the environment to encourage physical activity included 25 studies, 19 of which were studies aimed at encouraging the use of stairs (Foster et al., 2006). Whilst encouraging the use of stairs is undoubtedly a

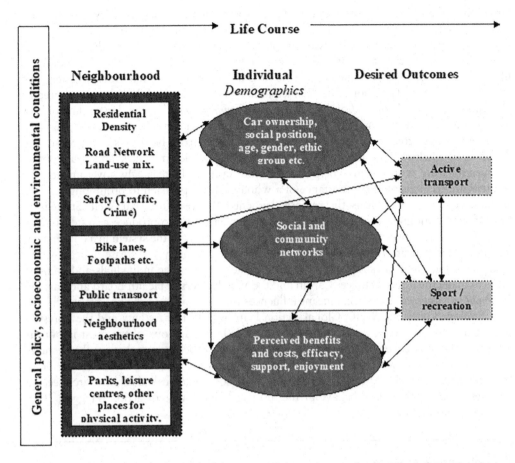

Figure 6.6 Evidence-informed model of the potential determinants of sport/physical acitivity: Source Adapted from Tackling obesities: future choices – obesogenic environments – evidence review, Government Office for Science (Jones, A., Bentham, G. Foster, C., Hillsdon, M. and Panter, J. (2007) Reproduced under the terms of the Click-Use Licence.

worthwhile venture, it is unlikely to increase the physical activity of any single individual by more than 10 minutes a day. The initial focus on encouraging stair use, often by decisional prompts, may reflect the difficulties with both instigating and evaluating more major changes to the environment. For instance, changing the environment to facilitate walking or cycling to work might require the building of cycle paths and the provision of showers, lockers, and bicycle sheds. Such major changes to the built environment have not been well evaluated in the past but more recent developments are beginning to be instigated and evaluated (Celis-Morales et al., 2017; Department of Health, Physical Activity, Health Improvement and protection, 2011; Sloman et al., 2010; Townsend & Lake, 2017; Department of Transport, 2020).

In 2007 Jones et al. concluded that the influence of the environment on overall physical activity is limited and the mechanisms for effect unclear. However, what is clear is the actual environment is less important than the way people perceive it (Maddison et al., 2009). Jones et al. (2007) raised concerns that improving the environment by building more cycle paths, safe places to walk etc. may have its main effects on those who are already active rather than the sedentary. They argued that it doesn't matter how many cycle paths you build if people do not see themselves as able to use them. Initially, many cycle paths were simply marked sections on roads with no physical barrier from cars. The development of protected cycle tracks does appear to encourage new cyclists. Cycling on London's Blackfriars Bridge rose by 55% in the 6 months after a protected bike track was installed (The Department of Transport, 2020). Since Jones et al. (2007) published the seminal report *'Tackling Obesities: Future Choices – Obesogenic Environments'* our understanding of how to promote active transport has improved considerably. Many cities are developing safe, continuous direct routes for cycling physically separated from both cars and pedestrians. Better cycle shelters, tax incentives to purchase bikes, electric bikes and many other interventions are working in synergy to promote cycling. Increasingly governments and councils are recognising the importance of a whole system approach to promoting physical activity. A recent example is the recently launched 'Move More, Eat Well' Strategy in Cardiff where multiple organisations have come together to co-produce a systems-based strategy and action plan to work collaboratively with all parts of the system in a community, including at the heart the people who live in that community, to create a healthy and sustainable food and physical activity environment, to encourage individuals and communities to make the healthy choice (Cardiff and the Vale University Health Board and partners 2020–2023, accessed 2023). Significant influences on this plan, and the process in which it was developed were the WHO Global Action Plan for Physical Activity and the Foresight Report on Obesity (Jones et al., 2007; WHO, 2018). Perhaps one of the most important aspects of the physical environment is its ability to 'trigger' behaviours that are then enacted with little conscious awareness in response to a specific set of conditions or contextual cues (Hagger, 2019). Environmental restructuring also sometimes called 'choice architecture' involves making the desired behaviour the most effective course of action (Hagger, 2019; Landais et al., 2020).

Applying this to Dafydd

Dafydd uses his car to commute to work and to transport his children to extra curricula activities. In this way the obesogenic environment that makes car use the easiest method of transport is negatively impacting on his lifestyle. Environmental and work-place initiatives to encourage cycling to work could enable Dafydd to achieve the recommended levels of physical activity. Cardiff have built a segregated cycle path along Dafydd's route to work that passes by his children's school along the way. The school is encouraging children to cycle and have put in a covered cycle rack. The children are very keen to cycle to school and so Dafydd can see a way he can incorporate more physical activity into his working day.

Psychological factors

Many different individual factors have been postulated to underpin physical activity behaviours; some of the key factors are presented in Table 6.5. The basic tenet of most traditional health promotion campaigns is to present either the risk of an unhealthy behaviour and/or the benefits of a healthy behaviour. Traditionally health promotion has assumed that individuals will weigh up the costs and benefits of physical activity and make a decision about whether to take up physical activity. However, understanding that lack of physical activity is bad for your health has not been found to predict physical activity (Harrison et al., 2002).

Table 6.5 Psychosocial factors implicated in behavioural change

Psychosocial factor	*Potential to increase physical activity*
Perception of the risk of physical inactivity	Minimal
Belief in the effectiveness of physical activity to improve health	Minimal
Objective barriers to physical activity	Minimal
Perceived behavioural control – perceived ability to overcome recognised barriers	Good
Social norms	Minimal as currently measured, but may be more useful if measured as perceived peer levels of activity
Self-efficacy	Good
Self-regulation	Good
Social support	Good

It would appear that perceptions and beliefs about the health risks and benefits of physical activity play only a small part in explaining variations in physical activity behaviours. Some authors have argued that they may be necessary but are not sufficient to promote physical activity change (Zeidi et al., 2021). However, studies such as Blue (2007) and Liu et al. (2022), which found no relationship between risk perception and activity levels, raise the question as to whether a perception of risk is necessary at all. It would seem that investing time or money in informing people about the costs of being sedentary and the benefits of being physically active is unlikely to generate widespread increases in physical activity.

Barriers to performing physical activity, such as lack of access to resources or lack of time, have some relationship to whether people are active but perceived behavioural control over such barriers has been found to be a better predictor of physical activity than the actual barriers themselves (Ayotte et al., 2010; Zeidi et al., 2021). Individuals often cite a list of barriers to physical activity as an explanation for remaining sedentary. Working with them to look at how they can overcome these barriers and increase confidence in their own ability to control these external factors is more likely to generate change than changing the barriers. If barriers are removed, perhaps by improving leisure facilities in the local area, such strategies are more likely to be utilised if their implementation is supported by psychological support for uptake of the new behaviour.

Applying this to Dafydd

Time in the day was a significant barrier for Dafydd being physically active but the new segregated cycle path helps him overcomes that barrier because he can cycle to school with the children now he is confident they will be safe. Cycling to school and on to work fits into his working day.

Social norms refer to what is both acceptable and practiced behaviour in the majority of an individual's peer group. Measures of social norms for physical activity have consistently failed to predicted significant variation in physical activity, but usually measure perceptions of what significant others think is acceptable behaviour (injunctive social norms) rather than perceptions of peer behaviour itself (Priebe & Spink, 2011). This has led some authors to argue that social influences on intentions to exercise and exercise behaviour are less important than individual factors. However, Priebe and Spink (2011) reported that descriptive norms were highly correlated with individual physical activity. Currently an accurate perception of peer physical activity for most groups in the population will be one of low levels of physical activity. Jones et al. (2007, p. 38), in their extensive review of obesogenic environments for the influential Foresight project remain convinced that *'capturing the concept of social norm and modifying that norm is one of the major public health challenges'*.

There is considerable evidence to suggest that social support plays an important role in adherence to physical activity (Kouvonen et al., 2012; Mama et al., 2015; Xiao et al., 2019). The Whitehall II Study, which followed over 5000 working people from a baseline assessment between 1997 and 1999 to a follow-up assessment between 2002 and 2004, found that high emotional and practical social support could help individuals remain physically active. High levels of practical social support also supported positive changes in physical activity (Kouvonen et al., 2012). The Whitehall II study is important because it is one of the few longitudinal studies reporting factors that can make a positive and sustained impact on levels physical activity. A systematic review of reviews by Greaves et al. (2011) evaluating factors associated with increased effectiveness of physical activity interventions also found that social support was a consistent factor in successful physical activity interventions. This was confirmed in a subsequent systematic review of psychosocial factors in physical activity in minorities (Mama et al., 2015). The evidence for social support being a key factor in both increasing and maintaining physical activity levels is robust. Greaves et al. (2011) recommend, based on their review, that future interventions should encourage participants to engage others who are important to them (such as family, friends and colleagues) in planned changes in physical activity.

Applying this to Dafydd

Dafydd has a clear idea of what the benefits of activity would be for him. Currently, he perceives that he lacks social support for taking up exercise and he sees the lack of support from his partner and his long working day as barriers to undertaking physical activity. Seeking social support from his partner, his children and also from his workplace for his planned changes to his physical activity may increase Dafydd's likelihood of making a change and sustaining it.

Probably, the most important psychological factor to emerge from research into physical activity behaviour is the concept of self-efficacy (Maddison et al., 2009; Ashford et al., 2010; Ayotte et al., 2010; Zeidi et al., 2021). Self-efficacy refers to internal aspects of control such as perceived ability and self-confidence for specific activities. Ayotte et al. (2010) found that both middle-aged and young-old individuals who reported higher levels of exercise self-efficacy were more likely to be physically active Self-efficacy predicts both the adoption and maintenance of physical activity (Ashford et al., 2010). Self-efficacy has been argued to be enhanced by personal accomplishment or mastery, vicarious experience, or verbal persuasion. According to Ayotte et al. (2010) people with high self-efficacy are more likely to utilise self-regulatory strategies, which in turn exert a large total effect on physical activity. Self-regulatory strategies include goal setting, self-monitoring, planning and problem solving. The impact of self-regulatory strategies on self-efficacy are likely to be through the positive feedback achieved from setting and achieving goals, highlighting the importance of setting short-term, challenging but achievable targets. The value of effective self-regulatory techniques have been established by Greaves et al. (2011) in their review of reviews of effective physical activity interventions which concluded that using self-regulatory techniques was associated with increased intervention effectiveness. Strobach et al. (2020) argue that there are inter-individual differences in the ability to self-regulate with people with higher levels of trait self-regulation demonstrating higher levels of physical activity.

Self-efficacy is not unrealistic optimism as it is based on experience, so in consequence realistic goals and plans that an individual can achieve are essential to increase self-efficacy (Ashford et al., 2010; Zeidi et al., 2021).

Applying this to Dafydd

Dafydd has low self-efficacy about his ability to increase his physical activity. Helping him increase his self-efficacy through self-regulatory techniques such as specific goal setting, prompting self-monitoring and providing feedback on performance will increase his chances of achieving his goals.

Stages of change

A key concept that has emerged from process models of change such as the Transtheoretical Model (TTM) is the idea that changing lifestyle behaviours is not a one-off decision, but a continuous process and that people move between different motivational states (see Chapter 4). Identifying where individuals are in terms of stages of change may well result in more effective interventions to support the uptake of physical activity (Table 6.6).

Different types of psychological support are more likely to be effective at different stages. When individuals are in the pre-contemplation stage, they may need education and motivational interventions to encourage them to move into the contemplation stage. Individuals who are contemplating or preparing to change may need to be helped to build self-efficacy for the proposed change. Individuals who are in the action or maintenance stage will need support to stay motivated, again through increases in self-efficacy and in self-regulation. They need to ensure that their new physical activity behaviour becomes a habitual behaviour that they can maintain without constant cognitive effort (Verplanken & Melkevik, 2008; Strobach et al., 2020).

Table 6.6 The stages of change in relation to achieving the government recommendations for physical activity

Stages of change	Behavioural and motivational characteristics
Pre-contemplation	Individuals are sedentary and have no intention of doing 30 minutes of physical activity five times a week in the next 6 months
Contemplation	Individuals are sedentary but intend to take up physical activity to the level of the government recommendations within 6 months
Preparation	Individuals are taking some physical activity and intend to achieve acceptable levels of activity within 6 months
Action	Individuals have taken up physical activity and are exercising for at least 30 minutes five times each week. This is the least stable stage and relapse is likely
Maintenance	Individuals have been regular exercisers for 6 months or more and are unlikely to relapse

Habitual behaviour

Past physical activity is an important predictor of future physical activity (Hirvensalo & Lintunen, 2011; Verplanken & Melkevik, 2008) which suggests that developing physical activity habits are key to promoting long-term positive changes in physical activity. The relationship between past behaviour and future behaviour (Verplanken & Melkevik, 2008) adds support to the argument that being physically active is an ongoing process. Consistent patterns of behaviours are often referred to as habits. However more contemporary theorists define habits as behaviours that are carried out with little conscious awareness or reflection in response to a specific set of associated conditions or contextual cues (Hagger, 2019; Gardner, 2015). Physical activity is usually a complex set of behaviours which has led some commentators to question whether theories of habit formation can be useful for health practitioners (Gardner, 2015). However, distinguishing between initiation and performance helps to understand how habitual physical activity behaviours can be promoted (Gardner, 2015). For example, a person who 'habitually' cycles to work may automatically get on their bike to go to work but negotiating the journey may require conscious cognitive thought. Gardner (2015) has argued there are three possible types of habitual behaviour: those that are habitually initiated but consciously performed (e.g., bicycle commuting), those that are consciously initiated but habitually performed (e.g., exercising in the gym) or habitually initiated and habitually performed (e.g., taking the stairs at work).

The reasons why people take up physical activity may be different from the reasons why people maintain the behaviour. Starting something new is a conscious choice but maintaining the behaviour may be habitual. So, what supports the development of a habit? As discussed previously the physical environment can support the formation of habitual behaviour and most active transport strategies are focused on 'choice architecture' or 'nudging' in order to support people to cycle or walk rather than drive (Landais et al., 2020). Once individuals have made the conscious choice to cycle or walk, well-lit pavements, separate cycle paths and other factors can be instigated to support the on-going behaviour.

Aarts et al. (1997) suggested that enjoyment is an essential aspect of habit formation. Strobach et al. (2020) have suggested that more complex vigorous physical activity behaviours such as playing team sports are more likely to remain explicitly regulated while less complex light-to-moderate activities such as active transport might be more likely to become habitual. Traditional approaches to health behaviours have been negatively focused, looking predominantly at why people don't exercise. Consequently, enjoyment as a moderator of physical activity choices is seldom investigated. Nevertheless, studies that do consider enjoyment report that individuals who are regular long-term exercisers report positive emotions during and following physical activity (Hagberg et al., 2009; Schneider & Cooper, 2011).

Interventions to increase physical activity

Interventions to increase physical activity have been many and varied in many different settings with many different sections of society (Greaves et al., 2011; Department of Health, Physical Activity, Health Improvement and Protection, 2011; Department of Health and Social Care, Llwodraeth Cymru Welsh Government, Department of Health Northern Ireland and The Scottish Government 2020). It is increasingly acknowledged that to make a significant impact on physical activity levels, interventions will need to both at the level of the community and individual (Department of Health, Physical Activity, Health Improvement and Protection, 2011; Department of Health, 2009; UK Chief Medical Officers, 2019).

Individual-level interventions

Individualised interventions for the purposes of this text refer to interventions to increase physical activity that are aimed at individuals or at a small group of individuals. Interventions such as these can be delivered in primary care and are frequently provided by public and commercial leisure centres and gyms. Walking and cycling groups are run by most councils and there are a plethora of independent groups that organise group level physical activities. Recently there has been a rapid growth in personal trainers who offer support for physical activity to both individuals and small groups. Individualised interventions are usually either information, or behavioural or frequently a combination of both. Unfortunately, in terms of evaluation, research often only evaluate short-term interventions of between 8 and 12 weeks which frequently demonstrate changes in physical activity behaviours immediately after the intervention which are not sustained in the long term (Pavey et al., 2011). Behavioural change requires long-term support if it is to be sustained (Hardcastle & Hagger, 2011; Hagger, 2019). Strategies for providing long-term support for physical activity are required if we are going to achieve any longer-term population changes in physical activity levels. Referring people into short-term exercise programmes that then cease is not an effective strategy as individuals then need to locate and integrate into another activity group, which they may or may not have the psychological, practical or financial resources to achieve.

It should be noted that many individualised interventions are part of wider-scale community initiatives to increase physical activity. So for example the exercise referral scheme is a UK-wide intervention to increase physical activity, but it is delivered through individualized programmes (Pavey et al., 2011). Many pedometer studies are highly individualized in that individuals get given a pedometer, advice, and any follow-up feedback on a one-to one basis but are frequently part of a wide-scale scheme to encourage walking within an organisation or community (Naylor & McKay, 2009).

Exercise or physical activity referral schemes

Exercise referral schemes have been prevalent across the UK, since the early 1990s, with an estimated 600 schemes currently running (Rowley, 2019). These schemes have the opportunity to provide many of the psychological support strategies described earlier, such as social support and goal setting which are known to promote physical activity. A 2010 randomized controlled trial (RCT) of the Welsh National Exercise Referral Scheme (NERS) found that all participants in the scheme had higher levels of physical activity than those in the control group, with this difference being significant for those patients referred for coronary heart disease risk factors. They also reported positive effects on depression and anxiety, particularly in those referred for mental health reasons. A particularly interesting aspect of this trial was it included an economic evaluation which concluded for those who adhere to the full programme the scheme is likely to be marginally cost saving (Murphy et al., 2010). In 2011 a systematic review with meta-analysis of exercise referral schemes was published in the British Medical Journal (Pavey et al., 2011) which concurred with the findings from the Murphy et al. (2010) RCT trial. The review found some evidence of a short-term increase in physical activity and a reduction in levels of depression in sedentary individuals who participated in the scheme compared with usual care but no evidence of sustained increases in physical activity. Pavey et al. (2011) concluded that there was support for the potential role of exercise referral schemes to increase physical activity and consequently improve public health but that one of the major limitations of the referral scheme is its focus on short-term interventions (typically 10 to 16 weeks) and the predominance of referrals into gym-based programmes. This is an issue of resourcing with many exercise referral schemes lobbying for funds for longer term support schemes (Personal Communication. Wyatt-Williams, 2013). Exercise referral schemes are also expanding their repertoires of activities with 'green' exercise opportunities now available and also links with walking schemes that are permanent programmes (Rowley, 2019). Social prescribing is a new framework for health referral programmes and is developing in its both popularity and availability across the UK (Griffiths et al., 2022). Social prescribing programmes provide a more holistic option for health referral programmes in primary care. Social prescribing is still in its infancy and its prevalence and connectedness to existing exercise referral schemes within the UK remains patchy. As mentioned earlier referring individuals into short-term programmes with no transition into long-term programmes is not effective. Participants need long-term support to sustain changes in physical activity and Social Prescribing has the potential to provide this.

Pedometers

One thing that has emerged from work on goal setting and physical activity is that positive feedback about the successful achievement of goals is key to continued success (Nigg et al., 2008; Watkinson et al., 2010). Regular professional feedback requires significant input from a health professional, so the possibility of feedback through self-monitoring using a relatively cheap monitoring system such as a pedometer has generated a lot of interest. Pedometers have recently become commonplace and the target of 10,000 steps a day is well understood (Slack, 2006; Bennett et al., 2006). Research has demonstrated that pedometers can be used successfully as part of a goal-setting programme to increase both the number of steps taken daily (Normand, 2008;

Baker et al., 2008; Fitzsimons et al., 2012) and the pace at which individuals walk (Johnson et al., 2006). However, the problem of setting goals that are both challenging and realistic remains, and the general goal of 10,000 steps a day would appear to have been too challenging for many individuals and resulted in failure to meet the daily target, loss of self-efficacy and giving up on the walking programme. In 2012 NICE revised their guidance to recommend the use of pedometers to encourage walking but only as part of a package which included support to set realistic goals (NICE, 2012). These guidelines were reviewed in 2019 due to the publication of new research on pedometer-based walking interventions (Harris et al., 2019) (see Box 6.1) and NICE concluded that the recommendation to use pedometers only as part of a package remained valid.

BOX 6.1 Applying Research in Practice

Effect of pedometer-based walking interventions on long-term health outcomes: Prospective 4-year follow-up of two randomised controlled trials using routine primary care data (Harris et al., 2019)

This longitudinal study evaluated the long-term impact of two primary care 12-week pedometer-based walking interventions in adults and older adults (PACE and PACE-Lift) and it was designed to evaluate the impact of the 12-week programmes in the long-term. A criticism of previous research of 12-week intervention programmes is the long-term impact is seldom evaluated and physical activity needs to be long term to deliver maximum health benefits.

1001 PACE participants, aged 45–75 and 296 PACE-Lift participants, aged 60–75 were followed up from primary care data for a 4-year period. New events such as cardiovascular issues, incident diabetes, depression, fractures and other relevant events were counted.

Both interventions were associated with significant increases in moderate-to-vigorous physical activity levels and with significant decreases in both cardiovascular events (heart attacks, strokes et) and fractures at 4 years.

This study is important because it was methodologically rigorous; participants were randomised to the intervention and because it is one of the few pedometer studies to assess the impact of an acute intervention in the longer term.

Some of the limitations of the study were the low number of events and only events recorded in primary care records were counted; however, any under-recording would not have differed by intervention status and so should not have led to bias.

Informational interventions

Hillsdon et al. (2005) in their evidence briefing to the Health Development Agency reported that brief advice from a health professional supported by written materials was likely to produce modest short-term (12 weeks or less) increases in physical activity. Information given on an individual basis can be seen as directly relevant to the individual, who cannot ignore their own susceptibility as easily as they can information from media-based campaigns. However, Kinmonth et al. (2008) reported no change in physical activity behaviour in sedentary individuals with a family history of type diabetes in response to a motivational advice leaflet when assessed at 6 months and 1 year post intervention. They conclude that personal education alone is unlikely to increase physical activity in an environment when there are plentiful inducements to keep still. However, a recent scoping review also revealed that while it is unlikely to address global inactivity on its own, physical activity messaging may still play a role improving population physical activity levels. However, it is a complex and multidimensional concept and greater understanding is still needed (Williamson et al., 2020). It is to be hoped as the environment changes to support active transport and other wider system-based public health interventions embed themselves into society over the coming years that personal interventions will have more chance of success.

Behavioural and psychosocial interventions

Behavioural and psychosocial interventions include strategies such as persuasion, motivational interviewing, self-regulation and social support. In 2005 Hillsdon *et al.* concluded that interventions that taught behavioural skills and were tailored to individual needs were associated with more long-term changes than interventions without such psychological support. More recently Greaves et al. (2011) in their review of reviews concluded that intervention effectiveness was increased by using well-defined/established behavioural change techniques. Further support for the value of psychologically based behavioural change programmes comes from Ogilvie et al. (2007), who found that targeted behavioural change programmes were the most effective way to promote walking. Howlett et al. (2018) carried out a systematic review of physical activity interventions for healthy inactive adults and found that behaviour change programmes could promote a change in physical activity in this important segment of the population, currently well but 'at risk' of ill health in the future. Psychologically orientated behavioural change programmes can work through a number of different psychological mechanisms. Perhaps most importantly they can provide regular contact with a health or physical activity practitioner who, seen regularly, can provide social support. Greaves et al. (2011) found that increased contact with the intervention provider was associated with increased effectiveness. Furthermore, an exercise specialist can set appropriate goals that foster and develop self-efficacy. Good behavioural change interventions include advice and help with goal setting, overcoming obstacles and developing social support, which facilitate uptake and maintenance of physical activity by increasing self-efficacy (Greaves et al., 2011; Ayotte et al., 2010).

Motivational interviewing or brief interventions

Motivational interviewing (MI) aims to increase an individual's motivation to consider change rather than showing them how to change. If a person doesn't want to change then it is irrelevant if they know how to do it or not. However, if a person is motivated to change then the interventions aimed at changing behaviour can begin. MI can therefore be viewed as the first stage of a process that moves people towards being physically active. The key aspects of MI are presented in Chapter 4. Hardcastle and Hagger (2011) found that participants in an MI intervention to increase physical activity found regular consultations with the MI practitioner helped facilitate lifestyle change. The participants also felt that on-going monitoring and continued support was paramount in their maintenance of any physical activity changes. This requirement for on-going support resonates throughout the literature and suggests that regardless of the intervention, be it one-to-one MI or exercise referral interventions, it must be long term, perhaps not at initial intensity but nevertheless sustained (Greaves et al., 2011; Hardcastle & Hagger, 2011).

Applying this to Dafydd

Working with Dafydd in a client-centred way, using motivational interviewing techniques, is more likely to result in increased physical activity than giving him advice about the risks of inactivity and benefits of physical activity.

Goal setting

The key to successful goal setting is setting challenging but realistic goals that enable people to feel they have achieved a goal and gives them confidence that they can achieve the next sub-goal on their way to a healthy level of physical activity. Getting goals right is a tricky task and requires understanding the physical capacities of an individual, their level of skill and their self-efficacy for the various activities that may be involved. Goal setting should place a strong emphasis on the characteristics, needs, preferences and goal setting styles of individuals (Jeong et al., 2021) Consequently, it requires the skilled input of a health or exercise specialist. It is not enough to set appropriate individualised goals—individuals need to get regular feedback, which may be provided by the health professional or alternatively it may be possible for an individual to self-monitor performance and receive feedback in that way (Jeong et al., 2021). The key strategies for successful goal setting in relation to physical activity are presented in Table 6.7.

Table 6.7 Effective strategies in goal setting to increase physical activity

Strategy	*Example*
Explore client motivation. This might be done using the stages of change paradigm. Pre-contemplation clients are not ready for goal setting	A middle-aged women refers herself to you to increase her physical activity levels to help her lose weight. Clearly, she is motivated to be more physically active. You need to explore the overarching goal. A weight loss goal may be less achievable than a stress reduction goal
Break down long-term goal into a series of short-term sub-goals and create an action plan	You might set the client a series of short-term goals, such as increasing weekly steps or getting off the bus two stops earlier to walk to work
Attempt where possible to set behavioural goals rather than physiological goals	If your client has an overarching aim of weight loss you should nevertheless encourage them to set behavioural goals rather than physiological 'pounds lost' targets
Evaluate client self-efficacy for the various behaviours involved in goal achievement	There are many different types of physical activity and the more confident the client is about performing an activity the more likely they are to achieve it

(*Continued*)

Table 6.7 (Continued)

Strategy	Example
Tailor sub-goals to client to ensure they are challenging but realistic and perceived as such by the client	Your client may wish to set goals that are unrealistic; rapid weight loss is attractive to most individuals wishing to lose weight. You need negotiate a goal for which you are likely to be able to deliver positive feedback
Provide regular feedback to the client or provide a mechanism for the client to self-monitor performance and receive Feedback	Feedback needs to be regular, supportive and reflect behavioural achievements and physiological achievements if appropriate
Goal adaptation	For long term complex change the short term sub-goals may need to be reviewed and renegotiated as the client's physiological status and self-efficacy change in response to behavioural adaptation

It has been argued that setting behavioural goals, such as attending an exercise class, rather than physiological goals, such as weight loss, are more effective goals to set because the individual has more direct control over behaviour. Furthermore, Segar et al. (2008) found that middle-aged women who had weight loss goals participated in less physical activity than their contemporaries who had physical activity goals focused on well-being and stress reduction. For inactive individuals' performance goals of any type, behavioural or physiological maybe detrimental to the desired outcomes. Swann et al.' 2021) have proposed learning goals maybe more useful for individuals who are attempting to move from being inactive to active. A performance goal would be to run or jog for 15 minutes every day. A learning goal would be to find three ways of fitting a 15-minute run or jog into your day.

Applying this to Dafydd

To increase Dafydd's self-efficacy about his ability to be more active, he needs to be encouraged to set himself challenging but achievable goals that he can review regularly. Dafydd is currently inactive so he may benefit from initial learning goals around how to adapt his lifestyle before any performance targets.

Social support

One advantage of goal setting, as described previously, is that it requires sustained input from a health specialist and this in itself can provide social support for physical activity. Such behavioural-specific social support has also been demonstrated to support physical activity when provided by friends and peers (Greaves et al., 2011; Kouvonen et al., 2012; Scarapicchia et al., 2017). Exercise groups can also provide social support for maintaining physical activity (Gruber, 2008). Furthermore, there is evidence from older women that exercise groups can develop over time to provide not only specific social support for maintaining physical activity, but also more general emotional support as the relationships made within the group develop (Bidonde et al., 2009). Consequently, encouraging individuals to participate in exercise groups has the potential to benefit health both through the increased levels of physical activity and also through the social support networks that individuals may develop over time.

Applying this to Dafydd

Dafydd's social support network is mainly based on his family, both his partner and his children. Will their general emotional support provide the support for his proposed change in physical activity, or will he require further specific social support?

Community-level interventions

Community-based interventions can involve environmental changes to remove barriers to physical activity, they can be informational or behavioural (Table 6.8). Many interventions at the level of the community are complex involving a range of strategies. Consequently, evaluating complex and often simultaneous community-level interventions can be difficult. However, evidence is emerging about effective ways to evaluate complex interventions that mean more recent interventions such as 'Smarter Choice Programmes in Sustainable Transport Towns' have been more effectively evaluated (Sloman et al., 2010).

Table 6.8 Physical activity interventions in community settings

Type of intervention	Aims
Information-based	To change knowledge and attitudes about the benefits and opportunities for physical activity within a community
Behavioural	To assist people in the development of behavioural management skills that enable them to adopt and maintain behavioural change and/or to create social environments that facilitate and enhance behavioural change
Environmental/policy	To change the structure of physical and organisational environments to provide safe, attractive and convenient places for physical activity

Environmental interventions

Public health policy addressing physical activity is increasingly focused on the obesogenic environment by integrating health and transport strategies to promote active transport (Department for Transport, 2020; NICE, 2008b; Department for Health, Physical Activity, Health Improvement and Protection, 2011). Evidence is just starting to emerge that such policies and associated interventions can make an impact.

In 2004 the Department for Transport launched its sustainable transport towns project to see whether intensive town-wide smarter choice programmes could significantly influence travel behaviour and traffic. The projects involved changes to the infrastructure, informational and persuasive communications. 3 towns were selected to run the projects; Darlington, Peterborough and Worcester. All three programmes aimed to increase more use of non-car options specifically bus travel, cycling and walking but did not necessarily all use the same strategies. In their review of the projects Sloman et al. (2010) report that cycling increased substantially by between 26% and 30% compared to a decline in similar medium sized towns. Walking also increased, although not as dramatically, by between 10% and 13%. Again this should be seen in the light of a decline in walking elsewhere. Sloman et al. (2010) conclude that the evidence supports expanding the project wider in the UK. It is important to recognise that these sustainable town projects whilst making changes to the infrastructure and environment also included a range of other informational and supportive strategies. A whole systems approach to physical activity has subsequently been adopted in many cities across the UK. Evidence is emerging that systems-based approaches are being used for planning, implementation and evaluation of physical activity interventions (Cavill et al., 2020). The Department for transport strategy for active transport: '*Gear Change: A bold vision for cycling and walking*' builds on the slow but steady investment into our physical environment to encourage more walking and cycling. The increasing important of reducing our carbon emissions has added impetus to the delivery of the infrastructure required to support active transport. There is long overdue recognition that cars, cyclists, and pedestrians need to be segregated and that both cycling and walking need to be kept safe and accessible to all. Segregated cycle paths are now one of the most visible signs of change in many major cities (Department of Transport, 2020).

In the first edition of this book in 2010 we commented that there was no evidence that active transport schemes were impacting positively on physical activity levels but that this may have reflected the time it takes for such schemes to be implemented and take effect. The second edition in 2014 concluded that the UK still had the lowest levels of cycling and walking in Europe, and it was important therefore that the localised interventions and strategies were sustained and implemented more widely. This is now happening and in 2013 the UK was ranked 11th out of 28 for rates of daily walking and 24th for daily cycling (Hirst, 2020). So, whilst progress is undoubtedly modest there is evidence that investment into infra-structure and public health initiatives can and are making a difference. It is important to remember that small increases in physical activity can have marked health benefits and so modest population changes in physical activity behaviours could have a profound impact in the long term.

The interest in 'green' activities continues to grow. There is increasing evidence that taking part in outdoor physical activity in natural or 'green' environments is particularly beneficial for health and well-being (Hawkins et al., 2011). Such environments include nature reserves, woodlands, and gardens, but health benefits have also been found from physical activity conducted in more urban green spaces such as inner-city parks. Walking in green environments, gardening at home, allotment gardening and community gardening are all physical activities that are receiving increasing attention as potential health-giving activities as a result of the synergistic benefits of exercising and interacting with nature. Common gardening tasks have been shown to involve both moderate and low levels of physical activity for sustained periods (Park et al., 2008; 2011), so the impact of gardening on sedentary time can be considerable. Recently, it has been suggested that allotment gardening is particularly beneficial for health, and this may be because of the social interaction opportunities that the allotment site provides as well as the physical activity in a green environment (Hawkins et al., 2011).

There is increasing involvement and interest in blue environments and their impact on health. Whilst both green and blue spaces are natural environments it is starting to be established that the mechanisms of benefit from blue (water-based) spaces are distinct. Open water swimming also known as outdoor or wild swimming is a long established blue activity that increased in popularity during the Covid-19 lockdowns due to its outdoor accessibility (Overbury et al., 2023). It is postulated that benefits of physical activity for mental health are increased in 'blue activities' such as surfing or swimming due to their immersive nature. There is also increasing popular interest in the benefits of immersion in cold water, which has also generated some public health warnings about the associated risks of rapid entry into cold water. A recent scoping review of the open water swimming literature is helpful for practitioners to understand what we currently know and what further evidence is needed to understand the benefits of cold water swimming for different populations (see Box 6.2).

Box 6.2   Applying Research in Practice

Swimming in nature: A scoping review of the mental health and wellbeing benefits of open water swimming (Overbury et al., 2023)

This scoping review summarised the mental health and wellbeing benefits specific to Open Water Swimming (OWS). The authors note that interventions supporting human and ecological health together are increasingly popular and this is the first review to explore whether OWS may offer such multifaceted benefits.

OWS in this review was defined as any form of swimming-based activity (bathing included) that takes place in a natural body of water e.g., rivers, lakes, ponds, sea, reservoirs, and lochs. Mental health and wellbeing was as broadly defined as possible to include as many studies as possible. Nevertheless, despite a very thorough research strategy only 14 articles were identified that met the criteria. 5 were quantitative, 8 qualitative and there was 1 study that employed mixed methods. The majority of studies (10) were based on sea swimming.

The authors conclude that there is a range of qualitative and quantitative evidence that exists for the mental health and wellbeing benefits of open water swimming but that the quality assessment of the research indicates there are significant limitations particularly in the quantitative research and caution is needed in drawing any conclusions about the benefits of OWS. OWS can involve physical activity, social interaction as well as being outdoors and in the water; these interactions are difficult to evaluate. The authors conclude that:

OWS was shown to improve wellbeing and positive mood states and to reduce negative mood states.

Qualitative research demonstrated rich positive experiences of OWS

The authors also suggest that OWS is accessible, cheap and requires little specialist equipment. However, they also recognise that cleanliness and accessibility of suitable water is a barrier and that the studies that provided demographic information demonstrate its lack of diversity.

Perhaps the most exciting initiative to emerge in the last decade is the global phenomenon which is Parkrun (Reece et al., 2019). Parkrun started in the UK and is now in 20 countries worldwide. It is aimed at all ability levels and welcomes walkers, joggers, runners, and volunteers. It offers free weekly 2 and 5 km events in public spaces (often parks) and it adopts a whole system, collaborative approach. By 2019 over 230,000 parkrun events had taken place involving millions of runners and walkers. It breaks down barriers to participation and challenges what it looks and means to be physically active. It is a global movement, actioned locally by volunteers with huge potential to improve population health and wellbeing. While Parkrun may not be the 'silver bullet' to cure inactivity and its associated health risks, there is evidence that it can make an impact on the health of individuals. This is especially significant due to the relatively high re-attendance rate observed meaning more people are more likely to reap those benefits long term. As the demographic of Parkrun is ever changing, attracting more previously inactive people each year perhaps future research will elucidate the full effect that Parkrun can have on an inactive person's health (McIntosh 2021).

All the research indicates that environmental adaptations need to be supported by behavioural interventions to support adaptation to the environment and positive changes in physical activity or we run the risk of supporting only the physical activity behaviours of the currently active (Jones et al., 2007).

Information interventions

Community-level information interventions can be as short and simple as point-of-decision prompts at the bottom of a where a choice of the lift or the stairs is available, or a more complicated media campaign to encourage people to take up more leisure time activity (Lewis & Eves, 2012; Sloman et al., 2010). Decisional prompts at the base of buildings with a number of floors have been found to be effective in increasing the decision to take the stairs rather than the lift (Lewis & Eves, 2012), Information can be provided through the media in written form or through radio and television campaigns. Increasingly, information is provided through the internet, such as the change4life campaign (Department of Health, 2009). In social cognitive terms an information intervention usually attempts to increase people's perception of risk from inactivity. Alternatively, or as well as, an information campaign may highlight the benefits of exercise for health. Most physical activity campaigns will take such a health-orientated focus, although reference to social benefits or enjoyment is not uncommon. Wakefield et al. (2010) in their review of informational campaigns found no evidence that informational-only media-based campaigns were effective, which is what we would have predicted from the research evidence about communicating risk and benefits (Thirlaway & Upton, 2009). Multi-component interventions, such as the sustainable transport town projects, where media-based information plays a central part, are more likely to be successful at increasing physical activity (Sloman et al., 2010)

Working effectively with others

Physical activity has not traditionally had practitioners embedded into the health service. Dieticians are established Professionals Allied to Medicine whereas physical activity has remained firmly in the remit of local authorities and increasingly private gyms and personal trainers. The Welsh national exercise referral scheme (NERS) was the first wide-scale government scheme that attempted to provide a clear pathway from primary (and sometimes secondary care) into supportive physical activity outside of the health service. NERS comprises two distinct but inter-related elements:

1 Generic NERS sessions for 'low risk' population groups that need some support to increase fitness and reduce general risks of developing chronic conditions; these are 16 week programmes.
2 Specialist NERS sessions for population groups deemed to be 'higher risk' and needing to undertake tailored exercise sessions as part of their rehabilitation; these can be 16-to-48-week programmes depending on the condition.

Many exercise referral schemes (not only NERS) are now expanding their range of activities and individuals can be referred not only to gyms but to increasing diverse activities, including outdoor activities. This is often the first port of call for practice nurses, doctors, and other specialists such as community diabetic nurses who are trying to encourage physical activity as a preventative strategy. The downside of the scheme is that for some groups in the population uptake and adherence was low. For example the evaluation of the NERS found that those who owned a car were twice as likely to join the scheme than non-car owners (Murphy et al., 2010). Adherence to the scheme in different areas of Wales ranged from 11% and 62% suggesting that the scheme is not reaching all sectors in society equally (Murphy et al., 2010); although this has improved following a Motivational Interviewing Training Programme for the exercise professionals and the development of sustainable exit route opportunities within local communities. Evidence from a systematic review of 33 studies of Exercise Referral schemes suggests that support from providers, other attendees and family was an important facilitator of adherence and longer term commitment to physical activity (Morgan et al., 2016). For health professionals interested in promoting physical activity in their clients and patients Exercise Referral schemes offer a safe route into physical activity.

More recently the Welsh Government has launched a consultation into social prescribing. (Welsh Government, 2020). Social prescribing is a way of linking people to community-based, non-clinical support. It can help empower individuals to recognise their own needs, strengths, personal assets and to connect with their own communities for support with their own health and well-being. If initiated and supported by the Welsh Government it will interesting to see how social prescribing can work with exercise referral and community initiatives such as Parkrun to support physical activity.

Conclusion

Educational campaigns to increase physical activity have had little impact on population levels of physical activity. We live in an obesogenic environment which discourages physical activity. People need psychological support to enable them to become more physically active and this support will need to be long term if they are both to adopt and maintain healthy levels of physical activity. Currently, evidence suggests that self-regulation through goal setting, self-monitoring and feedback is the most effective way to promote physical activity. Well-set goals can build self-efficacy and support physical activity in the long term. It is clear that enjoyment is central to the long-term maintenance of physical activity, but it is not clear why some people enjoy physical activity and others do not. This is an area worthy of further research.

Applying this to Dafydd

Dafydd is one of the majority of people who understands that physical activity would improve his health and he would like to be more active, and he is trying to work out how he can overcome the barriers he perceives to being more physically active. He doesn't need any more information about his risk or the benefits of physical activity. He needs support in finding a solution that is appropriate to his personal situation. He needs to be encouraged to make small changes to his activity that will give him a sense of achievement and the self-efficacy to attempt further changes. If he wishes to utilise active transport as a strategy, he will need to understand the habitual nature of activities such as driving to work and attempt to break the bad habit of driving to work and establish the good habit of cycling to work. He is now more likely to achieve this because his local community is investing in supporting cycling. He will lack social support for physical activity if it reduces his time in the home, so utilising active transport will minimise the impact of increasing his physical activity on his family and increase the likelihood that his partner will be supportive.

Key points

- What makes physical activity so important for health outcomes is the strength of its effect over such a wide range of conditions.
- People generally understand the risks of being sedentary and the benefits of physical activity but still do not get active.
- Self-efficacy is one of the best predictors of successful increase in physical activity and can be built through the encouragement of self-regulatory techniques in individuals.
- Individuals attempting to increase their physical activity levels are most likely to succeed if they get practical and emotional social support from friends, family and/or the exercise programme.
- The establishment of good physical activity habits may be crucial in the promotion of physical activity.
- Perceptions of the environment may be more important than the objective environment for physical activity.
- Whole system approaches that bring all levels of intervention together are increasingly being developed in geographical areas.

Points for discussion

- As with other lifestyle activities physical activity interventions are not accessed equally by all members of a community. How can we promote physical activity in those experiencing high levels of deprivation?
- Being sedentary is associated with poorer health and well-being. Should we be encouraging people to reduce their sedentary time, with any level of physical activity or should we remain focused on at least moderate physical activity?
- How would you encourage a person who is currently overweight/obese to become more physically active? Which psychological factors must you be aware of when planning an intervention to promote a more active lifestyle for them and why?

Further resources

Dugdill, L., Crone, D., & Murphy, R. (2009). *Physical activity and health promotion.* Oxford: Wiley-Blackwell.

Bouchard, C., Blair, S., & Haskell, W. (2012) *Physical activity and health (2nd ed).* Leeds: Human Kinetics.

British Heart Foundation http://www.bhfactive.org.uk

Diabetes UK http://www.diabetes.org.uk

References

Aarts, H., Paulussen, T., & Schaalma, H. (1997). Physical exercise habit: On the conceptualisation and formation of habitual health behaviours. *Health Education Research, 21,* 363–374.

Ajzen, I. (1998). Models of human social behaviour and their application to health psychology. *Psychology and Health, 13,* 735–739.

Ashford, S., Edmunds, J., & French, D. P. (2010). What is the best way to change self-efficacy to promote lifestyle and recreational physical activity? A systematic review with meta-analysis. *British Journal of Health Psychology, 15,* 265–288.

Ayotte, B. J., Margrett, J. A., & Hicks-Patrick, J. (2010). Physical activity in middle-aged and young-old adults: The roles of self-efficacy, barriers, outcome expectancies, self-regulatory behaviours and social support. *Journal of Health Psychology, 15*(2), 173–185.

Baker G., Gray, S. R., Wright, A., Fitzsimons C., Nimmo M., Lowry R., & Mutrie, N. (2008). The effect of a pedometer-based community walking intervention "Walking for Wellbeing in the West" on physical activity levels and health outcomes: A 12-week randomized controlled trial. *International Journal of Behavioural Nutrition and Physical Activity, 5,* 44.

BBC News. (2007). *Exercise 'must be tough to work'. To be healthy, you really do need to break into a sweat when you exercise, say experts.* Available at: www.bbc.co.uk (accessed September 2007).

Bennett, G. G., Wolin, K. Y., Viswanath, K., Askew, S., Puleo, E., & Emmons, K. M. (2006). Television viewing and pedometer-determined physical activity among multi-ethnic residents of low-income housing. *American Journal of Public Health, 96,* 1681–1685.

Biddle, S. J. H., & Mutrie N. (2008). *Psychology of physical activity. Determinants, well-being & interventions.* 2nd Edn. Oxon: Routledge.

Bidonde, J. M., Goodwin, D. L., & Drinkwater, D. T. (2009). Older women's experiences of a fitness program: The importance of social networks. *Journal of Applied Sport Psychology, 21*(1), S86–S101.

Blue, C. L. (2007). Does the theory of planned behaviour identify diabetes-related cognitions for intention to be physical active and eat a healthy diet? *Public Health Nursing, 24*(2), 141–150.

Booth, F. W., Roberts, C. K., & Laye, M. J. (2012). Lack of exercise is a major cause of chronic diseases. *Comparative Physiology, 2*(2), 1143–1121. Doi: 10.1002/cphy.c110025

Cancer Intelligence Team (2022). *Overweight and obesity prevalence projections for the UK, England, Scotland, Wales and Northern Ireland, based on data to 2019/20.* Cancer Research UK. www.cancerresearchuk.org

Cairney, J., Dudley, D., Kwan, M., Bulten, R., & Kriellaars, D. (2019). Physical literacy, physical activity and health: Toward an evidence-informed conceptual model. *Sports Medicine (Auckland), 49*(3), 371–383. Doi: 10.1007/s40279-019-01063-3

Cavill, N., Richardson, D., Faghy, M., Bussell, C., & Rutter, A. (2020). Using system mapping to help plan and implement city-wide action to promote physical activity. *Journal of Public Health Research, 9*(3). Doi: 10.4081/jphr/

Celis-Morales, C. A., Lyall, D. M., & Welsh, P. (2017). Association between active commuting and incident cardiovascular disease, cancer and mortality; prospective cohort study. *British Medical Journal, 357,* j1456. Doi: 10.1136/bmj,j1456

Chastin, S. F. M., Cauwenberg, J. V., Maenhout, L., Cardon, G., Lambert, E. V., & Van Dyck, D. (2020). Inequality in physical activity, global trends by income inequality and gender in adults. *International Journal of Behavioral Nutrition and Physical Activity*, 17(142). Doi: 10.1186s12 966-020-01039-x.

Chin, S. H., Kahathuduwa, C. N., & Binks, M. (2016). Physical activity and obesity: what we know and what we need to know. *Obesity Reviews*, 17(12), 1226–1244. Doi: 10.1111/obr.12460

Crone, D., Heaney, L., & Owens, C. S. (2009). Physical activity and mental health. In L. Dugdill, D. Crone and R. Murphy (Eds). *Physical activity and health promotion*. London: Wiley-Blackwell.

Department of Health. (1999). *Saving lives: Our healthier nation*. London: The Stationery Office.

Department of Health (2004). *At least five a week*. London: The Stationary Office.

Department of Health (2009). *Be active, Be healthy*. London: HM Government

Department of Health (2011). *Healthy lives, healthy people: A call to action on obesity in England*. London: HM Government.

Department of Health, Physical Activity, Health Improvement and Protection (2011). *Start Active, Stay Active*. London: DoH.

Department of Health, Social Services and Public Safety (2011). *Health Survey Northern Ireland: First results from the 2010/11 survey*. Belfast: Department of Health, Social Services and Public Safety.

Department for Infrastructure (2022). *Active and sustainable travel in Northern Ireland 2020/21*. Northern Ireland Statistics and Research agency. www.datavis.nisra.gov.uk

Department for Transport (2020). *Gear change: A bold vision for cycling and walking*, London: DfT Publications. www.gov.uk/dfdt

Dudley, D., Cairney, J., Wainwright, N., Kriellaars, D., & Mitchell, D. (2017). *Critical considerations for physical literacy policy in public health, Recreation, Sport, and Education Agencies*. Quest. Doi: 10.1080/00336297.2016.1268967

Edwards, L. C., Bryant, A. S., Keegan, R., Morgan, K., & Jones, A. M. (2017). Definitions, foundations and associations of physical literacy: A systematic review. *Sports Medicine*, 47(3), 113–126.

Edwards, L. C., Bryant, A. S., Morgan, K., Cooper, S.-M., Jones, A. M., & Keegan, R. J. (2019). A professional development program to enhance primary school teachers' knowledge and operationalisation of physical literacy. *Journal of Teaching in Physical Education*, 38(2), 126–135. Doi: 10.1123/jtpe.2018-0275

Fitzsimons C. F., Baker G., Gray S. R., Nimmo, M. A., & Mutrie N. (2012). Does physical activity counselling enhance the effects of a pedometer-based intervention over the long-term: 12-month findings from the Walking for Wellbeing in the west study. *BMC Public Health*, 12, 206.

Foster, C., Hillsdon, M., Cavill, N., Bull, F., Buxton, K., & Crombie, H. (2006). *Interventions that use the environment to encourage physical activity: Evidence review*. London: NICE.

Fukuoka, Y., Haskel, W., & Vittinghoff, E. (2016). New insights in discrepancies between self-reported and accelerometer-measured moderate to vigorous physical activity among women – the mPED trial. *BMC Public Health*, 16, 761. Doi: 10.1186/s12889-016-3348-7

Gardner, B. (2015). A review and analysis of the use of 'habit' in understanding, predicting and influencing health-related behaviour. *Health Psychology Review*, 9(3), 277–295. Doi: 10.1080/1 747199.2013.876238

Greaves, C. J., Sheppard, K. E., Abraham, C., Hardeman, W., Roden, M., Evans, P. H., & Schwartz, P., The IMAGE Study Group (2011). Systematic review of reviews of intervention components associated with increased effectiveness in dietary and physical activity interventions. *Biomedical Central Public Health*, 11, 119.

Griffiths, C., Hina, F., & Jiang, H. (2022). *Social prescribing through primary care: A systematic review of the evidence*. Northampton Healthcare NHS Foundation Trust, Doi: 10.4236/ojpm. 2022.122003

Gruber, K. J. (2008). Social support for exercise and dietary habits among college students. *Adolescence, 43*(171), 557–575.

Guthold, R., Stevens, G. A., Riley, L. M., & Bull. F. C. (2018). Worldwide trends in insufficient physical activity from 2011 to 2016: A pooled analysis of 358 population-based surveys with 1.9 million participants. *Lancet Global Health, 6*, e1077-86. Doi: 10.1016/S2214-109X(18)30357-7

Hagberg, L. A., Lindahl, B., Nyberg, L., & Hellenius, L. (2009). Importance of enjoyment when promoting physical exercise. *Scandinavian Journal of Medicine and Science in Sport, 19*(5), 740–747.

Hagger, M. S. (2019). Habit and physical activity: Theoretical advances, practical implications, and agenda for future research. *Psychology of Sport and Exercise, 42*, 118–119.

Hardcastle, S., & Hagger, M. S. (2011). "You can't do it on your own": Experiences of a motivational interviewing intervention on physical activity and dietary behaviour. *Psychology of Sport and Exercise, 12*, 314–323.

Harris, T., Limb, E. S., Hosking, F., Carey, I., DeWilde, S., Furness, C., Wahlich, C., Ahmad, S., Kerry, S., Whincup, P., Victor, C., Ussher, M., Lliffe, S., Ekeland, U., Fox-Rushby, J., Ibison, J., & Cook, D. G. (2019). Effect of pedometer-based walking interventions on long-term health outcomes: Prospective 4-year follow-up of two randomised controlled trials using routine primary care data. *PLOS Medicine, 16*(6), e1002836. Doi: 10.1371.journal.pmed.1002836

Harrison, J. W., Mullen, P. D., & Green, L. W. (2002). A meta-analysis of studies of the health belief model with adults. *Health Education Research, 7*, 107–116.

Hawkins, J. L., Thirlaway, K., Backx, K., & Clayton, D. (2011). Allotment gardening and other leisure activities for stress reduction and healthy aging. *HortTechnology, 21*, 577–585

Hillsdon, M., Foster, C., Cavill, N., Crombie, H., & Naidoo, B. (2005). *The Effectiveness of Public Health Interventions for Increasing Physical Activity among Adults: A Review of Reviews*, 2nd Edn. London: Health Development Agency.

Hirst, D. (2020). Briefing paper 8615: *Active Travel: Trends, policy and funding*. www.parliament.uk/commons-librarypapers@parliament.uk @commonslibrary

Hirvensalo M., & Lintunen T. (2011). Life-course perspective for physical activity and sports participation. *European Review of Aging and Physical Activity, 8*, 13–22.

Howlett, N., Trivedi, D., Troop, N. A., & Chater, A. M. (2018). Are physical activity interventions for health inactive adults effective in promoting behavior change and maintenance, and which behavioural change techniques are effective? A systematic review and meta-analysis. *TBM, 9*, 147–157. Doi: 10.1093/tbm/iby010

Information Analysis Directorate (2021). *Health Survey (NI) First results (2020/21)*. Belfast:Department of Health: www.health.ni.gov.uk

Jeong, Y. H., Healy, L. C., & McEwan, D. (2021). The application of Goal Setting Theory to goal setting interventions in sport: A systematic review. *International Review of Sport and Exercise Psychology, 16*(1), 474–499. Doi: 10.1080/1750984X.2021.1901298

Johnson, S. T., McCargar, L. J., Bell, G. J., Tudor-Locke, C., Harber, V. J., & Bell, R. C. (2006). Distilling a complex prescription for type 2 diabetes management through pedometry. *Diabetes Care, 29*(7), 1654–1655.

Jones, A., Bentham, G., Foster, C., Hillsdon, M., & Panter, J. (2007). *Tackling obesities: Future choices – Obesogenic environments – Evidence review*. London: United Kingdom Government Foresight Programme, Office of Science and Innovation.

Khan, K. M., Thompson, A. M., Blair, S. N., Sallis, J. F., Powell, K. E., Bull, F. C., & Bauman, A. E. (2012). Sport and exercise as contributors to the health of nations. *The Lancet, 380*(9836), 59–64. Doi: 10.1016/S0140-6736(12)60865-4

Kinmonth, A., Wareham, N. J., Hardeman, W., Sutton, S., Prevost, T. A., Fanshawe, T., Williams, K. M., Ekeland, U., Speigilhalter, D., & Griffin, S. J. (2008). Efficacy of a theory-based behavioural intervention to increase physical activity in an at-risk group in primary care (ProActive UK): A randomized trial. *The Lancet, 371*, 41–48.

Kouvonen, A., De Vogli, R., Stafford, M., Shipley, M., Marmot, M. G., Cox, T., Vahtera, J., Vaananen, A., Heponiemi, T., Singh-Manoux, A., & Kivimaki, M. (2012). Social support and the likelihood of maintaining and improving levels of physical activity: the Whitehall II Study. *European Journal of Public Health*, 22, 514–518. Doi: 10.1093/eurpub/ckr091.

Landais, L. L., Damman, O. C., Schoonmade, L. J., Timmermans, D. R. M., Verhagen, E. A. L. M., & Jelsma, J. G. M. (2020). Choice architecture interventions to change physical activity and sedentary behaviour: A systematic review of effects on intention, behavior and health outcomes during and after intervention. *International Journal of Behavioral Nutrition and Physical Activity*, 17(47). Doi: 10.1186/s12966-020-00942-7.

Lewis, A., & Eves, F. (2012). Prompt before the choice is made: Effects of a stair-climbing intervention in university buildings. *British Journal of Health Psychology*, 17(3), 631–643. Doi: 10.1111/j.2044-8287.2011.

Liu, J., Zeng, M., Wang, D., Zhang, Y., Shang, B., & Ma, X. (2022). Applying social cognitive theory in predicting physical activity among Chinese adolescents: A cross-sectional study with multi-group structural equation model. *Frontiers in Psychology*, Volume 12. PMC 8965556. Doi: 10.3389/fpsyg2021.695241

Maddison, R., Vander Hoorn, S., Jiang, Y., Ni Mhurchu, C., Exeter, D., Dorey, E., Bullen, C., utter, J., Schaaf, D., & Turley M. (2009). The environment and physical activity: The influence of psychosocial, perceived and built environmental factors. *International Journal of Behavioural Nutrition and Physical Activity*, 6, 19.

Mama, S. K., McNeill, L. H., McCurdy, S. A., Evans, A. E., Diamond, P. M., Adamus-Leach, H. J., & Lee, R. E. (2015). Psychosocial factors and theory in physical activity studies in minorities. *American Journal of Health Behaviour*, 39(1), 68–76. Doi: 10.5993/AJHB.39.1.8

Mandolesi, L., Polverino, A., Montuori, S., Foti, F., Ferraiolo, G., Soreentino, P., & Sorrention, G. (2018). Effects of physical exercise on cognitive functioning and wellbeing: Biological and psychological benefits. *Frontiers in Psychology*, 9(509). Doi:10.3389/fpsyg.2018.00509

McIntosh , T. (2021). Parkrun: A panacea for health and wellbeing? *Journal of Research in Nursing*, 26(5), 472–477.

McKinney, J., Lithwick, D. J., Morrison, B. N., Nazzari, H., Isserow. S. H., Heilbron, B., & Krahn, A. D. (2016). The health benefits of physical activity and cardiorespiratory fitness. *BMC Medical Journal*, 58(3) 131–137.

Morgan, F., Battersby, A., Weightman, A. L., Searchfield, L., Turkey, R., Morgan, H., Jagroo, J., & Ellis, S. (2016). Adherence to exercise referral schemes by participants – what do providers and commissioners need to know? A systematic review of barriers and facilitators. *BMC Public Health*, 16, 227. Doi 10.1186/s12889-016-2882-7

Morgan, K., Bryant, A. S., & Edwards, L. C. (2022). Appreciative inquiry as a methodological approach to collaboration between different sporting organisations in Wales to promote physical literacy. *Sport, Education and Society*, 27(1), 27–40. 10.1080/13573322.2020.1822311

Mulchandani, R., Chandrasekaran, A. M., Shivashanker, R., Kondal, D., Agrawal, A., Panniyammakal, J., Tandon, N., Prabhakaran, D., Sharma, M., & Goenka, S. (2019). Effect of workplace physical activity interventions on the cardio-metabolic health of working adults: Systematic review and meta-analysis. *International Journal of Behavioral Nutrition and Physical Activity*, 16, 134. 10.1186/s12966-019-0896-0

Murphy, S., Raisanen, L., Moore, G., Tudor Edwards, R., Linck, P., Hounsome, N., Williams, N., Ud Din, N., & Moore, L. (2010). *The evaluation of the National Exercise Referral Scheme in Wales*. Cardiff: Welsh Government.

Naylor, P. J., & McKay, H. A. (2009). Prevention in the first place: Schools a setting for action on physical inactivity. *British Journal of Sports Medicine*, 43, 10–13.

Ng, S. W., & Popkin, B. M. (2012). Time use and physical activity: A shift away from movement across the globe. *Obesity Review*, 13(8), 659–680.

NICE (2007). *Behavioural change at population, community and individual levels*. London: NICE.

NICE (2008a). *Promoting and creating built or natural environments that encourage and support physical activity.* London: NICE.

NICE (2008b). *Workplace health promotion: How to encourage employees to be physically active.* London: NICE.

NICE (2008c). *Occupational therapy interventions and physical activity Interventions to promoting the mental well-being of older people in primary care and residential care.* London: NICE.

NICE (2009). *Depression: The treatment and management of depression in adults.* London: NICE.

NICE (2011). *Preventing type 2 diabetes: population and community level interventions in high risk groups and the general population.* London: NICE.

NICE (2010). *Prevention of cardiovascular disease at population level.* London: NICE.

NICE (2012). *Physical activity: Walking and cycling.* London: NICE. www.nice.org.uk.guidance/ph41.

Nigg, C. R., Borrelli, B., Maddock, J., & Dishman, R. K. (2008). A theory of physical activity maintenance. *Applied Psychology: An international review, 57*(4), 544–560.

Normand, M. P. (2008). Increasing physical activity through self-monitoring, goal setting and feedback. *Behavioural Interventions, 23,* 227–236.

Ogilvie, D., Foster, C. E., Rothnie, H., Cavell, N., Hamilton, V., Fitzsimons, C. F. M., & Mutrie, N. (2007). Interventions to promote walking: Systematic review. *British Medical Journal Online, 33,* 1204. Doi: 10.1136/bmj.39198.722720.BE

Overbury, K., Conroy, B. W., & Marks, E. (2023). Swimming in nature: A scoping review of the mental health and wellbeing benefits of open water swimming. *Journal of Environmental Psychology, 90.* Doi: 10.1016/j.envp.2023.102073

Park, S., Lee, K., & Son, K. (2011). Determining exercise intensities of gardening tasks as a physical activity using metabolic equivalents in older adults. *HortScience, 46,* 1706–1710.

Park, S. A., Shoemaker, C. A., & Haub, M. D. (2008). Can older gardeners meet the physical activity recommendation through gardening? *Horttechnology, 18,* 639–643.

Pate, R. R., Yancey, A. K., & Kraus, W. E. (2010). The 2008 physical activity guidelines for Americans: Implications for clinical and public health practice. *American Journal of Lifestyle Medicine, 4*(3), 209–217.

Pavey, T. G., Taylor, A. H., Fox, K. R., Hillsdon, M., Anokye, N., Campbell, J. L., Foster, C., Green, C., Moxham, T., Mutrie, N., Searle, J., Trueman, P., & Taylor, P. S. (2011). Effect of exercise referral schemes in primary care on physical activity and improving health outcomes: Systematic review and meta-analysis. *British Medical Journal, 343.* Doi: 10.1136/BMS.d6462.

Priebe, C. S., & Spink, K. S. (2011). When in Rome: Descriptive norms and physical activity. *Psychology of Sport and Exercise, 12,* 93–98.

Reece, L. J., Quirk, H., Wellington, C., *et al.* (2019). Bright spots, physical activity investments that work: Parkrun; a global initiative striving for healthier and happier communities. *British Journal of Sports Medicine, 53,* 326–327.

Rejeski, J. W., & Brawley, L. R. (1998). Defining the Boundaries in Sport Psychology. *The Sport Psychologist, 2*(3), 231–242.

Roetert, & Ortega, C. (2019). Physical literacy for the older adult. *Strength and Conditioning Journal, 41*(2), 89–99. Doi: 10.1519/SSC.0000000000000430

Rowley, N. (2019). Exercise Referral Schemes in the UK. *ACSM's Health and Fitness Journal, 23*(6), 6–8. Doi: 10.1249/FIT00000000000000514

Saris, W. H. M., Blair, S. N., van Baak, M. A., Eaton, S. B., Davies, P. S. W., Di Pietro, L., Fogelholm, M., Rissanen, A., Schoeller, D., Swinburn, B., Tremblay, A., Westerterp, K. R., & Wyatt, H. (2003). How much physical activity is enough to prevent unhealthy weight gain? Outcome of the IASO 1st Stock Conference and consensus statement. *Obesity Reviews, 4,* 101–114.

Scarapicchia, T. M., F., Amireault, S., Faulkner, G., & Sabiston, C. M. (2017). Social support and physical activity participation among healthy adult: A systematic review of prospective studies. *International Review of Sport and Exercise Psychology*, 10(1), 50–83.

Schneider, M., & Cooper, D. M. (2011). Enjoyment of exercise moderates the impact of a school-based physical activity intervention. *International Journal of Behavioural Nutrition and Physical Activity*, 8, 64.

Segar, M. L., Eccles, J. S., & Richardson, C. R. (2008). Type of physical activity goal influences participation in healthy midlife women. *Women's Health Issues*, 18, 281–291.

Shepard, R. J. (2003). Limits to the measurement of habitual physical activity by questionnaires. *British Journal of Sports Medicine*, 37, 197–206.

Slack, M. K. (2006). Interpreting current physical activity guidelines and incorporating them into practice for health promotion and disease prevention. *American Journal of Health System Pharmacy*, 63, 1647–1653.

Sloman, L., Cairns, S., Newson, C., Anable, J., Pridmore, A., & Goodwin, P. (2010). *The effects of smarter choice programmes in the sustainable travel towns: Summary report*. London: DfT.

Sport England (2022). *Active Lives Adult Survey November 2020–21 report*. Sport England. Sportengland.org

Stensel, D. J., Hardman, A. E., & Gill, J. M. R. (2021). *Physical activity and health: The evidence explained* 3rd Edn. London. Routledge.

Strobach, T., Englert, C., Jekauc, D., & Pfeffer, I. (2020). Predicting adoption and maintenance of physical activity in the context of dual-process theories. *Performance Enhancement and Health*, 8(1), 100162.

Swann, C., Rosenbaum, S., Lawrence, A., Vella, S. A., McEwan, D., & Ekkekakis, P. (2021). Updating goal setting theory in physical activity promotion: A critical conceptual review. *Health Psychology Review*, 15(1), 34–50. Doi: 10.1080/17437199.2019.1706616

Teychenne, M., White, R. L., Richards, J., Schuch, F. B., Rosenbaum, S., & Bennie, J. A. (2020). Do we need physical activity guidelines for mental health: What does the evidence tell us? *Mental Health and Physical Activity*, 18. Doi: 10.1016/j.mhpa2019.100315

The Scottish Government (2011). *The Scottish Health Survey 2010, Volume 1: Main report*. Edinburgh: The Scottish Government. Available at: http://www.scotland.gov.uk/Publications/2011/09/27084018/91

The Scottish Government (2020). *The Scottish Health Survey 2019, Volume 1: Main report*. Edinburgh: The Scottish Government. www.gov.scot

Thirlaway, K. J., & Upton, D. (2009). *The Psychology of Lifestyle: Promoting Healthy Behaviour*. London: Routledge

Thompson, W. R.; Gordon, N. F., & Pescatello, L. S. (2009). *ACSMs guidelines for exercise testing and prescription*. Philadelphia PA: Lippincott Williams & Wilkins.

Toppa, S. (2015). Need a reminder to get out of your seat? There's an apple watch for that. *Time*, February 2015.

Townsend. T., & Lake, A. (2017). Obesogenic environments: Current evidence of the built and food environments. *Perspectives in Public Health*, 137(1), 38–44. Doi: 10.1177/1757913916679860

Transport Scotland (2020). *Active Travel Framework*. Glasgow. Transport Scotland. www.transport.gov.scot

UK Chief Medical Officers (2019). *UK Chief Medical Officers Physical Activity Guidelines 2019*. Department of Health and Social Care, Llwodraeth Cymru Welsh Government, Department of Health Northern Ireland and the Scottish Government (2019). www.gov.uk/dhsc

US Department of Health and Human Services (2008). *Physical Activity Guidelines Advisory Committee Report, from the Physical Activity Guidelines Advisory Committee*. US Department of Health and Human Services.

Verplanken, B., & Melkevik, O. (2008). Predicting habit: The case of physical exercise. *Psychology of Sport and Exercise*, 9, 15–26.

Wainwright, N., Goodway, J., Whitehead, M., Williams, A., & Kirk, D. (2018). Laying the foundations for physical literacy in Wales: The contribution of the Foundation Phase to the development of physical literacy. *Physical Education and Sport Pedagogy, 23*(4), 431–444. Doi: 10.1080/17408989.2018.1455819

Wakefield, M. A., Loken, B., & Hornik (2010). Use of mass media campaigns to change behaviour. *The Lancet, 367,* 1261–1271.

Warburton, D. E. R., Whitney, N. C., & Bredin, S. S. D. (2006). Health benefits of physical activity: The evidence. *Canadian Medical Association Journal, 174,* 801–809.

Watkinson C., van Sluijs E. M. F., Sutton S., Marteau T., & Griffin S. J. (2010). Randomised controlled trial of the effects of physical activity feedback on awareness and behaviour in UK adults: The FAB study protocol. *BMC Public Health, 10,* 114.

Welsh Government (2011). *Health Trends in Wales 2011.* Cardiff: WAG.

Welsh Government (2011a). *Welsh Health Survey 2010.* Assessed from: http://www.wales.gov.uk/statistics

Welsh Government (2020). *National Survey for Wales 2019-20.* Cardiff: Welsh Government. https://gov.wales/nationalsurvey-wales-population-health

Welsh Parliament (2022). *Active travel research briefing.* Cardiff: Welsh Parliament. www.research.senedd.wales.

Wen, C. P., Wai, J. P. M., Tsai, M. K., Yang, Y. C., Cheng, T. Y. D., Lee, M., Chan, H. T., Tsao, C. K., Tsai, S. P., & Wu, X. (2011). Minimum amount of physical activity for reduced mortality and extended life expectancy: A prospective cohort study. *Lancet, 378,* 1244–1253.

Whitehead M. (2013). Definition of physical literacy and clarification of related. *ICSSPE Bull Journal of Sport Science and Physical Education, 65,* 28–33.

WHO (2013). *Global action plan for the prevention and control of noncommunicable diseases 2013-2020.* Geneva: World health Organisation.

WHO (2018). *Global action plan on physical activity 2018–2030. More active people for a healthier world.* Geneva: World Health Organisation 2018: CC BY-NC-SA 3.0 IGO.

WHO (2020). *Fact sheet: Physical activity.* www.who.int

WHO (2020) *WHO guidelines on physical activity and sedentary behaviour.* Geneva: World Health organisation; 2020. Licence: CC BY-NC-SA 3.0 IGO.

WHO (2022). *The global health observatory: Physical inactivity.* World Health Organisation 2022. www.who.int

Williamson, C., Baker, G., Mutrie, N., Niven, A., & Kelly, P. (2020). Get the message? A scoping review of physical activity messaging. *International Journal of Behavioural Nutrition and Physical Activity, 17,* 51. Doi: 10/1186/512986-020.00954-3

Wyatt-Williams, J. (2013). *National exercise referral coordinator, Welsh Local Government Association.* Personal Communication.

Xiao, Y., Wang, H., Zhang, T., & Ren, X. (2019). Psychosocial predictors of physical activity and health-related quality of life among Shanghai working adults. *Health and Quality of Life Outcomes, 17,* 72. Doi: 10.1186/s12955-019-1145-6

Zeidi, I. M., Morshedi, H., & Shokohi, A. (2021). Predicting psychological factors affecting regular physical activity in hypertensive patients: Application of health action process approach model. *Nursing Open, 422–452.* Doi: 10.1002/nop2.645

Zhao, M., Veeranki, S. P., Magnussen, C. G., & Xi. B. (2020). Recommended physical activity and all cause and cause specific mortality in US adults: Prospective cohort study. *British Medical Journal, 370,* m2031. Doi: 10.1136/bmj.m2031

7   Sensible drinking

LEARNING OBJECTIVES

At the end of this chapter you will:

- Understand the extent of risky and heavy episodic drinking in different communities.
- Have reviewed government recommendations for low-risk drinking.
- Understand the health, economic, and social consequences of drinking alcohol.
- Appreciate the psychosocial factors that influence people to drink more than is healthy.
- Have evaluated the available interventions to help people reduce their drinking.

Case study

Olivia is a 35-year-old marketing executive who works in a large advertising company. She has worked in the firm since graduating from university and has been regularly promoted. Much of her work involves networking with clients. Olivia drank heavily as a student and, unlike many of her contemporaries, has not reduced her drinking. Drinking is part of her work culture. Olivia travels with her work, staying in expensive hotels and drinking late with colleagues and clients. Olivia is proud of her ability to drink on a par with her male colleagues and to get up early after a long night and work well. Olivia takes a lot of exercise and considers that the exercise she takes offsets the alcohol she consumes.

Olivia and her partner are considering starting a family but have so far been unable to conceive. They have come to see you for advice about assisted conception. Olivia's partner is clearly concerned about her drinking and thinks she should cut down. Olivia is less concerned and thinks she will be able to 'cut down a bit' once she is pregnant. Olivia says she doesn't drink all that much, probably around the government guidelines unless there is a special occasion. She goes on to imply that she thinks government recommendations are rather stringent and that on the continent they are far more relaxed about drinking. You suspect that Olivia drinks over the weekly recommended limits and may be a dependent drinker.

DOI: 10.4324/9781003471233-7

Introduction

Alcohol is a chemical compound, ethyl alcohol, often called ethanol. Ethanol produces intoxication through its action on the brain and is a legal psychoactive drug. Intoxication leads to impairments in psychomotor control, reaction time and judgement. Intoxication also influences mood and reduces social inhibitions (Babor et al., 2010).

The amount of alcohol in any drink depends on the concentration of alcohol in the beverage and how much of it you consume. The alcoholic content of drinks is usually stated on the container as percentage volume, sometimes followed by the abbreviation ABV (alcohol by volume) or simply by 'vol'. The quantity of liquid is also mandatory. Some manufacturers will state the actual amount of alcohol in a product. For example, for UK market Guinness states the quantity, 440 ml, percentage volume of alcohol, 4.1% and the units, 1.8 (UK units) on the side of its cans of Guinness. However, other manufacturers only give the percentage volume. In the UK pure alcohol is measured in units (Drinkaware, 2022). One UK unit of liquid contains 8 grams of pure alcohol. However, globally 10 grams is the most common size for a drink (WHO, 2018). Spirits used to be served in 25 ml measures, which are generally 1 unit of alcohol, but pubs and bars now serve 35 ml and 50 ml measures. Standard sizes of wine in pubs and bars have also increased with a large glass holding 250 ml which could be 3/4 UK units (24/32 grams) of alcohol in one drink. However, many beers and wines are stronger, having higher percentage volumes of alcohol than those cited in Figures 7.1 and 7.2.

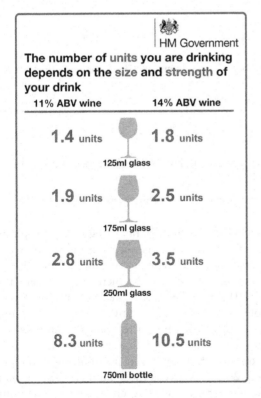

Figure 7.1 UK units of alcohol in wine. Taken from UK Chief Medical Officers Low Risk Drinking Guidelines (2016).

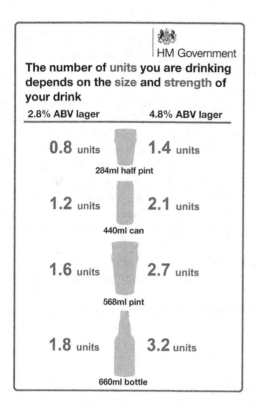

Figure 7.2 UK units of alcohol in lager & beer. Taken from UK Chief Medical Officers Low
Risk Drinking Guidelines (2016).

Applying this to Olivia

If Olivia is drinking large glasses of wine, or strong lagers, then she could easily be
underestimating her alcohol consumption.

People can be easily categorised as smokers or non-smokers but categorising people as
drinkers or non-drinkers, although just as straightforward, is not as useful. Smoking is
bad for you, with no positive aspects whatsoever. The majority of the UK population,
similarly to all Western societies, do not smoke. However, the picture is different for
alcohol. The Office for National Statistics (2018) reported that 57% of people aged over
16 reported drinking alcohol in the previous week. The 2019 Health Survey for England
(2020) reported that 20% of adults had not drunk alcohol in the last 12 months. The
2019 Scottish Health Survey (2020) reported 17% had not drunk alcohol in 2019. It is
safe to say that the majority of adults in the UK drink some alcohol, even if only
occasionally (Alcohol Change UK accessed, 2022). Whereas most smokers wish to quit
only 18% of people who drink in the lower risk ranges wish to change their behaviour
(HM Government, 2012). Whilst drinking a lot is accepted as bad for you, drinking

moderately has been thought to have some health benefits (Lee et al., 2009; Williams et al., 2007; PMC., 2000). However, latest research indicates that the benefits for cardiovascular health are less clear than previously thought. There is considerable controversy about the potential benefits, if any, of moderate drinking for cardiovascular health (Oppenheimer & Bayer, 2020). However, there is consensus that any protective effects are from drinking considerably less than the 14 units per week UK guidelines. Indeed, early in 2023 Canada reduced its weekly guidelines to less than 6 standard drinks a week (Paradis et al., 2023). UK data suggests that only women over 55 see a reduction in the risk of death from moderate drinking of less than 5 units a week (Department of Health, 2015).

Eleven countries have a total ban on alcohol but policy in most countries, the UK included, is to promote 'low risk drinking', not total abstinence (UK Chief Medical Officers, 2016; WHO, 2018; Health Survey for England, 2020). Until 2016 the UK government had defined drinking behaviours as sensible, hazardous, or harmful (HM Government, 2007, 2012). In 2016 the UK Chief Medical Officers moved to a risk-based approach. They based this change of approach on the premise that it is for individuals to make their own judgements about the risks they are willing to accept when they drink alcohol. The 2016 guidance also moved from daily guidelines to weekly guidelines because most people do not drink every day. The UK Chief Medical Officers (2016) advice to keep health risks low is:

not to drink more than 14 units a week on a regular basis
　　　　　(UK Chief Medical Officers' Low Risk Drinking Guidelines, 2016, p. 4)

Furthermore, they advise:

If you regularly drink as much as 14 units per week it is best to spread your drinking over 3 or more days

The 2016 guidelines no longer have different recommendations for men and women about low-risk drinking. However, men are considered to be drinking at a level which increases their risk if they consume between 14 and 50 units a week. If men drink more than 50 units a week, they are considered high risk drinkers. Women are considered high risk drinkers and at particular risk of alcohol-related health problems if they drink more than 35 units a week (Health Survey for England, 2020). The new Canadian guidelines are considerably more risk adverse than the UK guidelines (Paradis et al., 2023).

The phrase 'binge drinking' was originally used by health professionals to describe a prolonged drinking spree lasting at least 2 or 3 days. However, the term is now more broadly applied to describe a single drinking session that leads to drunkenness (Plant and Plant, 2006; HM Government, 2007, 2012). Binge refers to the time frame of drinking. It reflects the importance of the pattern in which alcohol is consumed for health and social outcomes. In 2007, binge drinking was described by the government as:

drinking too much alcohol over a short period of time, e.g., over the course of an evening and it is typically drinking that leads to drunkenness. It has immediate and short-term risks to the drinker and to those around them.
　　　　　　　　　　　　　　　　　　　　　　　(HM Government, 2007, p. 3)

In the UK Chief Medical Officers' guidelines (2016) binge drinking is now referred to single episode drinking, and the risks of single occasion drinking episodes are recognised to be particularly high when between 5 to 7 units are drunk in a 3–6 hour period. However, they do not advise on a specific number of units for single episode drinking, arguing that the differences in short term risks faced by different people drinking the same amount can be so wide. Previously binge drinking has been defined as males who exceed 8 units of alcohol in 1 day and females who exceed 6 units in 1 day (Office for National Statistics (2018). The World Health Organisation (WHO) uses the term heavy episodic drinking instead of binge drinking and defines it as 60 or more grams (7.5 UK units) on at least one single occasion at least once a month.

In summary, the UK guidelines for drinking alcohol have changed quite significantly since the second edition of this text was published in 2011. The weekly recommendations for low risk drinking for men are a third lower than the previous sensible drinking levels. The advice for women remains the same. The focus on binge drinking has lessened; there are no longer daily recommendations but instead a recommendation that weekly units are spread over a number of days. These changes indicate a focus more on the longer-term health implications of alcohol consumption and less on the social and acute consequences of heavy episodic drinking.

Alcohol use disorder and volitional drinking

Until 2013, the American Psychiatric Association recognised two separate disorders: alcohol abuse and alcohol dependence but in the DSM-5 classifications, first published in 2013, they were integrated into a single disorder called alcohol use disorder (AUD) with mild, moderate, and severe sub-classifications. The AUD criteria have 11 criteria and anyone meeting two of the criteria receives a diagnosis of AUD with the severity depending on the number of criteria met. The revised International Classification of Diseases-11 published in June 2019 continue to identify a separate condition alcohol dependence in addition to alcohol use disorder (Saunders et al., 2019).

Criteria that distinguish between volitional and dependent drinking are notoriously hard to establish as the authors of the latest revisions acknowledge (Saunders et al., 2019), although it is reasonable to assume that as intake increases dependency is more likely. There is a lack of reliable data on the prevalence of alcohol dependence because UK general population surveys don't include questionnaires that fit the ICD-11 diagnostic criteria for alcohol dependence. The health harm from drinking above the guidelines for low-risk drinking is the same whether the drinking is volitional or dependent; consequently, the value of delineating between dependent and volitional excessive drinking for purposes of public health/primary care treatment and intervention is limited. Primary care is the place where most AUDs should be treated but the ICD-11 is not relevant at the lower end of the alcohol use spectrum and is more useful in defining the most severe end of the spectrum (Rehm et al., 2019).

The new broad-spectrum diagnosis of AUD DSM-5 fits better with the risk-based assessment of drinking behaviour adopted by the UK Chief Medical Officers' (2016) and removes any need for a diagnosis of dependency to access services. There is no doubt that some people have a physiological dependency on alcohol that they develop over time and there is evidence that some people are more susceptible to becoming dependent than others (Grant et al., 2009; Kalsi et al., 2009; Barr et al., 2010). Alcohol interacts with neurotransmitter systems, which reinforces drinking behaviour through their influence on the positive outcomes from drinking—feeling euphoric, relaxed, etc. Individuals differ greatly in their neurophysiological and psychological responses to alcohol and therefore in their risk of developing a dependency. However, most people who drink more alcohol than is healthy do not become dependent drinkers. In 2001, Orton reported that 7.5% of men and 2.1% of women in Britain in the 1990s could be classified as having a clinical dependency on alcohol. Eight years later McManus et al. (2009) reported that 8.7% of men and 3.3% of women could be classified as being dependent on alcohol, indicating a slight increase in dependency levels. Interestingly, they also report that levels of dependency in young men (aged between 16 and 24) who have the highest dependency levels in the population had dropped from 11.5% in 2000 to 9.3% in 2007. In 2014, Drummond et al. estimated that the proportion of adults drinking at harmful or dependent levels was 3.6% and highest in young men (aged between 16 and 24) at 6.6%. Alcohol dependency in the UK appeared to be reducing, even acknowledging the differing ways it can be measured and estimated. However, somewhat worryingly in 2021 the UK Government reported that there were 602,391 adults with alcohol dependency in need of specialist treatment in 2018–2019. This is a rise of 2.6% and the first time these estimates have risen since 2015–2016 (Office for Health Improvement and Disparities, 2021). Perhaps most worrying is that only 18% of adults in need of specialist treatment were receiving it (Office for Health Improvement and Disparities, 2021).

Significant public health messaging should mean that most people recognise the health consequences of moderate, volitional drinking (Dixon et al., 2015). However, in 2022 Seidenberg, Weisman and Klein reported that more than 50% of U.S adults reported not knowing how alcohol affected cancer risk. UK surveys show similar low levels of accuracy in understanding the broad health risks from alcohol consumption (Public Health England, 2016). Epidemiological studies have made it clear that there are a host of problems related to drinking that are not associated with excessive or dependent drinking, including the well understood increased risk of developing liver disease, cancer, cardiovascular disease, and a range of other chronic diseases (Rehm et al., 2009; French & Zavala, 2007, Seidenberg et al., 2022, WHO, 2018). Furthermore, intoxication is a major factor in many social problems such as disorderly behaviour, violence, and crime. Intoxication is possible without dependence (Babor et al., 2010). Alcohol related deaths in the UK rose for the first time in 2 decades, rising 20% in England and Wales between 2019 and 2020 to the highest annual total since 2001(Office of National Statistics, 2021).

Applying this to Olivia

Based on the UK Chief Medical Officers Guidelines (2016), it is likely that Olivia would be considered as someone who is drinking at a level that will increase her risk of harm (UK Chief Medical Officers' Guidelines, 2016) but she is unlikely to meet any criteria for dependency.

Whilst less than half of the world's adults consumed alcohol in 2017 the global burden of disease caused by its harmful use is significant (WHO, 2018). Across the UK nations the measurement of alcohol consumption is not consistent with England and Wales using the new low risk, increased and high-risk categories whilst Scotland continues to use sensible, hazardous, and harmful definitions. In 2019, 19% of adults in England and Wales reported drinking at levels that put them at increased risk with 4% drinking at high risk levels of above 35 units a week for women or 50 units a week for men (Health Survey for England, 2020; Welsh Health Survey, 2020). In Scotland, 24% of adults reported drinking at hazardous or harmful levels with men twice as likely to be drinking at this level compared to women (Scottish Health Survey, 2020). Self-report is known to be inaccurate, and people are generally understood to be optimistic about lifestyle behaviours, underestimating drinking and overestimating fruit and vegetable consumption (Scottish Government, 2011).

Age-related patterns of drinking have changed over the last decade in the UK. People aged between 16 and 24 were previously the most likely to be drinking (Welsh Government, 2011; Scottish Government, 2011; Department of Health, Social Services and Public Safety, 2011; Department of Health, 2010). However, in 2019 the proportion of young adults drinking alcohol was 74% compared to 85% of 55 to 74-year-olds. The pattern of alcohol consumption being highest in the middle aged is mirrored across the UK (Health Survey for England, 2020; Welsh Health Survey, 2020; Health Survey (NI) 2021; Scottish Health Survey, 2020). If this generation of 16 to 24-year-olds maintain their drinking patterns as a cohort they may experience fewer alcohol related health conditions as they age.

Men drink more alcohol than women and remain more likely to exceed government recommended guidelines particularly now the guidelines for low-risk drinking are the same for men and women. In 2006/7, concerns were articulated in about the increasing levels of drinking in young British women compared to previous generations (Plant and Plant, 2006; HM Government, 2007; News, 2007). Emslie et al. (2009) reported, in their cross-sectional study of 3 generations from the West of Scotland, that across the generations the youngest cohort had had the smallest difference between levels of drinking in men and women. In 2019, McCaul et al. reported that the gender gap was closing with a decline in young men drinking heavily and an increase in younger women drinking heavily. However, the most recent surveys in England, Wales and Scotland do not show any significant trend of women consuming more alcohol over time (Health Survey for England, 2020; Welsh Health Survey, 2020; Health Survey (NI) 2021; Scottish Health Survey, 2020). Drinking patterns are fluid and subject to a myriad of physiological, psychological cultural and economic influences which makes the picture of gender-related drinking in the UK difficult to interpret.

There is some evidence in the UK that drinking levels are reducing, particularly in younger people (Health Survey for England, 2020; Welsh Health Survey, 2020; Health Survey (NI) 2021; Scottish Health Survey, 2020). However, too many people still drink more than is healthy. Even in England and Wales, where the lowest levels of drinking in the UK are reported, about 1/5 of men report drinking over the weekly recommended units and for men in Scotland that proportion is closer to ¼ (Table 7.1). In 2016, Public Health England reported that over 10 million people in the UK were drinking at levels that increased their risk of health harm (Public Health England, 2016).

Table 7.1 Drinking prevalence rates in men and women in the UK

Source of data	% of men reporting exceeding weekly limits	% of women reporting exceeding weekly limits
Health Survey for England 2019: Adult health-related behaviours (Health Survey for England, 2020) England 2012	30%	15%
Scottish Health Survey, 2019 (Scottish Health Survey, 2020)	32%	16%
National Survey for Wales 2019/20. (Welsh Health Survey, 2020)	25%	14%
Health Survey (NI): First results 2020/21 (Health Survey (NI), 2021)	No data on proportion drinking above weekly guidelines	No data on proportion drinking above weekly guidelines

Applying this to Olivia

Olivia thinks it is acceptable for her to drink above the government guidelines and has not yet reduced her drinking as she ages. She does acknowledge that she should reduce her drinking if she were to become pregnant. The average age of pregnancy has risen considerably, so if pregnancy does trigger a reduction in drinking in women it will be coming far later for the current generation of women.

Hurcombe et al. (2010) reviewed the research on alcohol and ethnicity in the UK since 1995 and concluded that, despite diversity within and between different groups, most UK minority ethnic groups had higher levels of abstinence and lower levels of drinking than those reported by white people living in the UK. In particular abstinence is high in people from Muslim groups. In the most recent survey in 2014, white British people were still more likely to drink at high levels than all other ethnic groups (Institute of Alcohol Studies, 2020). What is concerning is that when people from these generally abstinent groups do drink, they tend to drink heavily; these groups have similar levels of alcohol dependency and are less likely to seek support and advice from professionals for their drinking (Hurcombe et al., 2010; Institute of Alcohol Studies, 2020). In some minority ethnic groups, being in a high-income group is associated with lower likelihood of abstinence and higher levels of drinking. It is possible that drinking is under-reported in some young people and women from ethnic minorities where their drinking is proscribed (Hurcombe et al., 2010).

Socio-economic effects on patterns of drinking reverse the trends seen in smoking which is more common in lower income households. In England the proportions of men and women who reported drinking over 14 units of alcohol weekly increased with household income and was 44% in the highest income groups compared to 22% in the lowest income households (Health Survey for England, 2020). The pattern was similar in Wales, Scotland, and Northern Ireland although they used area of deprivation rather than income to measure socio-economic impact on drinking patterns (Welsh Health Survey, 2020; Health Survey (NI) 2021; Scottish Health Survey, 2020). These differences appear to be caused by drinking at increased risk/hazardous levels rather than high risk/harmful drinking levels. Abstinence is highest in the lowest income & most deprived groups (Health Survey for England, 2020; Welsh Health Survey, 2020; Health Survey (NI), 2021; Scottish Health Survey, 2020). However, despite these patterns' alcohol-related mortality is considerably higher (3 to 8-fold higher in some age groups) in the most deprived areas.

Government recommendations

Low risk drinking

Since 2016 the Chief Medical Officers' guidelines for both men and women are that:

- *To keep health risks from alcohol to a low level it is safest not to drink more than 14 units a week on a regular basis.*
- *If you regularly drink as much as 14 units per week, it is best to spread your drinking evenly over 3 or more days. If you have one or two heavy drinking episodes a week, you increase your risks of death from long term illness and from accidents and injuries.*
- *The risk of developing a range of health problems (including cancers of the mouth, throat, and breast) increases the more you drink on a regular basis.*
- *If you wish to cut down the amount you drink, a good way to help achieve this is to have several drink-free days each week.*

(UK Chief Medical Officers, 2016, pg 4)

This return to weekly guidelines of 14 units a week for men and women reflect the government view that daily guidelines are not useful as most adults do not drink every day.

Single occasion drinking episodes

The Chief Medical Officers' advice for men and women who wish to keep their short-term health risks from single occasion drinking episodes to a low level is to reduce them by:

- *Limiting the total amount of alcohol you drink on any single occasion.*
- *Drinking more slowly, drinking with food, and alternating with water*
- *Planning ahead to avoid problems e.g., by making sure you can get home safely or that you have people you trust with you.*

(UK Chief Medical Officers, 2016, pg 6)

Although the new guidelines do not set a single episode limit (which they did previously) they comment that the risks of injury to a person have been found to increase by two and five times when 5–7 units are drunk in a 3–6-hour period. However, it must be acknowledged that many individuals would not consider 6–8 units in an evening to constitute binge drinking, particularly if it doesn't result in them feeling particularly drunk (Plant & Plant, 2006). On the other hand, more than 6 or 8 units are enough to significantly increase your risk of cardiovascular events (O'Keefe et al., 2007).

Trends in binge drinking are usually identified in surveys by measuring those drinking over 6 units a day for women or 8 units a day for men. In practice, many binge drinkers are drinking substantially more than this level or drink this amount rapidly, which leads to the harm linked to drunkenness.

(HM Government, 2007, p. 3)

Applying this to Olivia

In common with many other people, Olivia considers the government recommendations for single episode drinking to be rather stringent and probably erring on the side of caution.

Consequences of Drinking

Social consequences of drinking

People under the influence of alcohol are more likely to be aggressive and behave violently, hurting other people and themselves (HM Government, 2007, 2012; Hughes et al., 2007; Room et al., 2005; Plant & Plant, 2006). In 2014–2016 in England and Wales, alcohol-related violent incidents made up 67% of all violent incidents that took place at the weekend and 68% of those which took place in the evening and at night (Alcohol Change UK accessed, 2022). In 2007, the HM Government (2007) reported that amongst young people who binge drink a quarter become involved in anti-social or disorderly behaviour (HM Government, 2007; McManus et al., 2009). In 2012, the HM Government recognised the role that 'preloading' plays in binge drinking and anti-social behaviour. Individuals who drink before going out were found to be four times more likely to drink in excess of 20 units on one night out and 2.5 times more likely to have been involved in a fight (HM Government, 2012; Hughes et al., 2007). Lower socioeconomic groups experience higher prevalence rates of all forms of alcohol related violence, including domestic and acquaintance violence and anti-social behaviour despite lower proportions of drinking alcohol (Bryant & Lightowlers, 2021). Drinking also has the potential to make people more vulnerable to crime (Nicolas et al., 2008; Bryant & Lightowlers, 2021).

People who are intoxicated are also more likely to have accidents. 29% of all alcohol-attributable deaths are caused by unintentional accidents (Drinkaware accessed, 2022). 21.9% of car accidents worldwide are alcohol related (Vissers et al., 2018). In the UK in 2019, 5% of road casualties and 13% of all road fatalities occurred when someone was drink-driving (Department of Transport, 2021). In the UK, where drink-driving laws are relatively stringent, from 1980 to 2019 the number of people killed or seriously injured annually in drink-driving incidents fell from 9,000 to 2,050, which is a significant reduction in alcohol-related incidents. However, the number of people killed or seriously injured in drink-driving incidents over the past 10 years has stabilised and new strategies to reduce such unnecessary fatalities are warranted (Department of Transport, 2021).

Health consequences of drinking

Alcohol has been found to increase the risk of over 60 medical conditions including mouth, throat, stomach, liver and breast cancers, high blood pressure, cirrhosis of the liver and depression (Room et al., 2005). The relationship between alcohol consumption and cardiovascular health is not linear; it is J-shaped with those who drink no alcohol appearing to have a greater risk of alcohol-related death than moderate drinkers (Public Health England, 2016). This has led to a widely held belief that moderate drinking is good for health. However, more recent research has demonstrated that any potential protective effects seem mainly relevant to older age groups, particularly women, with the peak of any protective effect achieved at very low levels of consumption, no more than 1 unit a day (Holmes et al., 2016). Often it is the pattern of drinking that is important. Heavy episodic drinking has been linked to an increased risk of coronary heart disease, stroke, and diabetes even when the overall volume of alcohol intake is low (Room et al., 2005; O'Keefe et al., 2007; Piano et al., 2017). The J-shaped relationship between drinking and total mortality illustrates that people who drink a small amount of alcohol each week have the lowest mortality rates (lower than adults reporting no drinking at the point of asking) rising steadily as alcohol intake increases. It is important to recognise that people who state they drink nothing are not a homogeneous group; they include former drinkers, occasional drinkers and people who have never consumed alcohol (Figure 7.3). Whilst the validity of the J-shaped curve is not in question the reasons for the curve are hotly contested and the debate about whether moderate drinking is

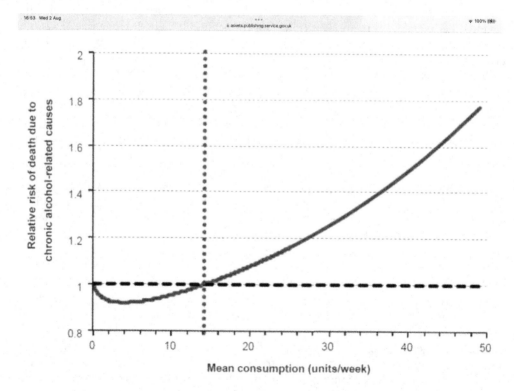

Figure 7.3 The relationship between average weekly alcohol consumption and the risk of dying from a chronic alcohol related disease: Taken from Public Health England, 2016.

protective or whether moderate drinking is a confounding factor that is masking other causal factors in health outcomes continues (Oppenheimer & Bayer, 2020).

In some diseases a linear relationship between alcohol consumption and disease does exist. Breast cancer risk increases linearly with increased alcohol consumption. Compared to zero consumption any level of alcohol consumption is associated with an increased risk with 10 grams of alcohol a day increasing the relative risk of breast cancer by 9%. A daily consumption of between 30 and 60 grams a day increases the relative risk by 41% (Chen et al., 2011; Public Health England, 2016).

Mental health is adversely impacted by alcohol. Depression, epilepsy, and alcohol addiction can all be caused by excessive drinking (Room et al., 2005; Balakrishnan et al., 2009; HM Government, 2007; Plant and Plant, 2006; Public Health England, 2016). Furthermore, drinking can make existing psychological conditions such as depression or anxiety worse.

The disorders most people think of as being caused by alcohol are liver diseases, and liver disease is responsible for 86% of directly attributable mortality from alcohol in the UK. The rate of hospital admissions due to alcoholic liver disease has risen continuously since 1970 (Public Health England, 2016). In 2001, there were 9,231 deaths from liver diseases and in 2020 there were 10,127, a rise of over 20%. Although not all these deaths are alcohol related, alcoholic liver disease is the most common cause of liver disease death (Effiong et al., 2012; Public Health England, 2016).

In England and Wales, alcohol-related injury or illness admissions have been steadily increasing and have accounted for over 1 million admissions in 2014/15, of which for more than 300,000 alcohol was the main reason for admission (Public Health England, 2016). In 2020 there were 8,974 alcohol-related deaths (14 per 100,000) in the UK an 18.6% increase compared with 2019. Since 1991, alcohol-related deaths have increased from 6.9% to 14.0% per 100,000 (Office of National Statistics, 2021). A summary of hospital admissions by disease and injury conditions related to alcohol is presented in Figure 7.4.

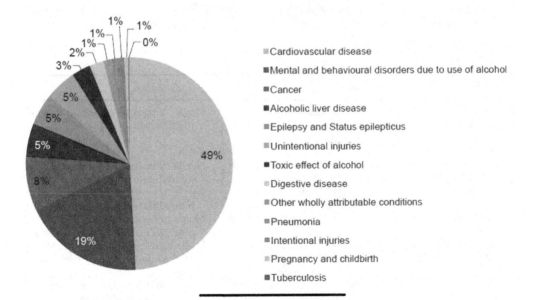

Figure 7.4 The percentage of hospital admissions by disease, injury or condition in 2014/15. Taken from: Public Health England (2016).

One area of concern is the number of people living with chronic diseases who regularly drink above the sensible drinking guidelines. Many people with diseases such as diabetes, coronary heart disease and hypertension where alcohol is implicated in the aetiology and progression of the disease continue to drink beyond their diagnosis (Pham et al., 2019).

Assessment of Drinking

Population levels of drinking can be estimated from per capita consumption, which is basically an estimate of all the alcohol produced (minus all alcohol exports) and imported into a country divided by the number of adults living there. Per capita consumption is a crude measure that is useful for international comparisons and for monitoring population consumption over time. However, it tells us little about who is drinking within that population or anything about how they drink. Collecting data from individuals provides more useful information about drinking. Physiological measures such as a urine test provide an objective measure of alcohol levels and some indication about drunkenness, but individual differences in alcohol tolerance will influence the levels of drunkenness displayed. Surveys are probably both the most common and also the most problematic way to collect data about drinking. Surveys can tell us a lot about who is drinking and about patterns and volume of consumption. Surveys facilitate comparisons over time providing a useful way of evaluating the effectiveness of alcohol intervention strategies. However, non-response bias is a potential problem for drinking surveys, which usually achieve response rates of about 60%. It is plausible that the types of people who do not complete surveys about drinking are different in their drinking from the types of people who do complete surveys, and this introduces a serious bias. Furthermore, it is well established that people completing surveys about their drinking tend to underestimate the amount of alcohol that they consume (Plant & Plant, 2006; Public Health England, 2016). Nevertheless, survey estimates of alcohol consumption predict alcohol-related conditions, which suggest that they do at least place people in an appropriate place in the drinking continuum (Room et al., 2005). A summary of the strategies available to measure drinking is provided in Table 7.2.

Table 7.2 Methods to measure drinking

Method	Advantages	Disadvantages
Per capita consumption	Enables international comparisons and monitoring of population drinking over time	Crude, subject to error and fails to identify who is drinking
Breathalyser tests	An objective, acute measure of alcohol levels	Needs to be immediate, gives only limited data about drunkenness
Urine tests	An objective, acute measure of alcohol levels	Needs to be immediate, gives only limited data about drunkenness
Blood samples	An objective, acute measure of alcohol levels	Needs to be immediate, gives only limited data about drunkenness
Questionnaire surveys of drinking habits	A quick and easy way of accessing data from a large sample. Can provide information about drinking patterns over time	Prone to response biases. People tend to underestimate their drinking in surveys. Response rates to drinking surveys are usually about 60%, so information cannot be said to be representative

(*Continued*)

Table 7.2 (Continued)

Method	Advantages	Disadvantages
Interviews about drinking habits	Provides in-depth data about drinking habits	Prone to response biases. Not practical for large-scale surveys
Direct Observation	Free from response biases. Unlikely to provide data about drinking patterns over time	Difficult to achieve reliable results in drinking situations. Not practical for large-scale surveys

---

Applying this to Olivia

It would be possible to get an accurate measure of how much Olivia drank at any one point by taking a blood sample whilst she was drunk. However, this is not likely to occur unless she is arrested. Asking Olivia to self-report on her drinking is likely to be biased as she may well adapt her answers to reflect what she knows are recommended drinking levels.

Why do people drink more alcohol than is sensible?

People in the UK and many other countries have always drunk alcohol, sometimes sensibly and sometimes not, so fundamentally nothing has changed. Overall, the majority of adults drink at least occasionally, and most people drink moderately with few harmful effects. There are many reasons why people drink: because they enjoy the taste, because they like the disinhibiting effects of alcoholic drinks and because consuming them is a sociable thing to do in their culture (HM Government, 2012; WHO, 2018). Young people often start to drink as part of their transition into adulthood (Measham & Ostergaard, 2011). In the UK, drinking is a symbolic behaviour that facilitates social bonding and peer status in adolescents. Some authors have argued that alcohol can provide young people with a seemingly adult status (Paglia & Room, 1999) In 2010, Kuntsche and Copper reported that enhancement motives (seeking fun and excitement) predict weekend drinking behaviour in young people more than other psychosocial factors. However, in 2021 MacLean et al. reported that in many Western countries including Australia, the UK, Nordic Countries and North America young people have, on average, been drinking less than their parents did at a similar age. MacLean et al. (2021) suggest that uncertainty and worry about the future, concerns about health, changes to technology and leisure and shifting relationships with parents have influenced these changes to drinking behaviours in young people. Somewhat controversially Maclean et al. (2021) suggest that declining alcohol consumption in young people may have more to do with the wider context of their lives than any policies that their governments may have implemented.

Despite a reduction in young people drinking the majority do still drink alcohol and it continues to serve an important social function in many people's lives. It enhances social integration and facilitates the development of relationships (Kuther & Timoshin, 2003). It is hardly surprising that people start to drink at a period in their lives which is normally associated with the development of stable adult relationships (Paglia & Room, 1999). Increased levels of drinking in newly divorced people may in part be due to the breakdown of stable relationships and the desire to establish new relationships (HM Government, 2007). Social isolation is a key factor in poor health outcomes (York et al.,

2009). Alcohol can be argued to have a positive social function of enabling people to develop social relationships in some cultures.

Applying this to Olivia

Olivia started to drink a lot at University, where she felt that drinking enabled her to make friends and cope with the transition from adolescence to adulthood.

Socio-economic factors

The relationship between socio-economic factors and drinking is not simple. There is increasing evidence that people living in deprivation are more likely to binge drink, develop alcohol dependency and die from conditions caused by excessive drinking even though regular consumption at levels above the recommended limits is more likely in people from higher socio-economic groups (Craig & Mindell, 2008; Welsh Assembly Government, 2009). This has led to what has been called the 'alcohol harm paradox' whereby disadvantaged populations who drink the same or lower levels of alcohol, experience greater alcohol-related harm than more affluent populations (Public Health England, 2016, Probst et al., 2020). Explanations for this paradox include more heavy episodic drinking (Craig & Mindell, 2008; Probst et al., 2020), lower resilience and/or compounding effects with other risk factors prevalent in lower socio-economic groups (Katikireddi et al., 2017) and differential access to health services. However, Angus et al. (2019) found that people from lower socio-economic groups were more likely to report having received a brief intervention for drinking. Given the evidence that patterns of heavy episodic drinking play a role in the alcohol harm paradox it is a concern that the UK government no longer provides guidelines for amount of alcohol that can be 'safely' consumed in a single episode of drinking (Probst et al., 2020).

Applying this to Olivia

Olivia is one of the new generation of professional women who drinks at risky levels, illustrating that excess drinking, unlike smoking, is common in higher socio-economic groups.

Psychological factors

Many different psychological factors have been used to explain why people drink. Initially, it was believed that educating people about the risks of excessive alcohol consumption would change their behaviour. However, similarly to other lifestyle behaviours, there is little evidence that perceptions of risk can explain much if any of the variation in drinking behaviour (Moss et al., 2009; Gray et al., 2021). Nevertheless the World Health Organisation WHO 2010) continues to recommend that public policy on alcohol should ensure that there is:

broad access to information and effective education and public awareness pro-grammes among all levels of society about the full range of alcohol-related harm

Whilst providing information and education may not directly change health behaviour the WHO (2010) believe it is the right of individuals to understand the consequences of alcohol consumption regardless of whether it results in a change of behaviour. Furthermore, it may influence public opinion and help the adoption of more stringent and effective policies for alcohol consumption.

In the first 2 decades of the twenty-first century a number of social cognitive variables were identified as predicting alcohol use. Kuther and Timoshin (2003) found that self-efficacy for controlling drinking predicted self-reported drinking. Those who believed they could control their drinking drank less. Gilles et al. (2006) demonstrated that alcohol expectancies and self-efficacy are related to drinking behaviour. Williams et al. (2007) found that self-efficacy was a key factor in predicting improved drinking habits in individuals identified as drinking unhealthily in the primary care setting. Similarly, Murgraff et al. (2007) found that improving self-efficacy for the ability to control their drinking resulted in a reduction in binge drinking in young women. However, the mechanisms by which self-efficacy can be improved have proved hard to establish. Increasingly, evidence demonstrate that coping skills are key mechanisms in successful cognitive behavioural therapy and consequently, increases in self-efficacy which arise from achieving a positive change in drinking behaviours (Magill et al., 2020).

Applying this to Olivia

As a woman working in an industry with a culture of drinking Olivia may not feel able to refuse a drink when she is out with clients and colleagues.

Social norms have been consistently related to drinking behaviour (Norman et al., 2019). Studies that report strong relationships between social norms and drinking behaviour ask individuals how much they think their peers are drinking (descriptive norms). Kuther and Timoshin (2003) looked at both descriptive peer norms and descriptive parental norms and found that both were associated with levels of drinking in students, although the relationship was stronger for peer norms. The impact of descriptive social norms represented through virtual social networks rather than traditional social networks has also been demonstrated (see Box 7.1). It is clear that for young people at least we establish what is typical and appropriate group normative behaviour from both actual and virtual interactions (Litt & Stock, 2011). Both Mcalaney et al. (2007) and Bertholet et al. (2011) have demonstrated that college students typically overestimate the amount of alcohol consumed by their peers. Similarly, in the workplace the descriptive drinking norms within that organisation and among colleagues were strongly associated with drinking behaviours both within and outside the working environment (Barrientos-Gutierrez et al., 2007). The relationship between perceptions of peer drinking norms and individual drinking has influenced interventions to reduce drinking. An individual could overestimate the acceptability of drinking among his or her peers or may underestimate the practice of health behaviours (Ramos & Perkins, 2006). Consequently, a number of interventions have attempted to challenge individual

---

Box 7.1   Applying research in practice

Adolescent Alcohol-Related Risk Cognitions: The Roles of Social Norms and Social Networking Sites (Litt & Stock, 2011)

This paper examined the impact of socially based descriptive norms on willingness to drink alcohol, prototype favourability, perceived vulnerability for alcohol related consequence, and affective-based attitudes towards alcohol use.

Descriptive norms were manipulated by having 189 young adolescents view experimenter-created profile pages from the social networking site Facebook, which either showed older peers drinking or not.

Findings found that Facebook profiles portraying alcohol use as normative among older peers significantly impacted on willingness to use, attitudes towards use, and perceived vulnerability.

The authors concluded that adolescents who perceive that alcohol use is normative, as evidenced by Facebook profiles, are at higher risk for cognitions shown to predict alcohol use than adolescents who do not see alcohol use portrayed as frequently on Facebook. This research is important because it demonstrates how perceptions of peer normative behaviour are influenced by virtual social networks, at least in young people. Young people who use social network sites will usually be 'friends' with a far larger number of individuals than they regularly interact with in 'real' settings.

---

perceptions of normative drinking behaviours amongst their peers and have met with some success (Ramos & Perkins, 2006; Delong et al., 2006).

The evidence that understanding stage of change is useful or important in changing drinking behaviours is not conclusive with some authors arguing that the Transtheoretical model of behavioural change cannot help in predicting drinking behaviour (Callaghan et al., 2007; Williams et al., 2007). Williams et al. (2007) found that measures of readiness to change did not predict either future heavy episodic drinking or future overall consumption in 312 primary care patients who drank unhealthily. They found that self-efficacy for controlled drinking predicted lower consumption and less heavy episodic drinking and concluded that interventions that support self-efficacy, such as motivational interviewing, might have greater utility than stage-based interventions for promoting behavioural change in people who drink unhealthily. Conversely, Heather et al. (2009) and Schulz et al. (2012) found some evidence that different factors are relevant for individuals at different stages of change. In particular, Schulz et al. (2012) found that participants in the action stage of change reported higher self-efficacy across social, emotional, and routine self-efficacy measures.

Since the second edition of this book interest has increased exponentially in mindfulness-based interventions for a range of psychiatric conditions including alcohol use disorder (Sancho et al., 2018). Mindfulness has been described as paying attention in the present moment without judgement. The core goal of programmes such as mindfulness-based relapse prevention programmes across a range of behaviours such as drinking, gambling, etc., is to cultivate an understanding of internal (emotions) and external (environmental) cues related to the behaviour (Schwebel et al., 2020). The intention is to create opportunities to address triggering situations rather than instinctively reacting to them. Cognitive behavioural therapies focus on reduction of the occurrence or the intensity of craving emotions whereas mindfulness approaches don't aim to dispel or alter craving thoughts or feelings but focus on attending to the cravings so that the individual can learn about their usual tendency to respond reflexively to urges. One suggestion is that through developing this understanding the link between feelings of craving and behaviour becomes increasingly conscious and under the control of intention (Kamboj et al., 2017). There is some evidence that mindfulness can be as effective as cognitive behavioural therapy and motivational interviewing in changing volitional drinking behaviours (Byrne et al., 2019) but all authors recognise that the evidence is weak and further research is needed. Mindfulness interventions appear to be linked to reduced craving and reductions in co-morbidities such as anxiety, depression and stress that can be associated with relapse (Cavicchioli et al., 2018).

Many different alcohol interventions have been found to be effective to some degree with no one approach, motivational, social cognitive or mindfulness consistently more effective than any other. This may reflect that many interventions include elements of a number of different approaches. NICE in their 2011 guideline (National Collaborating Centre for Mental Health, 2011, updated 2022) acknowledge the pivotal role of the therapist/health practitioner delivering the intervention to its success. The social support element that is inherent in all interventions is a key factor in the change process, the therapeutic alliance, collaborative care visits, and non-judgemental ongoing relationships with health practitioners can all provide a catalyst for change that supports effective change across different types of interventions (Glass et al., 2017; National Collaborating Centre for Mental Health, 2011 – updated 2022).

In conclusion, there is some evidence that social cognitive factors can predict sensible drinking in populations. In particular, social norms, measured as descriptive social norms, are important in understanding drinking behaviour. As with other lifestyle behaviours, risk perception appears to have little or no value in predicting drinking behaviour. Similarly to other lifestyle behaviours, the role of self-efficacy in promoting drinking behavioural change looks promising and increasingly the mechanism of coping skills, and supportive relationships appear to be critical elements of many different interventions for sensible drinking. Mindfulness techniques have become popular in behavioural change interventions, including alcohol management but their role within a toolkit of alcohol use control interventions is still to be established.

Applying this to Olivia

The social norms in Olivia's workplace clearly support her current drinking behaviours and currently she is not motivated to try and change her habitual drinking patterns.

Interventions to reduce drinking

The Nuffield Council on Bioethics (2007) have argued that public health policies should be about enforcement, and they propose an 'intervention ladder' as a useful way of conceptualising public health interventions and their impact on an individual's choice (Table 7.3).

Table 7.3 The intervention ladder: Adapted from Nuffield Council on Bioethics (2007)

Level	Description	Drinking example
Eliminate choice	Introduce laws that entirely eliminate choice	Prohibition
Restrict choice	Introduce laws that restrict the options available to people	Remove alcohol from supermarkets
Guide through disincentives	Introduce financial or other disincentives to influence behaviour	Increase taxes of alcohol via taxation
Guide through incentives	Introduce financial or other incentives to influence people's behaviour	Fund alcohol-free events
Guide choices	Change the default policy	Recommend sensible levels of alcohol consumption
Enable choice	Help individuals to change their behaviour	Provide drinking cessation schemes

Until recently, for drinking, current government policies have been firmly focused on strategies from the final two rows of the table, guiding choices and enabling choices, although certain limited strategies from higher in the table, such as taxation on alcohol and limited legal restrictions on drinking in some contexts (driving), have been in place for some time. However, the latest government alcohol strategy (HM Government, 2012) does commit to tackling the availability of cheap alcohol by introducing a minimum unit price (MUP) which is believed by many practitioners to be (if set high enough) a highly cost-effective strategy to reduce harm from alcohol (Anderson et al., 2009; Wagenaarr et al., 2009; Public Health England, 2016). Public Health England (2016) suggest that MUP is a highly targeted measure which ensures tax increases are passed on to the consumer and improves the health of the heaviest drinkers who are experiencing the greatest amount of harm. A minimum price of 50 pence per unit of alcohol has been implemented in Wales and Scotland but not in England (Woodhouse, 2020). There is limited evidence as yet of the impact of MUP on drinking behaviour, although Public Health England (2016) have suggested that the 50 pence per unit may be too low to have a significant impact.

Many interventions to encourage sensible drinking are aimed at adolescents and young people with the goal of preventing the establishment of unhealthy drinking habits. There is an assumption that 'bad leads to bad' as studies indicate that alcohol misuse in adolescence places individuals at increased risk for adult alcohol abuse and related problems (Byrnes et al., 2019; Fiellin et al., 2013). Although it should be remembered that it only increases the risk, and bad beginnings do not always have bad ends. Many people who experiment with excessive drinking in their youth are not excessive drinkers in their mid-to late 20s (Masten et al., 2008). Nevertheless, it is indisputable that it is in adolescence that drinking begins, so encouraging sensible drinking in this cohort continues to be high on public health agendas.

Individual level interventions

Early drinking interventions

There are a great many school, university and community-based programmes focused on preventing the early onset of drinking and promoting sensible drinking (Anderson et al., 2009). In 2003, Foxcroft et al. reviewed the effectiveness of programmes designed to prevent excessive drinking in young people and, worryingly, found very little evidence that any of these programmes were effective. In 2019, NICE reported that the evidence for targeted alcohol interventions in secondary and further education remained weak but there was enough evidence for them to continue to recommend targeted interventions for young people at risk of alcohol misuse along side universal school-based alcohol education interventions (NICE, 2019).

In line with increased confirmation from genetic studies that certain individuals have an increased genetic risk for developing addictions to alcohol and/or other substances (Barr et al., 2010; Grant et al., 2009; Kalsi et al., 2009), the efficacy of personality-targeted interventions have been investigated (see Box 7.2). It is encouraging to see that initial research indicates that personality targeted interventions may be useful (O'Leary-Barrett et al., 2010; Conrod et al., 2011). However, it also raises ethical issues as the genetic underpinning of these 'at risk personality factors' start to be understood (Barr et al., 2010; Clarke & Thirlaway, 2011; Grant et al., 2009; Kalsi et al., 2009). Dependency and addiction are complex conditions and are multi-factorial, undoubtedly influenced by a number of different genes and also by a range of environmental factors. Genetic risk is highly personal, sensitive, complex, and potentially discriminating information. As we start to understand genetic risk for complex multi factorial behaviours such as drinking alcohol the potential benefits of using such information will have to be carefully considered in light of the considerable costs (Clarke & Thirlaway, 2011). However, the latest evidence suggests that encouraging young people to develop personality-specific coping skills that can be applied across different situations, rather than focusing on alcohol use alone is a less contentious approach to recognising individual differences in young people without linking it to any one specific deleterious behavioural coping strategy (Newton et al., 2022).

Box 7.2   Applying research in practice

Effect of Selective Personality-Targeted Alcohol Use Prevention on 7-year Alcohol-Related Outcomes Among High Risk Adolescents: A Secondary Analysis of a cluster randomised clinical trial (Newton et al., 2022)

A cluster randomised clinical trial evaluated the effectiveness of the personality-targeted PreVenture programme to reduce risky alcohol use through early adolescence to early adulthood. Participants included grade 8 students attending 14 secondary schools across New South Wales and Victoria, Australia in 2012 who screened as having high levels of 1 to 4 personality traits: anxiety sensitivity, negative thinking, impulsivity and sensation seeking. 7 schools were randomised to the PreVenture group and 7 schools to the control group. Whilst the primary study concluded in 2014 this study extended the follow-up period to 7 years post baseline.

The PreVenture intervention is a two session, personality targeted intervention designed to upskill adolescents to cope better with their emotions and behaviours. The impact of the intervention was measured using self-reported monthly binge drinking, alcohol related harms and hazardous alcohol use using the Alcohol Use Disorders Identification Test-Concise Consumption Screener.

This study is particularly important because it followed up on the short-term impact to see what the longer-term benefits of the intervention were for participants. 54% of the original participants participated in the 7-year follow-up. It is difficult to retain participants in longitudinal research and this level of drop out is comparable to other studies. However, it does require caution in interpretation of the findings. The 54% of young people who were available for the follow-up evaluation may not be representative of the whole group. Nevertheless, it is impressive that a 2-session intervention was still associated with reduced odds of any alcohol related harm and a greater mean reduction in the frequency of alcohol-related harms at the 7-year follow-up. The findings of an earlier exploratory analysis suggest that PreVenture was effective in reducing annual odds of monthly binge drinking and hazardous alcohol use from the 5.5-year follow-up, but this was not sustained 7 years on when participants had reached early adulthood.

This is an important study because it has such a long follow-up period and suggests that encouraging young people to develop generic personality-specific coping skills, rather than focusing on alcohol alone can provide a scalable intervention to reduce alcohol harm in adolescents that continues to impact through to early adulthood. This supports the continued investment into evidence-based prevention programmes in schools.

Family-based interventions

There have been some promising family-based interventions in the US, including the Iowa Strengthening Families (ISF) Programme and the Preparing for Drug Free Years (PDFY) Programme (Spoth et al., 2004). Both programmes aimed to develop prosocial bonds within the family and coping skills of the adolescent. Spoth et al. (2004) reported that both interventions delayed the initiation of drinking and reduced current use compared to the control group and that these differences persisted for four years past baseline. The different legal position and promotion of abstinence until 21 in the US compared to the promotion of sensible drinking in the UK may mean that successful strategies in the US may not be successful in the UK. In 2019, Gilligan et al. carried out a systematic review of 46 studies of family-based interventions based in the US or European countries for alcohol use in young people and found no clear benefits for these programmes over standard care or individual interventions. They concluded that the heterogeneity of the studies prevent any conclusions about intervention effects and additional studies are required to strengthen the evidence and clarify the marginal effects observed to date. Percy et al. (2011) suggest in their report for the Joseph Rowntree Foundation that parental attempts to restrict teenagers' contact with alcohol are seldom effective, although the parental attempts they describe are pre-dominantly around injunctive norms, i.e., the setting of rules and expectations. Interestingly in the Joseph Rowntree Foundation report, the most effective parental strategy was not to drink or to drink very little themselves (Percy et al., 2011). In this way the Rowntree study supports the growing body of literature which suggests that injunctive norms and expectations about what is acceptable drinking behaviour do not influence drinking, whereas descriptive norms (what people believe their peers or influential others are actually drinking) are important. Whilst adolescents are living at home their parents will form part of their regular social circle and provide evidence about what is acceptable drinking for their children. Care is needed to identify the mechanism of interventions, given the many programmes that fail to deliver long-term change. It would seem that increasing the skills of young people and improving their social support networks are key to enabling them to avoid or resist peer pressure to take up drinking.

Student interventions

In 2007, Carey et al. published a review of individual-level interventions to reduce college student drinking which included 62 studies and nearly 14,000 participants. They reported that participants in risk reduction interventions drank significantly less relative to controls over follow-up intervals of up to 6 months. Whilst this is a review of a very specific group of young people it is nevertheless very positive that interventions to reduce drinking in this group, where drinking is endemic, can reduce the amount of alcohol consumed. The review indicates that individual, face-to-face interventions using motivational interviewing and personalised normative feedback result in the greatest reductions in alcohol-related problems. However, interventions to reduce heavy episodic drinking that is a common behaviour in students have proven less successful. Norman et al. (2019) found that although Theory of Planned Behaviour-based messages about heavy episodic drinking reduced student intentions to drink heavily, it did not influence their actual behaviour.

Face-to-face individualised interventions are a resource intensive intervention and young people do not often seek help for their drinking behaviour (Bewick et al., 2010). The internet has the potential to provide some level of personalised feedback and interaction whilst being a less resource intensive intervention. It may also be a more acceptable way for young people to look for help with their drinking. A multi-centred study in four universities in the UK demonstrated that web-based interventions for student drinking can be effective (Bewick et al., 2010). In this instance, similarly to the study with adolescents described in Box 7.1, the intervention was based in social normative theory with participants receiving both personalised feedback and social norms information. Interestingly, the control group in this study were monitored on their drinking without receiving the intervention but their drinking still reduced. This indicates that monitoring has an impact on drinking, possibly because it encourages self-regulation (see Chapter 4 for more on self-regulation).

Established drinking interventions

Intervening in primary care is the most common way for behavioural interventions to reach their audience of established drinkers (Mulvihill et al., 2005). In Britain, brief counselling interventions in primary care settings are the most common way that people who volitionally drink too much will receive support (Mulvihill et al., 2005; Public Health England, 2016). However, brief interventions to reduce drinking have also been delivered in accident and emergency departments, criminal justice settings, schools, and pharmacies. It is likely that many people who are clinically dependent on alcohol and who perhaps warrant more intense intervention are also treated in this way, and so the effectiveness of these interventions for volitional drinkers may be underestimated if participants with a serious addictive disorder are included.

Alcohol brief interventions (ABI)

Brief interventions for alcohol use are well researched. They have many advantages. They are acceptable to individuals with less severe drinking problems for whom more intensive treatment would not be acceptable. They can be administered by a wide range of health professionals in many settings and are inexpensive (NICE, 2010). Perhaps most importantly they have consistently been found to reduce hazardous/risky and harmful/ high risk alcohol. The 2018 Cochrane review of 69 ABI studies found that Brief Interventions reduced hazardous and harmful drinking by an average of 20 grams of alcohol/2.5 UK units per week. Brief interventions, although varied have similar theoretical underpinnings in motivation and social cognitive theory (Beyer et al., 2019). They have been described by Moyer et al. (2002) as having the six features in Table 7.4.

Table 7.4 Key features of brief interventions

1	A goal of reduced or non-problem drinking rather than abstinence
2	Delivered by a health professional as opposed to an addiction specialist
3	Directed at volitional rather than dependent drinkers
4	Addressing individuals' level of motivation to change drinking habits
5	Being self (as opposed to professionally) directed, and/or
6	Having the following ingredients: feedback of risk; encouraging responsibility for change; advice; menu of options; therapeutic empathy; enhancing self-efficacy

Importantly, they have a component structure commonly referred to as FRAMES:

Feedback about existing consumption
Responsibility for change
Advice about practical strategies to reduce drinking
Menu of options for behaviour change
Empathic delivery
Self-efficacy building

Brief interventions, while following this basic framework, can vary, and, in particular, the length of a brief intervention, although intuitively short, can range from one 5-minute session to brief multi-contact interventions. Many studies have found that brief interventions can reduce drinking (Nilsen, 2008; Mulvihill et al., 2005; Williams et al., 2007; NICE, 2010; Beyer, 2019, Public Health England, 2016) Mulvihill et al. (2005) in their review conclude that multi-contact brief interventions are more effective than single very brief sessions. However, the 2018 Cochrane review concluded that short advice-based interventions can be as effective as extended counselling based interventions (Beyer, 2019). Most trials reported at 6 or 12 months there was no decay in the impact of the intervention over the first 12 months. However, longer term follow-up would be of value.

Level of motivation derives from the stage of change concept which acknowledges the importance of the individual's motivational state (Table 7.4). Self-efficacy is another key social-cognitive variable which has been consistently found to predict behavioural change. Consequently, the theoretical underpinnings of such an approach are clear. Interestingly, Williams et al. (2007) found that readiness to change did not predict reduction of drinking in their cohort of people identified in primary care as drinking unhealthily, whereas levels of self-efficacy did predict a reduction in drinking. Williams et al. (2007) argue that in the busy primary care setting, formal assessment of readiness to change may not be necessary.

As ABI have become an established method of addressing hazardous and high risk drinking the settings in which the intervention is delivered have started to be considered. NICE encourages and recommends that all appropriate health care professionals should deliver ABI as part of Making Every Contact Count (MECC), an initiative in the NHS to encourage health professionals to raise and address lifestyle issues with their patients (Figure 4.2, Chapter 4) (Public Health England, 2016). In particular, the efficacy of the intervention within accident and emergency departments is being considered (NICE, 2010; Nilsen, 2008). Intervening when individuals are in the NHS as a result of their hazardous drinking may capture more people for whom the intervention is appropriate than is achieved within primary care settings. There is some evidence that intervening with a brief intervention within accident and emergency settings can be effective and reduce drinking levels (Nilsen, 2008). However, the capacity for accident and emergency staff to deliver such brief interventions as a regular part of their role has not been established (NICE, 2010). Other settings that have been explored as suitable for brief interventions for drinking include the workplace (Webb et al., 2009).

Cognitive behavioural therapy

Cognitive behavioural therapy (CBT) remains one of the predominant approaches to the treatment of alcohol use disorders, either directly through CBT counselling or indirectly through CBT-influenced interventions (Magill et al., 2020; Mulvihill et al., 2005, Public Health England, 2016; Longabaugh et al., 2005). There is consistent evidence that CBT is an effective intervention for alcohol use disorders when compared to minimum or no intervention (Longabaugh et al., 2005; Magill et al., 2020; National Collaborating Centre for Mental Health, 2011, updated 2022). CBT is based on the premise that thought distortions and maladaptive behaviours play a role in the development and maintenance of psychological disorders and that symptoms and associated distress can be reduced by teaching new information-processing skills and coping mechanisms. It requires individuals to work collaboratively with a therapist to achieve agreed treatment goals. Whilst the effectiveness of CBT interventions for AUDs is well established the mechanisms by which the therapy works is less clear. Magill et al. (2020) have suggested that changes in self-regulatory coping skills seem to be the most effective change mechanism but that motivation and self-efficacy were clearly involved in the complex change process. Whilst CBT is predominantly a prescribed intervention for high risk/harmful drinking (National Collaborating Centre for Mental Health, 2011, updated 2022) its influence on ABI for less severe drinking behaviours is considerable (Public Health England, 2016).

Mindfulness

The National Collaborating Centre for Mental Health (2011, updated 2022) in their NICE guideline document for harmful drinking conclude that there is very limited evidence that mindfulness interventions are effective for reducing harmful drinking. There is some evidence that mindfulness interventions are useful for co-morbidities such as anxiety or depression that often accompany AUDs. Some reviews suggest there is evidence that mindfulness interventions are better than no treatment and comparable to effective treatments for AUDs (Byrne et al., 2019). Over the last decade, interest, and investment into mindfulness interventions for drinking has been considerable (Cavicchioli et al., 2018; Garland & Howard, 2018). It is possible that mindfulness interventions may be of value for less serious alcohol use disorders, either as a standalone treatment or as an adjunct to other therapies.

Community level interventions

There are certain groups in the UK who would support prohibition and the criminalisation of alcohol (Eliminate or restriction of choice in the intervention ladder, see Table 7.3) but these are a minority voice and there is no likelihood of prohibition becoming policy in the UK. However, alcohol is illegal for certain age groups in various countries. In the US, you cannot legally drink alcohol before you are 21, whereas in the UK you may drink alcohol in private from the age of 5 but may not purchase or drink alcohol in a public place until you are 18. Consequently, some interventions, particularly school-based interventions in the US, have a goal of total abstinence. The rationale for such a stance is not only to limit damaging drinking in young people in the 'here and now' but also to reduce the risk of problem drinking later, because the earlier a person starts to drink, smoke, or use illegal drugs the higher the risk of later abuse (Masten et al., 2008; Skidmore, Juhasz and Sucker, 2011, cited in Saunders and Rey (Eds) 2011). In the UK, where young people are legally allowed to drink before the age of 21, there is more of a problem with binge drinking in young people. However, many countries with equally lax laws about the age of drinking do not report the same incidence of binge drinking that is reported in Britain (HM Government, 2012). Nevertheless, there is evidence that increasing the minimum drinking age in the UK could reduce drinking in young people and importantly delay the onset of drinking. (Kaestner & Yarnoff, 2011.)

Taxation as a public health measure is a familiar practice in smoking (Guidance through disincentives, Table 7.7). It is only effective if people drink less in response to rising price. Some people have argued that it would only be worthwhile to increase taxes if people who are currently drinking hazardously or dangerously drank less in response to the rise in tax. In 1995 Manning et al. (1995) argued that moderate drinkers are more affected by price changes than heavy drinkers so taxation would not decrease the risk of alcohol disorders. However, in 2010, Black, Gill and Chick reported that amongst their cohort of individuals with serious alcohol problems the lower the price paid per unit the more units a patient consumed. In 2016, Public Health England concluded that policies that reduce the affordability of alcohol are the most effective approaches to prevention and health improvement. Wagenaar et al. (2009) also report that price affects drinking across the whole population of drinkers from light drinkers to heavy drinkers. Xu and Chaloupka (2011) suggest that adolescents are particularly responsive to the price of alcohol and that increasing the price of alcohol would be effective in reducing heavy drinking and related harm among this cohort. Research has shown that alcohol taxes in Scotland (and by default elsewhere in the UK) would need to increase by 28% to match the reductions in alcohol-related deaths that even a fairly modest 50 pence minimum unit price is expected to achieve (Institute of Alcohol Studies, 2016). The advantage of taxation to reduce affordability is that the government get the revenue and could invest it back into alcohol interventions.

The UK Government consulted on the proposal to introduce a minimum unit pricing (MUP) in 2012/13 and concluded that the evidence did not conclusively demonstrate that MUP would reduce problem drinking without penalising all those who drink responsibly. So MUP has not been introduced in England. However, in Wales and Scotland a minimum unit price of 50 pence per unit has been introduced. It is early days and the impact of this is yet to be established. However, evidence from other countries where MUP has been implemented have demonstrated reductions in hospital admissions for alcohol related illness and injury, reductions in crime and a reduction in alcohol related deaths (Public Health England, 2016).

Early drinking interventions

Many community level drinking interventions aimed at young people are educational in nature. In essence these are risk communication messages and the evidence from psychological research is that improving risk perceptions will have little impact on levels of drinking. Unsurprisingly then, there is little evidence that alcohol education and health promotion have any positive effect on drinking habits in the UK (Plant & Plant, 2006) or the US (Anderson et al., 2009; Martineau et al., 2013). These campaigns are heard and understood because knowledge about UK drinking guidelines in heavy and binge drinkers has been reported to be as high as 98% (Moss et al., 2009). When the new UK guidelines were published in 2016 a survey of nearly 1000 drinkers was conducted and 71% were aware of the new guidelines but only 8% knew what they were (Rosenberg et al., 2018). Communication of the new limits needs to be improved, particularly given the lowering of the weekly units guidelines for men. Worryingly in the past, there has been some evidence that educational programmes to reduce drinking can have the opposite effect and increase drinking (Duryea & Okwumabua, 1988; Wechsler et al., 2003). Anderson et al. (2009) reported that industry-funded educational programmes tend to lead to positive views about alcohol and the alcohol industry. It is possible that young people who may be attracted to unconventionality or rebelliousness could be attracted by the described risks that are intended to prevent initiation of drinking.

Wechsler et al. (2003) evaluated a social marketing-based intervention in two colleges in the US. The intervention involved a poster campaign that stated that most students had 5 drinks on a night out. The result of this was those students drinking less than 5 drinks increased their consumption whilst there was no impact on the drinking of those originally drinking more than 5 drinks. Wechsler et al. (2003) concluded that whilst social marketing strategies are an attractive solution to the problem of heavy drinking for the alcohol industry, they are at best ineffective and at worst counter-productive and tougher measures aimed at limiting access to alcohol and controlling the marketing practices of the beverage industry are more likely to be effective in reducing drinking. There are instances where social marketing-based campaigns have been effective. For example a social marketing campaign on drink-driving did reduce people driving over the alcohol limits (Janssen et al., 2013) but whether it was the social marketing techniques or other factors that produced the impact was not established.

Established drinking interventions

Many interventions to challenge established drinking are targeted at higher risk drinkers. Nevertheless, community level interventions to challenge less serious drinking exist. As predicted by psychological research, health promotion messages that inform people about the risks of drinking are as ineffective in established drinkers as they are in early drinkers (Room, 2004; Babor et al., 2010; Plant & Plant, 2006, Janssen et al., 2013; Public Health England, 2016). However, there is evidence that informational campaigns and, in particular, mass media campaigns and health warning labels do have a role to play in the promotion of sensible drinking. In multi-level campaigns where an informational message is supported by programmes to support sensible drinking, decreases in drinking levels have been reported (Paglia & Room, 1999; Janssen et al., 2013).

There is a significant body of work on workplace drinking norms that suggests that changing workplace drinking norms to support sensible drinking could be of value in changing drinking behaviours both in work and non-work contexts (Barrientos-Gutierrez et al., 2007). The challenge will be to develop interventions that can successfully change group-based norms. Challenging descriptive social norms in interventions with young people has been utilised with some success but usually as part of a more individualised intervention (Paglia & Room, 1999; Prochaska et al., 2004). Similar work-based interventions may well be a useful additional strategy for established drinkers. Webb et al. (2009) carried out a systematic review of workplace interventions and found 10 studies that reported on workplace alcohol interventions but all had methodological problems. The various study designs, types of interventions, measures employed and types of workplaces varied considerably, making comparison of results difficult. However, it appears from the evidence that brief interventions, interventions contained within health and lifestyle checks, psychosocial skills training and peer referral have potential to produce beneficial results. Ames and Bennett (2011) also reported that whilst workplace drinking interventions had some limited success they were varied and piecemeal and a more strategic approach that coordinated interventions effectively should be established. Whilst tackling drinking in the workplace may be identifying a particularly useful community setting in which to work, the interventions that appear to work are more individualised.

Applying this to Olivia

A work-based intervention would be particularly useful for Olivia as it is through work that most of her drinking occurs. A change in work culture would support her if and when she decides to change her drinking.

Working effectively with others

Sensible drinking advice ranges from universal prevention messages to specialist treatment. It is increasingly acknowledged that there is a wide-scale need for support with sensible drinking that goes further than public health-based health promotion but not is not specialist addiction treatment. Alcohol Brief Interventions (ABI) provide a middle level intervention to fill this gap (Burrell et al., 2006; Public Health England, 2016) and there are now a number of established brief interventions available and training packages for health professionals to deliver these interventions (Burrell et al., 2006; NICE, 2010, Public Health England, 2016). Unlike physical activity or weight-reduction, where primary care professionals can direct individuals to out of health-care settings for support, supporting sensible drinking remains very much a health care led activity. However, there is increasing interest in delivering brief interventions for drinking in sites outside of primary care and GP surgeries such as accident and emergency settings and also out of health care settings completely and into workplace settings (NICE, 2010; Public Health England, 2016). The move to intervening in emergency service settings is in response to evidence that brief interventions for drinking are most productive at a 'moment of crisis' (Burrell et al., 2006, pg 8). The idea is to carry out both the screening and the brief intervention within the same setting, although it is possible that individuals who are screened outside of primary care may also be referred to their GP for intervention.

Regardless of the move to deliver brief interventions in a range of non-GP settings, the GP surgery is likely to remain the first port of call for individuals who are actively looking for help with reducing their drinking. Consequently, many health professionals in primary care will require training in order to deliver such programmes and also in identifying when more specialist treatment from their colleagues in alcohol and addiction services is required.

Conclusion

Many people drink more alcohol than is good for them. It has been argued that reducing the availability and increasing the cost of alcohol are the best ways to reduce excess drinking but despite consulting on minimum unit pricing (MUP) only Wales, Scotland and Northern Ireland have introduced an MUP and at 50 pence a unit it is yet to be seen if that is a high enough unit price to have the health impact seen in other countries that have introduced MUP. Interventions that improve coping skills and in particular self-regulatory coping skills have been found to be the most effective mechanisms for supporting reductions in drinking. Improved self-efficacy, particularly for refusing alcohol is associated with less relapse. Initial research suggest that challenging perceived social norms for drinking are a good way to help people change their drinking habits, but more recent evidence suggests that interventions based in motivational or social cognitive theories are the most consistently effective. However, the role of social support be that from a specialist or general health practitioner or from peers or family is increasingly recognised as a critical component of all successful interventions.

Applying this to Olivia

It is going to be difficult to help Olivia until she recognises that she is drinking too much and is motivated to change. The stages of change concept would define her as at the pre-contemplation stage.

Motivational interviewing may be effective for Olivia. On the one hand she has the social support from her partner for change, on the other the challenges of a very pro-drinking culture at work. A change in working culture may increase the chances of successfully motivating Olivia to reduce her drinking. However, this is an unlikely scenario. If Olivia becomes motivated to reduce her drinking then she will need to develop her self-regulatory coping skills and through meeting self-regulatory goals build her alcohol refusal self-efficacy so that she can continue to network with clients and colleagues without drinking to excess.

Olivia is in the habit of drinking a lot. If she were to succeed in becoming pregnant this would be an ideal time to change this habit and develop new, healthier habits. A major life event such as becoming pregnant upsets routines and provides an opportunity to change habits. Mindfulness interventions at the point at which Olivia is making the transition may help with any cravings or distress that reducing her drinking creates. However, what is increasingly clear is that the health practitioner involved in delivering any intervention that Olivia engages with may be as important to the intervention success as the nature of the intervention.

Key points

- Alcohol contributes to a wide range of diseases.
- Many people in the UK drink more alcohol than is good for their health.
- Young people are the most likely to engage in heavy episodic drinking.
- Many people will have established drinking habits that are difficult to overcome without reaching and dependency criteria
- The availability and low cost of alcohol have been implicated in the early establishment of drinking.
- Brief interventions for alcohol use that have a goal of low-risk drinking, rather than abstinence, can be delivered by non-addiction specialists and have been proven to be effective in reducing drinking levels.
- Cognitive behavioural therapy and interventions that incorporate key CBT principles have been proven to be effective in reducing drinking levels.
- Improving coping skills and in particular self-regulatory coping skills are a key mechanism for successful reduction in drinking.
- The quality of the practitioner delivering any intervention has been found to be critical to its success.

Points for discussion

- What are the benefits and costs associated with identifying individuals with a genetic risk of becoming addicted to alcohol?
- Delaying the onset of drinking in adolescents and young people has been found to reduce the incidence of alcohol-related problems in later life. Should we consider raising the legal drinking age in public places to 21?
- Should we be introducing alcohol brief interventions to reduce problem drinking for everyone who visits an accident and emergency unit or is admitted to hospital due to a drink-related incident?
- How can we coordinate universal and targeted interventions across different settings to maximise impact?

Further resources

Alcoholics anonymous 0800 9177650 www.alcoholicsanonymous.org.uk/
Talk to FRANK 0300 1236600 www.talktofrank.com
Drink aware Trust www.drinkaware.co.uk/
Alcohol Change UK www.alcoholchange.org.uk/
NHS: Units of alcohol calculator www.nhs.uk

References

Alcohol Change UK: alcoholchange.org.uk accessed 2022.

Ames, G.M., & Bennett, J.B. (2011). Prevention Interventions of alcohol problems in the workplace. Alcohol Research & health, *34*(2), 175–187.

Anderson, P., Chisholm, D., & Fuhr, D.C. (2009). Effectiveness and cost-effectiveness of policies and programmes to reduce the harm caused by alcohol. Lancet., *373*(9682), 2234-2234.

Angus, C., Brown, J., Beard, E., Gillespie, D., Buykx, P., Kaner, E.F.S. Michie, S., & Meier, P. (2019). Socioeconomic inequalities in the delivery or brief interventions for smoking and excessive drinking: Findings from a cross-sectional household survey in England. BMJ Open, *9*, e023448 doi:10.1136/bmjopen-2018-023448.

Babor, T., Caetano, R., Casswell, S., Edwards, G., Giesbrecht, N., Graham, K., Grube, J., Gruenewald, P., Hill, L., Holder, H., Homel, R., Osterberg, E., Rehm, J., Room, R., & Rossow, I. (2010). Alcohol: No ordinary commodity. 2nd Edition. Oxford: Oxford University Press.

Balakrishnan, R., Allender, S., Scarborough, P., Webster, P., & Rayner, M. (2009). The burden of alcohol-related ill health in the United Kingdom. Journal of Public Health, *31*(3), 366–373.

Barrientos-Gutierrez, T. Gimeno, D. Mangione, T.W., Harrist, R.B., & Amick, B.C. (2007). Drinking social nomas and drinking behaviours: A multilevel analysis of 137 workgroups in 16 worksites. Occupational and Environmental Medicine, *64*, 602–608.

Barr, C.S. *et al.* (2010). Suppression of alcohol preference by naltrexone in the rhesus macaque: a critical role of genetic variation at the μ-opioid receptor gene locus. Biol. Psychiatry, *67*, 78–80.

Bertholet, N., Gaume, J., Faouzi, M., Daeppen, J.B., & Gmel, G. (2011). Perception of the amount of drinking by others in a sample of 20 year old men: The more I think you drink, the more I drink. Alcohol and Alcoholism, *46*(1), 83–87.

Bewick, B.M., West, R., Gill, J., O'May, F., Mulhern, B., Barkham, M., & Hill, A.J. (2010). Providing web-based feedback and social norms information to reduce student alcohol intake: A multisite investigation. Journal of Medical Internet Research, *12*(5), e59

Beyer, F.R., Campbul, F., Bertholet, N., daeppen, J.B., Saunders, J.B., Pienaar, E.D., Muirhead, C.R., & Kaner, E.F.S. (2019). The Cochrane 2018 review on brief interventnions in primary care for hazardous and harmful alcohol consumption: A distillation for clinicians and policy makers: 10.1093/alcalc/agz035

Black, H., Gill, J., & Chick, J. (2010). The price of a drink: Levels of consumption and price paid per unit of alcohol by Edinburgh's ill drinkers with a comparison to wider alcohol sales in Scotland. Addiction, *106*(4), 729–736.

Burrell, K., Sumnall, H., Witty, K., & McVeigh, J. (2006). Preston alcohol brief intervention training pack: Evaluation report. Centre for Public Health John Moores University.

Bryant, L., & Lightowlers, C. (2021). The socioeconomic distribution of alcohol-related violence and anti-social behaviour in England and Wales. PLoS ONE, *16*(2), eo243206. 10.1371/journal.pone.0243206.

Byrne, S.P., Haber, P., Baillie, A., Coata, D.S.J., Fogliati, V., & Morely, K. (2019) Systematic reviews of mindfulness and acceptance and commitment therapy for aochol use disorder: Should we be using third wave therapies? Alcohol and Alcoholism, *54*(2), 159–166. 10.1093/alcalc/agy089

Byrnes, H.F., Miller, B.A., Grube, J.W., Bourdeau, B., Buller, D.B., Wang-Schweig, M., & Woodall, W.G. (2019). Prevention of alcohol use in older teens: A randomised trial of an online family prevention programme. Psychology of addictive behaviours, *33*(1), 1–14. 10.1037/adb0000442.

Callaghan R.C., Taylor L., & Cunningham J.A. (2007). Does progressive stage transition mean getting better? A test of the Transtheoretical Model in alcoholism recovery. Addiction, *102*(10), 1588–1596.

Carey, K.B., Scott-Sheldon, L.A., Carey, M.P., & DeMartini, K.S. (2007). Individual-level interventions to reduce college student drinking: a meta-analytic review. Addictive Behaviour, *32*(11), 2469–2494.

Cavicchioli, M., Movalli, M., & Maffei, C. (2018). The clinical efficacy of mindfulness-based treatments for alcohol and drug use disorders: A meta-analytic review of Randomised and Non randomised Controlled Trials. European Addiction Research, *24*, 137–162. 10.1159/000490762

Chen, W.Y., Rosner, B., Hankinson, S.E., Colditz, G.A., & Willnett, W.C. (2011). Moderate alcohol consumption during adult life, drinking patterns, and breast cancer risk. JAMA, *306* (17), 1884–1890.

Clarke A., & Thirlaway K. (2011). Genetic counselling for personalised medicine. Human Genetics, *130* (1), 27–31.

Conrod, P.J., Castellanos-Ryan, N., & v Mackie, C.J. (2011). Long-term effects of a personality-targeted intervention to reduce alcohol use in adolescents. Journal of Consulting and Clinical Psychology, *79*(3), 296–306.

Craig, R., & Mindell, J. (2008). Health survey for England 2006. Volume 1: Cardiovascular disease and risk factors in adults. London: The Information Centre.

Delong, W., Schneider, S.K., Towvim, L.G., Gomberg, L., Murphy, M.J., Doerr, E.E., Simonen, N.R., Mason, K.E., & Scribner, R.A. (2006). A multi-site randomized trial of social norms marketing campaigns to reduce college student drinking. Journal of Studies on Alcohol, *67*(6), 868–879.

Department of Health (2010). Health survey for England, 2010. The NHS Information Centre, 2011. Available at: http://www.ic.nhs.uk/pubs/hse10report

Department of Health (2015). UK Chief Medical Officers' Alcohol Guidelines Review: Summary of the proposed new guidelines Department of Health.

Department of Health, Social Services and Public Safety (2011). Health Survey Northern Ireland: First results from the 2010/11 survey. Belfast: Department of Health, Social Services and Public Safety.

Department of Transport (2021). Reported Road Casualties in Great Britain, final estimates involving illegal alcohol levels: 2019 Annual Report. U Government.

Dixon, H.G., Pratt, I.S., Scully, M.L., Miller, J.R., Patterson, C., Hood, R., & Slevin, T.J. (2015). Using a mass media campaign to raise women's awareness of the link between alcohol and cancer: Cross-sectional preinternvention and post-intervention evaluation surveys. BMJ Open 11, *5*(3). 10.1136/bmjopen-2014-006511.

Drinkaware (2022). Facts about Alcohol. Drinkaware.co.uk accessed 2022.

Duryea, E.J., & Okwumabua, J.O. (1988). Effects of a preventive alcohol education programme after 3 years. Journal of Drug Education, *18*, 23–31.

Emslie C., Lewars H., Batty G.D., & Hunt K. (2009). Are there gender differences in levels of heavy, binge and problem drinking? Evidence from three generations in the west of Scotland. Public Health, *123*, 12–14.

Effiong, K. Osinowo A., Pring A., & Verne J. (2012) Deaths from liver disease: Implications for end of life care in England, March 2012. National End of Life Care Intelligence Network. 2012.

Fiellin, L.E., Tetrault, M., Becker, W.C., Fiellin, D.A., & Hoff, R.A. (2013). Previous use of alcohol, cigarettes, and marijuana and subsequent abuse of prescription opioids in young adults. Journal of Adolescent Health, *52*(2), 158–163.

French, M.T., & Zavala, S.K. (2007). The health benefits of moderate drinking revisited: Alcohol use and self-reported health status. American Journal of Health Promotion, *21*, 484–491.

Foxcroft, D.R., Ireland, D., Lister-Sharp, D.J., Lowe, G., & Breen, R. (2003). Longer-term primary prevention for alcohol misuse in young people: a systematic review. Addiction, *98*(4), 397–411.

Garland, E.L., & Howard, M.O. (2018). Mindfulness-based treatment of addiction: Current state of the field and envisioning the next wave of research. Addiction Science & Clinical Practice, *13*, 14. 10.1186/s13722-018-0115-3.

Gray. H.M., Wiley, R.C., Williams, P.M., & Shaffer, H.J. (2021). A scoping review of "Responsible Drinking" Interventions. Health Communications, *36*(2), 236–256. 10.1080/1 0410236.2020.1733226

Gilles, D.M., Turk, C.L., & Fresco, D.M. (2006). Social anxiety, alcohol expectancies, and self-efficacy as predictors of heavy drinking in college students. Addictive Behaviour, *31*, 388–398.

Gilligan, C., Wolfenden, L., Foxcroft, D.R., Williams, A.J., Kingsland, M., Hodder, R.K., Stockings, E., McFadyen, T.R., Tindall, J., Sherker, S., Rae, J., & Wiggers, J. (2019). Family-based prevention programmes for alcohol use in young people. Cochrane Database of Systematic Reviews, *3*(3), CD012287–CD012287. 10.1002/14651858.CD012287.pub2.

Glass, J.E., Andreasson, S., Bradley, K.A., Wallhed Finn, S., Williams, E.C., Bakshi, A., Gual, A., Heather, N., Tiburcio Saninz, M., Benegal, V., & Saitz, R. (2017). Rethinking alcohol interventions in health care; a thematic meeting of the International Network on Brief Interventions for Alcohol & Other Drugs (INEBRIA). Addiction Science and Clinical Practice, *12*(14). 10.1186/s13722-017-0079-8.

Grant, J.D., Agrawal, A., Bucholz, K., Madden, P. et al. (2009). Alcohol consumption indices of genetic risk for alcohol dependence. Biological Psychiatry, *66*(8), 795–800.

Health Survey England (2020). Health Survey for England 2019: Adult health-related behaviours. NHS Digital.

Health Survey (NI) (2021). Health Survey (NI): First results 2020/21. Public Health Information and Research Branch, Information Analysis Directorate.

Heather, N., Honekopp, J., & Smailes, D. (2009). Progressive stage transition does mean getting better: A further test of the Transtheoretical Model in recovery from alcohol problems. Addiction, *104*(6), 949–958.

HM Government. (2007). Safe. Sensible. Social. The next steps in the National Alcohol Strategy. London: Department of Health and The Home Office.

HM Government (2012). The government's alcohol strategy. London. The Home Office.

Holmes, J., Angus, C., Buykx, P., Abdallah, A., Stone, T., Meier, P. et al. (2016). Mortality and morbidity risks from alcohol consumption in the UK: Analyses using the Sheffield Alcohol Policy Model (v2.7) to inform the Chief Medical Officers review of UK lower risk drinking guidelines Final report. University of Sheffield. Available from: https://www.shef.ac.uk/polypoly_fs/1.538671!/file/Drinking_Guidelines_Final_Report_Published.pdf

Hughes, K., Quigg, Z., Bellis, M.A., van Hasselt, N., Calafat, A., Kosir, M., Juan, M., Duch, M., & Voorham, L. (2007). Alcohol, nightlife, and violence: The relative contributions of drinking before and during nights out to negative health and criminal justice outcomes. Addiction, *103*, 60–65.

Hurcombe, R., Bayley, M., & Goodman, A. (2010). Ethnicity and alcohol: A review of the UK literature. Joseph Rowntree Foundation.

Institute of Alcohol Studies (2016). Alcohol taxes would have to rise by 28% to match minimum unit pricing in Scotland. News. www.ias.org.uk

Institute of Alcohol Studies (2020). Alcohol Knowledge Centre Briefing: Ethnic Minorities and Alcohol. www.ias.org.uk

Janssen, M.M., Mathijssen, J.J., van Bon-Martens, M.J., van Oers, H.A., & Garretsen, H.F. (2013). Effectiveness of alcohol prevention interventions based on the principals of social marketing: A systematic review. Substance Abuse Treatment Prevention & Policy, *1*(8), 18.

Kaestner, R., & Yarnoff, B. (2011) Long term effects of minimum legal drinking age laws on adult alcohol use and driving fatalities. The Journal of Law and Economics, *54*(2), 325–363.

Kalsi G., Prescott C.A., Kendler K., & Riley B. (2009). Unravelling the molecular mechanisms of alcohol dependence. Trends in Genetics, *25*(1), 49–55.

Kamboj, S.K., Irez, D. Serfaty, S., Thomas, E., & Freeman, T.P. (2017). Ultra-brief mindfulness training reduces alcohol consumption in AT-risk drinkers: A randomised double-blind active-controlled experiment. International Journal of Neuropsychopharmacology, 20 (11), 936–947.

Katikireddi, S.V., Whitley, E., Lewsey, J., Gray, L., & Leyland, A.H. (2017). Socioeconomic status as an effect modifier of alcohol consumption and harm: Analysis of linked cohort data. Lance Public health, *2*(6), e267–e276.

Kuntsche, E., & Cooper, M.L. (2010). Drinking to have fun and to get drunk: Motives as predictors of weekend drinking over and above usual drinking habits. Drug and Alcohol Dependence, *110*(3), 259–262.

Kuther, T.L., & Timoshin, A. (2003). A comparison of social cognitive and psychosocial predictors of alcohol use by college students. Journal of College Student Development, *44*, 143–154.

Lee, S.J., Sudore, R.L., Williams, B.A., Lindquist, M.S., Chen, H.L., & Covinsky, K.E. (2009). Functional limitations, socioeconomic status and all-cause mortality in moderate drinkers. Journal of the American Geriatrics Society, *57*, (6), 955–962.

Litt, D.M., & Stock, M.L. (2011). Adolescent alcohol-related risk cognitions: The roles of social norms and social networking sites. Psychology of Addictive Behaviors, *25*(4), 708–713.

Longabaugh, R., Donovan, D.M., Karno, M.P., McCrady, B.S., Morgenstern, J., & Scott Tonigan, J. (2005). Active ingredients: How and why evidence-based alcohol behavioral treatment interventions work. Alcoholism: Clinical and Experimental Research, *29*(2), 235–247.

Magill, M., Scott Tonigan, J., Kiluk, B., Ray, L., Walthers, J., & Carroll, K. (2020). The search for mechanisms of cognitive behavioural therapy for alcohol or other drug use disorders: A systematic review. Behaviour Research and Therapy, *131* (103648).

MacLean, S.J., Pennay, A., Caluzzi, G., Holmes, J., & Torronen, J. (2021). Why are young people drinking less than their parents' generation did? The Conversation.

Manning, W.G., Blumberg, L., & Moulton, L.H. (1995). The demand for alcohol: The differential response to price. Journal of Health Economics, *14*, 123–148.

Martineau, F., Tyner, E., Lorenc, T., Petticrew, M., & Lock, K. (2013). Population-level interventions to reduce alcohol-related harm: An overview of systematic reviews. Preventative Medicine, *57*, 278–296.

Masten, A.S., Faden, V.B., Zucker, R.A., & Spear, L.P. (2008). Underage drinking: A developmental framework. Paediatrics,*121*, 2007–2243.

Mcalaney J., & McMahon J. (2007). Normative beliefs, misperceptions, and heavy episodic drinking in a British student sample. Journal of Studies on Alcohol and Drugs, *68*(3), 385–392.

McCaul, M.E., Roach, D., Hasin, D.S., Weisner, C., Chang, G., & Sinha, R. (2019). Alcohol and Women: A Brief Overview. Alcoholism: Clinical and Experimental Research, *43*(5), 774–779. 10.1111/acer.13985.

McManus, S., Meltzer, H., Brugha, T., Bebbington, P., and Jenkins, R. (2009). Adult Psychiatric Morbidity in England, 2007. Results of a household survey. Leeds: The NHS Information Centre for Health and Social Care.

Measham & Ostergaard (2011). Emerging drug trends in Lancashire: Night Time Economy Surveys: Phase One Report. Lancashire: Lancashire drug and alcohol action team.

Moss, A.C., Dyer, K.R., & Albery, I.P. (2009). Knowledge of drinking does not equal sensible drinking. The Lancet, *374*, 1242.

Moyer, A., Finney, J.W., Swearingen, E., & Vergun, P. (2002). Brief interventions for alcohol problems a meta-analytic review of controlled investigations in treatment seeking and non-treatment seeking populations. Addiction, *97*, 279–292.

Mulvihill, C., Taylor, L., Waller, S., Naidoo, B., & Thom, B. (2005). Prevention and reduction of alcohol misuse: evidence briefing, 2nd edn. London: Health Development Agency.

Murgraff, V., Abraham, C., & McDermott, M. (2007) Reducing Friday alcohol consumption among moderate women drinkers: Evaluation of a brief evidence-based intervention. Alcohol and Alcoholism, *42*, 37–41.

National Collaborating Centre for Mental Health (2011 – updated 2022). Alcohol Use Disorders: The NICE guideline on diagnosis, assessment and management or harmful drinking and alcohol guidance. National Clinical Practice Guideline 115 NICE https://www.nice.org.uk/guidance/cg115/evidence/full-guideline-136423405

News. (2007). Alcohol, breast and colorectal cancer. European Journal of Cancer, *43*, 1225.

Newton, N.C., Debenham, J., Slade, T. Smout, A., Grummitt, L., Sunderland, M., Barrett, E.L., Champion, K.E., Chapman, C., Kelly, E., Lawler, S., Castellanos-Ryan, N., Teeson, M.,

Conrod, P.J., & Stapinski, L. (2022). Effect of selective personality-targeted alochol use prevention on 7-year alcohol-related outcomes among high-risk adolescents. JAMA Network Open, *5*(11). 10.1001/jamanetworkopen.2022.42522

NICE (2019). Alcohol interventions in secondary and further education. NICE guideline NG135. London: NICE.

NICE (2010). Alcohol-use disorders: Preventing harmful drinking: NICE Public Health Guidance 24. London: NICE.

Nicolas, S., Kershaw, C., & Walker, A. (2008). Crime in England and Wales 2007/2008. Home Office. Available at: www.homeoffice.gov.uk/rds/pdfs08/hosb0708.pdf.

Nilsen, P., Baird J., Mello M.J. et al. (2008). A systematic review of emergency care brief alcohol interventions for injury patients. Journal of Substance Abuse Treatment, *35*(2), 184–201.

Norman, P., Webb, T.L., & Millings, A. (2019). Using the theory of planned behaviour and implementation intentions to reduce binge drinking in new university students. Psychology & Health, *34*(4), 478–496.

Nuffield Council on Bioethics. (2007). Public Health Ethical Issues. London: Nuffield Council. www.nuffieldbioethics.org

Office of National Statistics (2018). Adult drinking habits in Great Britain 2017. London: Office of National Statistics.

Office of National Statistics (2021). Quarterly alcohol-specific deaths in England and Wales: 2001 to 2019 registrations and Quarter 1 (Jan to Mar) to Quarter 4 (Oct to Dec) 2020 provisional registrations. Census 2021

Office for Health improvement and disparities (2021). Adult substance misuse treatment statistics 2020 to 2021: report. Gov,UK.

O'Keefe, J.H., Bybee, K.A., & Lavie, C.J. (2007). Alcohol and cardiovascular health. The razor-sharp double-edged sword. Journal of the American College of Cardiology, *50* (11), 1009–1014.

O'Leary-Barrett, M., Mackie, C.J., Castellanos-Ryan, N., Al-Khudhairy, N. & Conrod, P.J. (2010). Personality-targeted interventions delay uptake of drinking and decrease risk of alcohol-related problems when delivered by teachers. Journal of the American Academy of Child and Adolescent Psychiatry, *49* (9), 954–963.

Oppenheimer, G.M., & Bayer, R. (2020). Is moderate drinking protective against heart disease? The science, politics and history of a public health conundrum. The Milbank Quarterly, *98*(1), 39–56.

Orton, J. (2001). Excessive Appetites, 2ndedn. Chichester: John Wiley & Sons.

Paradis, C., Butt, P., Shield, K., Poole, N., Wells, S., Naimi, T., Sherk, A., and the Low-Risk Alcohol Drinking Guidelines Scientific Expert Panels (2023). Canada's Guidance on Alcohol and Health: Final Report. Ottawa, Ont: Canadian Centre on Substance Use and Addiction.

Paglia, A., & Room, R. (1999). Preventing substance use problems among youth: A literature review and recommendations. Journal of Primary Prevention, *20*, 3–50.

Percy, A., Wilson, J., McCartan, C., & McCrystal, P. (2011). Teenage drinking cultures. York: Joseph Rowntree Foundation.

Pham, T., Thu, L., Callinan, S., & Livingston, M. (2019). Patterns of alcohol consumptions among people with major chronic diseases. Australian Journal of Primary Health, *25*(2), 163–167.

Piano. M.R., Mazzuco, A., Kang, M., & Phillips, S.A. (2017). Cardiovascular consequences of binge drinking: An integrative review with implications for advocacy, policy and research. Alcoholism, clinical and experimental research, *41*(3), 487–496. 10.1111.acer.13329

Plant, M. & Plant, M. (2006). Binge Britain. Oxford: Oxford University Press.

PMC (2000). Health risk and benefits of alcohol consumption. Alcohol Research & Health, *24*(1), 5–11.

Prochaska, J.M., Prochaska, J.O., Cohen, F.C., Gomes, S.O., Laforge, R.G. and Eastwood, B.S. (2004). The Transtheoretical model of change for multi-level interventions for alcohol abuse on campus. Journal of Alcohol and Drug Education, *47*, 34–50.

Probst, C., Kilian, C., Sanchez, S., Lange,S., & Reham, J. (2020). The role of alcohol use and drinking patterns in socioeconomic inequalities in mortality: A systematic review. Lancet Public Health, *5*, e324–e332.

Public Health England (2016). The Public Health Burden of Alcohol and the Effectiveness and Cost-Effectiveness of Alcohol Control Policies: An evidence review. Public Health England. UK Government.

Ramos, D., & Perkins, D.F. (2006). Goodness of fit assessment of an alcohol intervention program and the underlying theories of change. Journal of American College Health, *55*, 57–64.

Rehm, J., Mathers, C., Popova, S., Thavorncharoensap, M. et al (2009) Global burden of disease and injury and economic cost attributable to alcohol use and alcohol-use disorders. The Lancet, 373, 2223–2233.

Rehm, J., Heiig, M., & Guai, A. (2019). ICD-11 for alcohol use disorders: Not a convincing ANSWER TO THE CHAllenges. Alcoholism: Clinical and Experimental Research, 43(11), 2296–2300.

Room, R. (2004). Disabling the public interest: Alcohol strategies and policies for England. Addiction, 99, 1083–1089.

Room, R., Babor, T., & Rehm, J. (2005). Alcohol and public health. Lancet, *365*, 519–530.

Rosenberg, G., Bauld, L., & Vohra, J. (2018). New national alcohol guidelines in the UK: Public awareness, understanding and behavioural intentions. Journal of Public Health, *40* (3), 549–556.

Sancho, M., De Gracia, M., Rodriguez, R.C., Mallorqui-Baque, N., Sanchez-Gonzalez, J., Trujols, J., Sanchez, I., Jimenez-Murcia, S., & Menchon, J.M. (2018). Mindfulness-Based Interventions for the treatment of substance and behavioural addictions: A systematic review. Frontiers in Psychology, 9(95). 10.3389/fpsyt.2018.00095.

Saunders, J., & Rey, J. (2011). Young People and Alcohol: Impact, Policy Prevention, Treatment. London: Wiley.

Saunders, J., Degenhardt, L., Reed, G., & Poznyak, V. (2019). Alcohol use disorders in the ICD-11: past, present and future. Alcohol Clin Exp Res, *43*, 1617–1631.

Schwebel, F.J., Korecki, J.R., & Witkiewitz, K. (2020). Additive behaviour change and mindfulness-based interventions: Current research and future directions. Current Addition Reports, 7, 117–124.

Schulz, D.N., Kremers, S.P.J., & de Vries, H. (2012). Are the stages of change relevant for the development and implementation of a web-based tailored alcohol intervention? A cross sectional study. BMC Public Health, *360*. 10.1186/1471-2458-12-360.

Scottish Government (2011). The Scottish Health Survey 2010, Volume 1: Main Report. Edinburgh: The Scottish Government. Available at: http://www.scotland.gov.uk/Publications/2011/09/27084018/91

Scottish Health Survey (2020). Scottish Health Survey 2019. The Scottish Government www.gov.scot

Seidenberg, A.B., Wiseman, K.P., & Klein, W.M.P. (2022). Do beliefs about Alcohol and Cancer Risk Vary by alcoholic beverage type and heart disease risk beliefs? Cancer Epidemiology, Biomarkers and Prevention. OF1–OF8. 10.1158/1055-9965EPI-22-0420

Skidmore, S. M., Juhasz, R. A., & Zucker, R. A. (2011). Early Onset Drinking. In Eds Saunder & Rey. Young People and Alcohol: Impact, Policy, Prevention and Treatment. Oxford: Wiley-Blackwell.

Spoth, R.L., Redmond, C., Shin, C., & Azevedo (2004). Brief family interventions effects on adolescent substance initiation: School-level growth curve analysis 6 years following baseline. Journal of Consulting and Clinical Psychology, *72*, 535–542.

UK Chief Medical Officers (2016). UK Chief Medical Officers' Low Risk Drinking Guidelines. Department of Health, Welsh Government, Department of Health Northern Ireland & Scottish Government. Crown Copyright.

Vissers, L., Houwing, S., & Wegman, F. (2018). Alcohol-related road casualities-official-crash-statistics. International Transport Forum. International Traffic Safety Data and Analysis Group.

Wagenaar, A.C., Salois, M.J., & Komro, K.A. (2009). Effects of beverage alcohol price and tax levels on drinking: a meta-analysis of 1003 estimates from 112 studies. Addiction, *104*, 179–190.

Webb G., Shakeshaft A., Sanson-Fisher R., & Havard A. (2009). A systematic review of workplace interventions for alcohol-related problems. Addiction, *104*(3), 365–377.

Wechsler, H., Nelson, T., Lee, J.E., Seibring, M., Lewis, C., & Keeling, R.P. (2003). Perceptions and reality: A national evaluation of social norms marketing interventions to reduce college students heavy alcohol use. Journal of Studies of Alcohol, *64*, 484–494.

Welsh Assembly Government. (2009). Welsh Health Survey 2008: Initial Headline Results. Cardiff: Welsh Assembly Government.

Welsh Government (2011) Welsh Health Survey 2010. Assessed from: http://www.wales.gov.uk/statistics

Welsh Health Survey (2020). National Survey for Wales 2019/20. Welsh Government.

Woodhouse, J. (2020). Alcohol minimum pricing. Briefing paper 5021. House of Commons library www.parliament.uk/commons-library.

WHO (2010). Global Strategy to reduce the harmful use of alcohol 2010 Available from: http://www.who.int/substance_abuse/msbalcstrategy.pdf

WHO (2018). Global Status Report on alcohol and health 2018. World Health Organisation Switzerland.

WHO (2010) ICD-10 Version: 2010. Mental and behavioural disorders F10-F19, Available at: http://apps.who.int/classifications/icd10/browse/2010

Williams, E.C., Horton, N.J., Samet, J.H., & Saitz, R. (2007). Do brief measures of readiness to change predict alcohol consumption and consequences in primary care patients with unhealthy alcohol use? Alcoholism: Clinical and Experimental Research, *31*, 428–435. www.alcoholandyou.org'

Xu, X., & Chaloupka, F.J. (2011). The effects of prices on alcohol use and its consequences. Alcohol Research and Health, *34* (2).

York Cornwell, E., & Waite, L.J. (2009). Social disconnectedness, perceived isolation and health among older adults. Journal of Health and Social Behavior, *50* (1), 31–48.

8 Smoking

LEARNING OBJECTIVES

At the end of this chapter, you will be able to:

- understand the current extent and demographics of tobacco smoking in the United Kingdom (UK) and other nations.
- appreciate the health and economic consequences of tobacco smoking.
- consider the potential benefits and drawbacks of e-cigarettes and how the increased prevalence of 'vaping' is changing the landscape of smoking.
- outline how the stages of change model can and has been applied to smoking and smoking cessation.
- explain the approaches to smoking cessation at an individual and community level while recognising how health professionals can aid cessation.
- apply the motivational interviewing (MI) technique to smoking cessation.
- explain the development of assessment, action and intervention plans for smoking.
- appreciate some of the difficulties faced when attempting to quit smoking and how to cope with them.

Case study

Yuri is a 53-year-old window cleaner currently running his own business but who is looking forward to retiring shortly. He has worked continuously since he started work when he left school without any qualifications at 14 years old. He has few hobbies but loves to play with his grandchildren in the back garden. However, recently, he has found himself getting breathless frequently and thus unable to enjoy playing with them as much as he would like. He does enjoy socialising and likes a couple of pints in the evening with his friends and family at the local working men's club.

Yuri has smoked cigarettes since he was a teenager and still smokes some 25–30 per day, with his first cigarette upon waking. He used to smoke more heavily but has recently cut down. Yuri has developed frequent chest and breathing problems—he often has bouts of bronchitis and recently suffered four cracked ribs

DOI: 10.4324/9781003471233-8

due to prolonged and severe coughing. In addition to his chest problems, he also suffers from early peripheral vascular disease and has a mild degree of lower limb neuropathy. Yuri knows that he has to stop smoking, but as he has been doing it for over 40 years, he feels he cannot stop.

He sees you in the clinic, and you realise that his behaviour severely compromises his health, and he must change it or suffer ever more serious consequences. Yuri reports that he only 'smokes now and again', although you think it is much more frequent than this. Yuri has now noticed that his grandson, Dmitry, has started acting like him, playing 'smoking cigarettes' and refusing to eat anything other than chips and bacon butties.

Applying this to Yuri

You have to be able to assess Yuri's smoking behaviour and work with him to reduce (and stop) his smoking. You also need to ensure that Dmitry does not start smoking.

Introduction

Surely everyone appreciates the health damage that cigarette smoking causes? It remains the most avoidable cause of death and disability in the UK and the Western world (Everest et al., 2022). According to the World Health Organization (WHO), over 8 million deaths yearly result from smoking, including exposure to second-hand smoke (WHO, 2021). If current trends continue, tobacco will kill one billion people in the twenty-first century (ASH, 2021). Despite the health effects of smoking being known for over 50 years and the health impact being publicised considerably, some 6.9 million individuals in the UK still smoke: 15.9% of men and 12.5% of women (ASH, 2021). However, the number of young people starting to smoke has decreased, with a decline of 26% since 1982; however, a core number of individuals still smoke (ASH, 2021).

Further, the increasing availability and usage of e-cigarettes ('vaping') should also be considered. The prevalence of vaping in young people aged 11–18 in 2021 was 8.6%. For adults, this figure was around 7%. It is now estimated that just under 2.5 million people in England use e-cigarettes. These figures have increased in recent years for both adolescents and adults. E-cigarettes are currently the most popular stop-smoking aid. While some research has shown e-cigarettes can be an effective smoking cessation tool, most people who vape are dual users (meaning they also smoke tobacco; Fadus et al., 2019). This indicates that e-cigarettes may not be effective in helping people quit smoking entirely but rather act as a complementary method for smoking reduction.

Moreover, the long-term health effects of e-cigarettes are not yet fully understood, and there is evidence suggesting that they may still pose health risks, particularly for young people and pregnant women. There is also a risk that e-cigarettes could act as a gateway to smoking for young people who have never smoked, as they may become addicted to nicotine through e-cigarettes and eventually switch to traditional cigarettes (Chaffee et al., 2018). As such, it is important to continue monitoring the efficacy and safety of e-cigarettes and implementing measures that protect public health. These implications are discussed in further detail throughout this chapter.

Trends in smoking prevalence across the four home countries in the United Kingdom

Across the four home countries, the prevalence of cigarette smoking in adults aged 18 years and above is lowest in England at 14.4%. Similar prevalence rates are observed for Scotland, Wales and Northern Ireland across the same period (16.3%, 15.9% and 15.5%, respectively). Smoking rates for men and women followed a similar trend for all home countries in 2019, with smoking prevalence slightly higher amongst males than females. Again, England demonstrates a lower prevalence of smoking in men and women compared to Scotland, Wales and Northern Ireland (see Table 8.1).

The prevalence of smoking is not the same in different groups: 23.4% of individuals in manual occupation groups smoke compared to 9.3% of the professional and managerial groups. Similarly, smoking is highest in the 25–34 age group (at 21.8%) and the lowest among the over 60 s (at 9.5%) (ASH, 2021). Individuals from lower socioeconomic backgrounds tend to be more at risk of mortality due to smoking. For instance, more than half of the socioeconomic status (SES) differences in mortality are due to smoking in men aged 35–69 (ASH, 2021). This may be partly because people from a lower socioeconomic background have different attitudinal beliefs regarding their health than those from higher socioeconomic backgrounds. For example, a cross-sectional study by Wardle and Steptoe (2003) revealed that respondents of a low SES were not as focused on future thinking and did not consciously engage in health-seeking/maintenance behaviours as often as those of a higher SES. Importantly, many of these attitudes related to a perceived lack of control regarding one's health. This lack of control has been found to relate to environmental and financial deprivation, social limitations and lower problem-solving skills (Faber et al., 2016). This difference in attitude is thought to contribute to the variance in smoking rates between SESs.

A related factor contributing to the variance in smoking rates is education level. For example, a recent population-based study revealed that in Europe, individuals with lower levels of education generally have higher mortality rates for tobacco-related cancers and infections, such as lung cancer, with a relative risk of mortality for less educated men and women of 2.4 and 1.8, respectively (ASH, 2021).

Socioeconomic status also interacts with several other social health determinants and disparities that influence smoking behaviour. For example, as can be seen throughout

Table 8.1 Smoking prevalence for men and women in the UK

Source of data	% of adults who currently smoke	% of men who currently smoke	% of women who currently smoke
Statistics on Smoking: England 2011 (The Health and Social Care Information Centre, 2011)	21%	22%	20%
Health Survey for Scotland 2010 (Bromley The Scottish Government 2011)	25%	26%	25%
Welsh Health Survey (ASH 2021)	23%	25%	22%
Health Survey Northern Ireland 2010/2011 (Department of Health, Social Services and Public Safety, 2011)	24%	25%	23%

this book, factors like ethnicity or the social marginalisation of certain communities (prisoners, LGBTQI+ individuals, people who use illicit drugs and those with mental illness) significantly impact health and lifestyle factors, and smoking is no exception (Brady, 2020). Therefore, addressing these social determinants is critical to reducing smoking rates and improving population health.

Applying this to Yuri

Yuri is in the lower socioeconomic class, which currently has the highest level of smoking in the UK. Many of his family and peers likely smoke, so the health care professional must be aware of his cultural and social background.

The WHO *Framework Convention on Tobacco Control* is an evidence-based treaty developed in response to the global tobacco epidemic (WHO, 2003). The WHO *Framework Convention on Tobacco Control* aims to reaffirm 'the right of all people to the highest standard of health'. One of the most widely embraced treaties in history, it has 168 signatories, including the European Union. In summary, the guiding principles consider the need to: a) protect everybody from exposure to tobacco smoke, b) prevent and decrease the consumption of tobacco products and support cessation, c) promote culturally appropriate programmes for indigenous individuals and their communities and d) address gender-specific risks when developing tobacco control strategies. In line with principles laid out by the WHO *Framework Convention on Tobacco Control*, the UK government (along with most other governments) is determined to reduce smoking across its population through health promotion and clinical 1:1 interventions. The UK government has set a target to make the country smoke-free by 2030, meaning less than 5% of the population will smoke. This goal is part of a wider plan to improve public health and reduce the burden of smoking-related illnesses. To achieve this target, the government has proposed a range of measures, including increasing funding for stop-smoking services, introducing legislation to ban smoking in outdoor public spaces and launching new public awareness campaigns to encourage people to quit smoking.

In the UK, the Department of Health's tobacco programme is split into 'strands', each of which, it is hoped, will contribute to an overall reduction in smoking. These strands include:

'Smoke-free' legislation: From March 2006 in Scotland, April 2007 in Northern Ireland and Wales and July 2007 in England, virtually all enclosed public places and workplaces in England became smoke-free, including all pubs, clubs, membership clubs, cafés and restaurants.

Reducing exposure to second-hand smoke: Legislation such as introducing smoke-free public buildings and workplaces has reduced the exposure to second-hand smoke.

Tobacco media/education programmes: A key strand of the government's tobacco control programme is delivering an ongoing media/education campaign.

Reducing the availability of tobacco products: Price increases have been a highly successful way of helping people quit smoking for good. UK budget changes to tobacco duty have been directed towards increasing the real cost of cigarettes, thereby increasing economic pressures on people who smoke.

NHS Stop Smoking Services and nicotine replacement therapies (NRTs): The government has established an NHS Stop Smoking Service. Services are now available across the NHS in the UK, providing counselling and support to people who smoke and want to quit, complementing the use of stop-smoking aids such as NRT and bupropion (Zyban).

Reducing tobacco advertising and promotion: The UK has a comprehensive ban, just like many other countries in Europe and beyond, on tobacco advertising and promotion, including displays at the point of sale.

Regulating tobacco products: This strand of the government's tobacco control programme concerns regulating the contents of tobacco products and labelling of packaging. According to the Tobacco Products Directive (2014/40/EU), cigarettes and other tobacco products must now include health warnings in the form of a text warning, information on stop-smoking services and one of 42 pictures from the European Union picture library of graphic health warning photos. The warnings must cover 65% of the front and back of the packages (European Commission, 2014).

Restricting the promotion and advertising of e-cigarettes: E-cigarettes are considered a potential tool to help achieve the UK's goal of being smoke-free by 2030. This is because e-cigarettes can be used as a smoking cessation aid for those trying to quit smoking tobacco. However, there are ongoing debates and discussions around the safety and regulation of e-cigarettes and their potential long-term health impacts (McNeill et al., 2022). To protect children and young people, the UK has imposed comprehensive regulation of e-cigarettes under the *Tobacco and Related Products Regulations 2016* (TRPR). The regulations cover a range of areas, including:

a Product safety and quality: e-cigarettes and e-liquids must meet certain safety and quality standards, including being child-resistant and tamper-evident.
b Packaging and labelling: e-cigarettes and e-liquids must be labelled with health warnings and information about their nicotine content and ingredients.
c Advertising and promotion: e-cigarettes and e-liquids cannot be advertised or promoted in a way that is misleading or encourages non-smokers to use them.
d Age of sale: selling e-cigarettes and e-liquids to anyone under 18 is illegal.
e Restrictions on use: e-cigarettes are banned in enclosed public places and certain workplaces, and there are restrictions on their use on public transport.
f The UK government also provides businesses with guidance on complying with the regulations.

The health consequences of smoking

The link between smoking and cancer has been appreciated since the seminal work of Doll and Hill (1952). This report has been followed by several studies highlighting the strong link between poor health and tobacco smoking. For example, in the UK, it is suggested that over 100,000 people die annually due to their smoking habit (ASH, 2021). Every year, tobacco smoking kills around 8 million people worldwide (WHO, 2021).

In 2021, deaths caused by tobacco smoking in the UK were higher than the number of deaths caused by road traffic accidents (1,558), other accidents (6,203), poisoning and overdose (4,859), alcoholic liver disease (5,608), suicide (6,319) and human immuno-deficiency virus infection (797). Almost half of all people who smoke regularly will be killed by their habit. A man who smokes cuts short his life by 13.2 years and a woman by 14.5 years (ASH, 2021).

Concerning morbidity, more than a quarter of all cancer deaths in the UK can be attributed to smoking (ASH, 2017). It has also been linked to a whole host of diseases and chronic conditions, including heart disease, throat cancer, stomach and bowel cancer, lung cancer, leukaemia, peripheral vascular disease, premature and low-weight babies, bronchitis, emphysema, sinusitis, peptic ulcers and dental hygiene problems. It can also worsen the effects of asthma and infections (see Table 8.2 and Figure 8.1 for an overview). Further, in light of the COVID-19 pandemic, evidence suggests that compared to people who have never smoked, people who currently smoke are at a higher risk of hospitalisation and mortality due to the virus (Clift et al., 2022).

Table 8.2 Illness associated with smoking

System	Illness
Cardiovascular	Aneurysm
	Angina (20 × risk)
	Beurger's disease (severe circulatory disease)
	Coronary artery disease
	Myocardial infarction (2–3 × risk)
	Peripheral vascular disease
	Stroke (2–4 × risk)
Musculoskeletal	Back pain
	Ligament injuries
	Muscle injuries
	Neck pain
	Osteoporosis
	Osteoarthritis
	Rheumatoid arthritis
	Tendon injuries
	Low bone density
	Hip fractures
Visual	Cataracts (2 ×risk)
	Posterior subcapsular cataract (3 × risk)
	Optic neuropathy (16 × risk)
	Macular degeneration (2 × risk)
	Nystagmus
	Ocular histoplasmosis
	Tobacco amblyopia
Genitourinary	Erectile dysfunction
	Impotence (2 × risk)
	Decreased fertility in women
	Pregnancy complications (e.g., premature rupture of membranes, placenta previa or placental abruption, miscarriage, still birth, low birth weight, reduced lung function in infants)
Digestive, metabolic	Gum disease
	Duodenal ulcer
	Colon polyps
	Crohn's disease
	Diabetes
	Stomach ulcer
	Tooth loss

(*Continued*)

Table 8.2 (Continued)

System	Illness
Respiratory	COPD
Cancers	Lung (90% associated with smoking)
	Mouth and throat (90% associated with smoking)
	Breast (60% increased risk)
	Pancreatic (2 × risk)
	Oesophageal cancer
	Stomach
	Liver
	Bladder (2–5 × risk)
	Kidney
	Cervical cancer
	Myeloid cancer
	Urinary tract cancer
Other conditions	Depression
	Psoriasis (2 × risk)
	Hearing loss
	Sudden Infant Death Syndrome (SIDS)
	Exacerbates:
	Asthma
	Chronic rhinitis
	Diabetic retinopathy
	Graves' disease
	MS
	Optic neuritis
	Coughing, sneezing, shortness of breath
	Common colds, influenza, pneumonia

Applying this to Yuri

Yuri is currently 53, and, given his current smoking pattern and the considerable ill health he suffers, he will be unlikely to live until he reaches his retirement at 65 years of age. Yuri needs to fully appreciate the consequences of his continued smoking.

Those who quit smoking by the age of 40 years retain almost the same life expectancy as lifelong non-smokers. Even those who quit upon diagnosis of early stages of lung cancer are thought to benefit from increased life expectancy (Jassem, 2019). In fact, a recent study showed that for people who quit, the average length of survival is 6.6 years compared to 4.8 years for those who do not quit smoking (Sheikh et al., 2021). Thus, quitting smoking at any age and health status brings health benefits.

Vaping versus smoking

There is contention surrounding using e-cigarettes as a replacement for combustible tobacco products, and opinions surrounding their relative safety and regulation can differ markedly by country. For example, Nargis et al. (2019) examined trends in e-cigarette use and attitudes towards e-cigarettes in Australia and the UK between 2010 and 2016. The

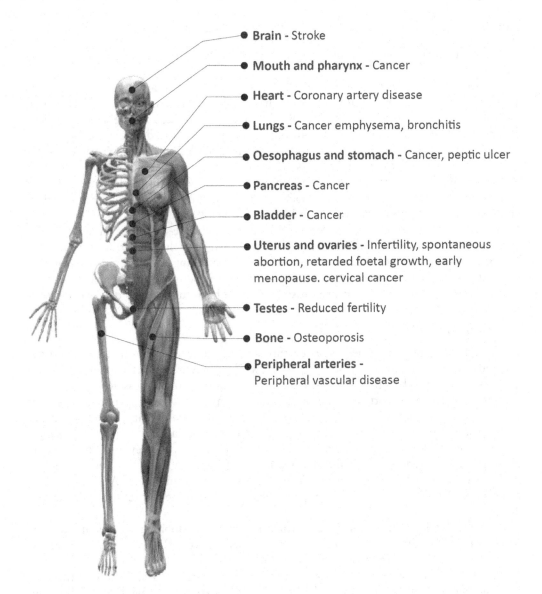

Brain - Stroke

Mouth and pharynx - Cancer

Heart - Coronary artery disease

Lungs - Cancer emphysema, bronchitis

Oesophagus and stomach - Cancer, peptic ulcer

Pancreas - Cancer

Bladder - Cancer

Uterus and ovaries - Infertility, spontaneous abortion, retarded foetal growth, early menopause. cervical cancer

Testes - Reduced fertility

Bone - Osteoporosis

Peripheral arteries - Peripheral vascular disease

Figure 8.1 Health impact of smoking.

data in this study was taken from the International Tobacco Control Four Country Smoking and Vaping Survey. This study found that awareness of e-cigarettes did increase during this time but that experimentation with e-cigarettes was more common in the UK compared to Australia. The authors suggested that this study showed no evidence that e-cigarettes were serving as a 'gateway' to smoking in either country. However, this study only focused on adult smokers and recent ex-smokers. Thus, the results may not apply to other groups, such as non-smokers or younger people.

Research by Gorukanti, Delucchi, Ling, Fisher-Travis and Halpern-Felsher (2017) found that adolescents perceive e-cigarettes to be less harmful and less addictive than traditional cigarettes, which may lead to increased experimentation and use of e-cigarettes. Adolescents were also more likely to perceive e-cigarettes as a socially acceptable behaviour, and peer influence played a significant role in their decision to use e-cigarettes.

Further, in a study by Chaffee et al. (2018), adolescents aged between 12 and 17 participated in the nationally representative Population Assessment of Tobacco and Health Survey. This longitudinal cohort study concerned tobacco use behaviour, beliefs and attitudes, and tobacco-related health outcomes among approximately 46,000 adults and youth in the United States. The study found that adolescents who experiment with e-cigarettes are more likely to progress to smoking tobacco than those who did not experiment with e-cigarettes. In any case, exposure to nicotine during adolescence can have long-lasting consequences on the developing brain, leading to impaired cognitive function and increased susceptibility to nicotine addiction (Leslie, 2020).

The message of these studies appears to be that while e-cigarettes may not be a gateway to smoking for adults, there is evidence to suggest that experimentation with e-cigarettes may increase the risk of progression to smoking tobacco among younger populations. This highlights the need for stronger regulation and prevention efforts targeting adolescents to prevent progression to more harmful patterns of tobacco use.

Assessment of smoking

Smoking behaviour can be best assessed through the subjective recording of cigarettes smoked during a defined period (usually 4 weeks); however, this can often be an underestimate, which must be considered when making your assessment. The most commonly used self-report measure of smoking behaviour is the Fagerström Test for Nicotine Dependence (Fagerström, 1978). People who smoke are asked a set of questions, and the answers are scored and added to provide a total score. A score of 6 or more is considered to indicate a high nicotine dependence. However, if an objective measure is required, a biochemical assessment of carbon monoxide levels can be performed (using 10 ppm as a cut-off level) with specialist equipment. A saliva sample can also be tested for levels of cotinine, a by-product of nicotine metabolism (Hall et al., 2018).

However, aside from whether a confirmed recording of smoking has taken place or whether the subjective record is accurate (which it usually is not), assessing the addiction history is most important (see Table 8.3). Obviously, the stronger the addiction, the harder it is to quit successfully. Consequently, there is a need to assess both motivation for smoking (see Table 8.4) and dependency on cigarettes (Table 8.5). These two elements should provide sufficient information for the practitioner to adequately assess the individual and determine appropriate interventions (e.g., the stronger the addiction, the more likely NRTs will be required).

Applying this to Yuri

Yuri needs a cigarette when he wakes up and has been smoking for a considerable time. He is likely heavily addicted. Although his motivation to quit is high, his current surroundings and numerous previous failed attempts count against him. Yuri would be classed as in the 'very high dependence' category (Table 8.4).

Therefore, his needs and support when attempting to quit will vary considerably from those who smoke but are classed in the 'low dependence' category. As Yuri has a very high dependence, it is important that NRTs are used in conjunction with behavioural therapies to support Yuri quitting.

Why do people smoke?

Before we explore how to get people to stop smoking, it is important to see how psychologists have explained why people smoke. People smoke for various reasons, and a myriad of explanations have been proposed from psychological, social and medical perspectives. The psychological explanations have been from both a behavioural and

Table 8.3 Assessment of addiction to smoking

1.	Do you smoke more than 15 cigarettes per day?
2.	Have you smoked for more than 1 year?
3.	Do you smoke low-tar cigarettes?
4.	Do you smoke alone mainly, or in company?
5.	Do you have a strong craving for cigarettes?
6.	Do you smoke the first cigarette of the day within 30 minutes of getting up in the morning?
7.	Have you tried more than twice to stop before?
8.	Do you think stopping will be difficult?
9.	Are you likely to encounter many situations where you are likely to be tempted to smoke?
10.	Are you attempting to stop smoking alone?

Previous attempts

1.	How many times in the past have you attempted to give up?
2.	How long in the past have you managed to give up for?
3.	What different methods have you tried?
4.	Which was the most successful?

Assess whether – very addicted
– moderately addicted
– mildly addicted

Table 8.4 Assessing motivation for smoking

1. What is your reason for smoking?
2. On a scale of 1–10, how much do you enjoy smoking?
1 – hate, 10 – enjoy very much
3. On a scale of 1–10, how much do you want to stop smoking?
1 – not at all, 10 – desperately keen
4. What are the negative and positive aspects of smoking for you?
5. How would you benefit from giving up?
6. How do you feel smoking affects your health?
7. How much would you pay/give up if it meant you could stop smoking?
Assess whether – highly motivated
– moderately motivated
– not motivated

Table 8.5 Fagerstrom dependence scale

1 How many cigarettes do you smoke daily?
10 or fewer (0)
11–20 (1)
21–30 (2)
30+ (3)
2 How soon after waking up do you smoke your first cigarette?
Less than 6 minutes (3)
6–30 minutes (2)
31–60 minutes (1)
60+ minutes (0)
Scoring
Add up questions 1 and 2
0–1 Low dependence: stopping smoking should be easy.
2 Moderate dependence: guidance and medication to reduce withdrawal symptoms may help.
3 High dependence: guidance and medication may be required.
4–6 Very high dependence: smoking cessation will be difficult and considerable support needed.
  Medication to reduce withdrawal symptoms will be required.

Source: Adapted from *British Medical Journal*, 328, pp. 338–39 (West, R. 2004), with permission from BMJ Publishing Group Ltd.

Table 8.6 Behavioural explanation of smoking development

Concept	Rules	Example
Classical conditioning	Behaviours acquired through associative learning	Having a cup of coffee and a cigarette equals relaxation
Operant conditioning	Behaviour is likely to increase if it is positively reinforced by the presence of a positive event, or negatively reinforced by the absence or removal of a negative event	Smoking is positively reinforced by social acceptance
Observational learning	Behaviours are learned by observing others	Parents or friends smoking
Cognitive factors	Other factors such as coping mechanisms or self-image may contribute	Belief that smoking looks 'cool'
Social learning perspective	Behaviour is learned by modelling and social reinforcement	Seeing parents and peers smoking—being reinforced as 'part of the gang'

social learning perspective (see Table 8.6 for how behavioural elements can help explain why people smoke). The information provided in Table 8.6 goes some way to explaining why people smoke and, on this basis, how we can help them quit.

Psychological models of smoking

Several psychological variables have been implicated in the continuance of smoking. Models of health behaviour such as the health belief model, the protection motivation theory, the theory of reasoned action and the health action process approach have been used to examine the cognitive factors contributing to smoking initiation. Obviously, the distinction between these models and the social explanation is somewhat tenuous. There is a clear overlap between these factors and attempting to explain smoking (or any) lifestyle behaviour monotheoretically is a flawed task.

Another approach is based on the theory of planned behaviour (TPB) (Ajzen, 1991), which appears to be one of the most popular and successful models for studying health behaviour (Armitage & Conner, 2001). The TPB has successfully predicted adolescent smoking (e.g., Smith et al., 2007; Tate et al., 2021). These studies provided good predictions of intentions and subsequent behaviours. According to the TPB, the proximal determinants of behaviour are the intentions to engage in the behaviour. Intentions reflect an individual's decision to exert effort to perform the behaviour. They are assumed to be a function of several related factors such as attitudes, subjective norms, perceived behavioural control and self-efficacy. Smoking can be assumed to be different from some of the other behaviours in this book. In particular, people who smoke might become addicted (whether psychologically or biologically) to cigarettes, but this should not suggest that they have lost control over their behaviour. However, it is a difficult behaviour to change in the sense that their perception of control over the behaviour appears incomplete. As we have seen, those at the highest risk of cigarette dependency (such as low SES groups) often report attitudes or feelings that they have little control over what determines their health or future. These considerations compound the difficulty many quitters face (see Wardle & Steptoe, 2003).

However, more recently, the limitations of this model have been highlighted. For example, the TPB has been criticised for being too simplistic and not considering other factors that may influence behaviour. It has been criticised for its focus on rational reasoning, exclusion of unconscious influences on behaviour and failure to consider emotions beyond anticipated affective outcomes. Crucially, empirical investigations of the TPB have been rare, and those conducted have not consistently supported the theory's assumptions (Sniehotta et al., 2014).

Biological factors associated with smoking

The biological model suggests that smoking results from individuals becoming physically dependent on nicotine and the many chemical substances in cigarettes. The nicotine entering the lungs from a cigarette is transported through the blood supply and to the brain, which activates the autonomic nervous system. Consequently, there is an increase in heat rate and blood pressure, which makes the body more aroused and alert. Once the person has stopped smoking, the nicotine level reduces, as do the 'positive' effects. From this, a model of nicotine regulation can be proposed: people who smoke continue to smoke to avoid withdrawal symptoms (Schachter et al., 1977).

However, some people stop smoking for several years (hence, all the nicotine disappears from their bodies) but then start smoking again. Further, some people who smoke are known as 'chippers'; they smoke a few cigarettes a day for a number of years but do not increase the amount they smoke (hence, they do not show tolerance). Because of these issues, it is recognised that biological theories are not the complete picture; there must be other social and psychological factors involved.

Social factors of smoking

The social context in which smoking develops and is maintained is key. The social factors implicated in the initiation of smoking behaviour (e.g., parents, siblings and peers) all play a part in maintaining this behaviour. Although the relative importance of these various groups has been debated, most research agrees that they do contribute.

Smoking is a social activity for many, but this can differ from individual to individual and from cigarette to cigarette. Thus, for somebody at work, smoking a cigarette may provide an opportunity to escape from the drudgery of the workplace and to have a break. In contrast, down the pub, sharing a cigarette can strengthen social bonds with friends. Positively enhancing their image is often cited as a reason for starting smoking among young children (Hrubá & Zaloudíková, 2010). While positive attitudes towards cigarette smoking in young people have reduced over the last decade, research shows that e-cigarettes are viewed relatively positively by adolescents. However, e-cigarettes tend to be viewed more favourably by adolescents who already use tobacco (Gorukanti et al., 2017). Researchers note that current public knowledge on using e-cigarettes as a smoking cessation device is insufficient. Researchers and policymakers stress the importance of placing e-cigarettes in the market as a quitting device and not promoting them as a substitute or supplement to tobacco cigarettes.

Applying this to Yuri

Yuri tends to smoke more at the pub (although he now has to go into the pub garden to do so) and when he is around people who are smoking. It is important to appreciate some of the triggers prompting Yuri's smoking behaviour, such as peer influence.

Interventions to reduce smoking

Evidence suggests that most people who smoke want to stop smoking (The Health and Social Care Information Centre, 2011). Indeed, of United States (US) respondents, up to 70% of people who smoke say they want to quit, and in 2016, 59% of people who smoked quit, an increase of more than 8% since 2005 (Truth Initiative, 2018). Just over half of those who smoke are successful in quitting smoking before they die, although for many, it is too late. It can be argued that every health care practitioner has a moral duty to try to encourage people to quit smoking. Research suggests that unplanned quit attempts are often successful, and health care professionals are in a good position to provide advice that could trigger a spontaneous quit attempt (Nabi-Burza et al., 2021).

Smoking cessation interventions in a health care setting have been shown to increase quit attempts and success rates for smoking cessation. WHO recognises the unique role of the health care provider in tobacco control (WHO, 2021). However, some research suggests clinicians may be missing opportunities to provide treatment for smoking cessation to all their patients regardless of their reason for presenting (Papadakis et al., 2020). Clearly, there is a need to change how health care practices target smoking cessation, ensuring that all tobacco users receive treatment as part of routine care.

The Ottawa model for smoking cessation (OMSC) has been at the forefront of implementing necessary changes within health care practices concerning the provision of smoking cessation treatment (UOHI, 2023). The OMSC combines education and organisational change practices to encourage smoking cessation treatment as part of routine care. It involves applying the 5 A's in a hospital setting: ask (do you smoke?), advise patients to quit smoking, assess readiness to quit, assist with the quit attempt and arrange follow-up (Mullen et al., 2017).

A real-world effectiveness study by Mullen et al. (2017) compared hospital patients who received OMSC treatment with those who received usual care. They found significantly lower rates of readmissions (smoking-related or otherwise) and fewer emergency room visits in the intervention group compared to the control group. Impressively, assessment at year one also showed a significant decrease in mortality rates in the group that received smoking cessation support. These findings stress the vital need for smoking cessation treatment to be incorporated into routine care in health care facilities.

Alternative strategies for intervention in a health care setting may involve very brief advice (VBA). The foundation of VBA interventions are the 3 A's (as opposed to 5): ask, advise and act (van Schayck et al., 2020). VBA is employed when multiple health professionals are involved or when the time to intervene is limited (Himelfarb-Blyth et al., 2021). While the VBA method does not assess readiness to quit, it assumes that if the intervention is repeated, the likelihood and rate of quit attempts will increase (Papadakis et al., 2020). In fact, evidence is starting to mount that suggests that quit attempts occur at the same rate regardless of the perceived readiness of the patient (Himelfarb-Blyth et al., 2021). As such, the traditional 'opt-in' approach of providing tobacco cessation to patients based on perceived readiness (i.e., the assess and assist steps of the 5 A's) may be limiting the number of patients who receive treatment to help them stop smoking. Himelfarb-Blyth et al. (2021) found that this kind of automatic referral of evidence-based cessation support in an outpatient oncology setting was an effective strategy for providing tobacco cessation treatment.

Thus, there are techniques, both medical and psychological, that can support people in smoking cessation attempts. The health care professional must be aware of these and how clients/patients can access them.

Although it undoubtedly has considerable health benefits, quitting can be fraught with difficulties, and many people report getting irritable, depressed, anxious and restless, and craving tobacco. There are methods that can help overcome some of these difficulties, and a range of pharmacological treatments has been developed to help relieve them. For example, sprays, chewing gum, patches and inhalers have proven benefits for people who smoke (Rigotti, 2022). E-cigarettes have also been suggested as a potential smoking cessation device (Bullen et al., 2013). However, the limited conclusive evidence surrounding their efficacy and safety means that e-cigarettes are not currently a first-line treatment for quitters (Splete, 2022). However, there is always a psychological element to cessation, and the health care professional is in a prime position to maximise motivation, technique and emotional and cognitive engagement with the cessation programme.

Vaping as a smoking cessation tool

Electronic cigarettes (e-cigarettes) have recently become increasingly popular as an alternative to traditional tobacco cigarettes. While e-cigarettes have been marketed as a safer alternative to smoking, their effectiveness as a tool for smoking cessation is still uncertain. Some studies suggest that e-cigarettes may help smokers quit or reduce their cigarette use (Goniewicz et al., 2018), while others argue that they may be a gateway to smoking or prolonging nicotine addiction (Soneji et al., 2018).

A recent Cochrane review by Hartmann-Boyce et al. (2021) aimed to provide a comprehensive evaluation of e-cigarettes' effectiveness as a smoking cessation tool and to determine any potential harmful effects associated with their use. The review included 50 randomised controlled trials involving over 12,000 participants. The review found moderate certainty evidence that using e-cigarettes increased the likelihood of quitting smoking compared to using no support or non-nicotine e-cigarettes. However, the evidence was less certain when comparing e-cigarettes to other smoking cessation aids, such as nicotine patches or gum. The review also found low-certainty evidence that using e-cigarettes may increase the risk of adverse events, such as throat and mouth irritation, nausea and headaches. However, the review found no evidence of serious adverse events, such as heart attacks, strokes or respiratory problems, associated with e-cigarette use.

A review conducted by the National Centre for Epidemiology and Population Health on the health effects of electronic cigarettes or 'vaping' commissioned by the Australian Department of Health highlights that the use of e-cigarettes is increasing and that over one-third of current e-cigarette users in Australia were aged under 25, with half aged under 30. This suggests that most e-cigarette use is not for smoking cessation, particularly among young users. The identified risks of e-cigarettes include addiction, intentional and unintentional poisoning, acute nicotine toxicity, burns and injuries, lung injury, indoor air pollution, environmental waste and fires, dual use with cigarette smoking and increased smoking uptake in non-smokers. Further, the review indicates that non-smokers who use e-cigarettes are three times as likely to go on to smoke combustible tobacco cigarettes as non-smokers who do not use e-cigarettes, supporting a 'gateway' effect. The review suggests that e-cigarettes are harmful for non-smokers, particularly youth, and there is limited evidence that e-cigarettes are an effective aid for quitting smoking when used in the clinical setting. The evidence for the effects of nicotine and non-nicotine e-cigarettes on most major health conditions is lacking, meaning their safety concerning these outcomes has not been established (Banks et al., 2023).

Stopping people smoking

Encouraging and enhancing smoking cessation is now recognised as an important part of public health and a key role of the health care practitioner. Mohiuddin et al. (2007) reported a reduction in total mortality due to an intensive smoking cessation programme compared to a usual care group. Other studies have also suggested that interventions to improve smoking result in beneficial changes in other health behaviours, such as exercise, which is routinely recommended as an aid to smoking cessation. The most recent Cochrane review on this topic suggests that the evidence for exercise as a cessation tool is mixed. Still, several factors may make it a helpful addition for some people wanting to quit smoking (Ussher et al., 2019). Cardiovascular exercise has been shown to reduce the withdrawal symptoms associated with quitting smoking and smoking cravings because exercise stimulates similar reward pathways in the brain as nicotine, which may also reduce weight gain and increase fitness levels. Thus, getting people to stop smoking can positively impact health behaviours other than smoking.

Individual-level interventions

Interventions aimed at the individual concerning smoking cessation can take many forms. In this section, a selection of the individual-level approaches, interventions and policies will be discussed. From this, it will be possible to understand the underlying theory behind them and how psychological principles can be used in addressing smoking cessation. Clinical smoking cessation includes (either alone or in combination) behavioural and pharmaceutical interventions, and they range from brief advice and counselling to intensive support and administration of medications that contribute to reducing or overcoming dependence in individuals and the entire population (Kotz et al., 2014).

Clinical interventions

The simplest individual interventions are brief interventions that most health care professionals can engage in without specific training. The Five A's model in Table 8.7 is promoted for all health care professionals. A flow diagram is presented in Figure 8.2, highlighting the process that health care professionals should follow when they are in a position to offer guidance and advice.

Table 8.7 The Five A's model for facilitating smoking cessation

Five A's	Example	Key points
Ask about tobacco use	Always include questions about tobacco use	Include questions about smoking in all consultations
Advise smokers to quit	Use clear, strong, and personalised language	'Quitting tobacco is the most important thing you can do to protect your health.'
Assess smokers' willingness to quit	Ask every tobacco user if he/she is willing to quit at this time.	'On a scale of 1–10, how ready are you to quit smoking?'
	• If willing to quit, provide resources and assistance • If unwilling to quit at this time, help motivate the patient: • Identify reasons to quit in a supportive manner. • Build patient's confidence about quitting.	
Assist the patient	• Set a quit date, ideally within 2 weeks.	Help the patient make a quit plan (see later)
	• Remove tobacco products from their environment. • Get support from family, friends and co-workers. • Review past quit attempts—what helped, what led to relapse? • Anticipate challenges, particularly during the critical first few weeks, including nicotine withdrawal. • Identify reasons for quitting and benefits of quitting. Give advice on successful quitting: • Total abstinence is essential—not even a single puff.	

Table 8.7 (Continued)

Five A's	Example	Key points
	• Drinking alcohol is strongly associated with relapse. • Allowing others to smoke in the household hinders successful quitting. Encourage use of medication: • Recommend use of over-the-counter nicotine patch, gum or lozenge; or give prescription for varenicline, bupropion SR nicotine inhaler or nasal spray, unless contraindicated.	
Arrange follow-up	Follow-up should occur.	Arrange for follow-up within a fortnight

Source: Adapted from Okuyemi et al. (2006).

Applying this to Yuri

Yuri has come to you and asked for support to give up smoking. Arrange to see Yuri within 7 days of your first appointment. This will enable you to fully assess, support and guide Yuri throughout his lifestyle behaviour change.

Methods for assisting people quitting

Obviously, the assist stage can vary, and these interventions are many and varied, with most (but not all) improving smoking cessation rates efficaciously. For example, these therapies include self-help methods, physician advice, telephone counselling, cognitive behaviour therapy, NRT and non-nicotine medication such as bupropion (Akanbi et al., 2019). These interventions will be explored in more detail later.

But are patients informed of all (or indeed, any) of these treatment options? Surveys showed that most people who smoke (55.3% in 2021) wanted to stop smoking, and 21.7% said they intended to quit in the next 3 months (Office for National Statistics, 2020). Although the percentage of unassisted quitting among smokers has decreased over time, it remains the most common method for smoking cessation in Australia. In 1998, 61% of smokers attempted to quit without assistance, compared to 40% in 2017. However, seeking help from a doctor for advice or support was the most popular assisted method in 2017, with 34% of smokers choosing this method, a significant increase from 18% in 1998.

Figures appear to vary depending on location; however, a study of 31 countries by Ahluwalia et al. (2021) showed that much support is under-utilised. For example, of those surveyed, only 7% employed counselling services to assist in quitting smoking, 6% used some form of NRT, 2% used prescription medications, and less than 1% utilised smoking Quitlines.

There is also evidence to suggest that many individuals, particularly those in the 'hard to reach groups' (see Chapter 3) where smoking prevalence is often greater, are less likely to have access to cessation programmes and are less likely to receive advice on quitting

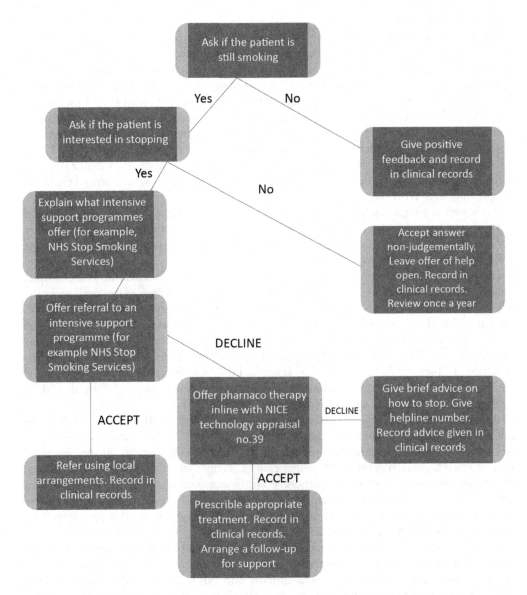

Figure 8.2 Brief intervention for people who smoke attending the clinic.

Source: National Institute for Health and Clinical Excellence (2006) Adapted from *Brief Interventions and referral for smoking cessation in primary and other settings.* London, UK: National Institute for Health and Clinical Excellence. Available from www.nice.org.UR/PH001. Reproduced with permission.

from primary care providers (Nargis et al., 2019). Alongside this, it is also understood that deprived individuals require a greater level of support when undertaking smoking cessation (O'Connell et al., 2022). However, a meta-analysis of smoking cessation behaviour in low- and middle-income countries suggests that individuals with a low SES are not necessarily less successful at quitting (Nargis et al., 2019). Nevertheless, all health care professionals should know about local services and facilitate access.

Pharmacological treatments

Pharmacological treatments (see Table 8.8) are popular methods for assisting individuals with quitting. These include five forms of NRT (gum, patch, nasal spray, inhaler and lozenge) and bupropion sustained release. In a recent review of 150 trials, Stead et al. (2012) surmised that all forms of NRT increase people's chance of quitting by 50 to 70%. NRTs can, in some circumstances, double the abstinence rate at over 5 months. A study by Jackson et al. (2019) modelled continuous abstinence rates of clinical trials of pharmacological interventions for smoking cessation over 52 weeks. The authors observed that for varenicline, bupropion and NRT, abstinence rates were 22.5%, 16.7%, and 13.0% at 52 weeks compared to a placebo (8.3%). Thus, evidence suggests nicotine replacement or other pharmacological interventions can significantly help some people quit long term.

Even with the pharmacological intervention, it is important to provide psychological support and encouragement for the individuals who smoke: the psychological factors involved in NRT use are considerable. Without continued motivation, the success of NRT will be compromised. Simply focusing on NRTs may be 'doomed to failure' because nicotine is only part of the explanation for smoking behaviour. For example, behavioural techniques or denicotinised cigarettes may be required to deal with the sensory-motor activities associated with smoking. Interestingly, e-cigarettes have also been positioned within the market as a smoking cessation device. Preliminary findings from a randomised control trial found that with or without nicotine, e-cigarettes were as effective as nicotine patches at helping people abstain from smoking cigarettes (Bullen et al., 2013). Nevertheless, research has suggested that pharmacological therapies can be considered a 'vital component' of smoking cessation programmes and thus should be available to all quitters (Cofta-Woerpel et al., 2007, p. 47).

Although NRTs successfully assist people to quit smoking, NRTs have not been as influential as predicted. It has been suggested that NRTs are less beneficial for individuals who wish to reduce the amount they smoke or partake in temporary abstinence than individuals who aim to make a permanent change. People who smoke but wish to reduce their consumption or partake in temporary abstinence were found to be using NRT in addition to a non-reduction in cigarette smoking (Beard et al., 2011). It could be suggested that individuals who do not aim to quit fully have less motivation; therefore, other methods should be suggested.

Consequently, the use of NRTs has not removed the need for psychological input into smoking cessation; rather, it has increased it. It is recognised that the most effective cessation technique combines personal support and NRT (Fiore, 2009). Many studies highlight that personal or telephone support with NRT increases quit rates (Hollis et al., 2007). This support works by increasing motivation for quitting and remaining tobacco-free. However, in England, most individuals attempting to quit do not use the National Health Service Stop Smoking Service (NHS-SSS), which is effective, free and combines behavioural and pharmacological approaches (Kotz et al., 2009). According to Song et al. (2020), success rates for attempts to quit were shown to be significantly higher with SSS support (15.1%) compared to attempts made without support (11.3%). Thus, when behavioural aspects of quitting are not addressed, individuals may not receive the required support and motivation to continue. There are several ways of assessing motivation, which will be explored in more detail in a later section. However, three simple questions can be used:

Table 8.8 Pharmacological interventions for smoking cessation

Intervention	Advantage	Disadvantage	Quit rates (%)
Bupropion	Non-nicotine Easy to use Can be used with NRT	Can cause insomnia, dry mouth, headache, tremors, nausea or anxiety	21–30
Nicotine gum • Use 4 mg if smoking 10 cigarettes or more • Use 2 mg if smoking fewer than 10 • Chew each piece slowly for 30 minutes when there is an urge to smoke • Max 15 per day. Reduce slowly over 3 months	Over the counter Flexible Quick delivery Different flavours Low compliance	No food or drink 15 minutes beforehand Frequent use required Jaw pain, mouth soreness, dyspepsia Under-dosing is common	7–10
Nicotine inhaler • 6–12 cartridges daily for 8 weeks • Reduce to half in next 2 weeks • Gradually stop over the next 2 weeks	Flexible dosing Mimics hand-to-mouth action of smoking Few side effects Comes in menthol flavour	Frequent dosing necessary May cause mouth and throat irritation Low compliance Under-dosing is common	23
Nicotine lozenge • 1 or 2 tabs per hour under the tongue • Maximum 40 per day • Continue for at least 3 months and then withdraw slowly until only 1 or 2 tabs needed per day	Over the counter Flexible dosing No food or drink 15 minutes beforehand Quick delivery Oral administration	Frequent dosing necessary May cause mouth soreness or dyspepsia Low compliance Under-dosing is common	24
Nicotine patch • 21 mg patch for 6 weeks • 14 mg patch for 2 weeks • 7 mg patch for 2 weeks • If smoking 10 cigarettes or fewer, start with the 14 mg patch and reduce after 6 weeks to the 7 mg patch for the last 2 weeks • Apply in the morning to non-hairy area of skin on trunk or upper arm • Replace in 24 hours • Use for 10 weeks maximum	Over the counter Daily application Overnight use	Less flexible dosing Slow delivery of nicotine May cause skin irritation or sleep problems Not good at treating acute cravings	8–21
Nicotine nasal spray • 1 spray to each nostril as required for 8 weeks	Flexible dosing Fastest delivery Reduces craving within minutes	Frequent dosing necessary May cause nose and eye irritation	30

(Continued)

Table 8.8 (Continued)

Intervention	Advantage	Disadvantage	Quit rates (%)
• Maximum 1 spray to each nostril twice per hour or 64 sprays per day • Reduce by half over the next 2 weeks • Stop gradually over the last 2 weeks • Maximum treatment is 3 months		Most addictive of the NRTs	

- Do you want to stop smoking for good?
- Are you interested in making a serious attempt to stop in the near future?
- Are you interested in receiving help with your quit attempt?

These provide a qualitative indicator of motivation to stop smoking (West, 2004).

Applying this to Yuri

Given Yuri's level of smoking and the number of years that he has been smoking, some form of NRT will probably be required. You should explore all the options with Yuri to see which one he feels most comfortable with. Discussing options with the client is important as they need to feel confident and comfortable with any changes they make.

Psychological approaches

Psychological approaches to smoking cessation are important, either alone or in conjunction with pharmacological approaches, and this has been recognised since the 1960s. There are, of course, several psychological intervention methods and Table 8.9 summarises the effectiveness of particular psychosocial treatment contents (adapted from US Surgeon General, 2008).

Applying this to Yuri

Yuri would benefit from additional social support: you could arrange for him to contact a Quitline or the local Stop Smoking clinic. You may also want to talk with his family so he obtains support from that quarter.

Table 8.9 Psychosocial content and abstinence rates

Psychosocial content	Estimated abstinence rate (95% CI)
No counselling (i.e., nothing)	11.2
Relaxation (muscle and imagery relaxation)	10.8 (7.8, 13.8)
Contingency contracting (e.g., 'If you give up smoking I will give you £10')	11.2 (7.8, 14.6)
Cigarette fading (reducing number of cigarettes smoked over specified time period)	11.8 (8.4, 15.3)
Intratreatment social support (support from practitioners during treatment)	14.4 (12.3, 16.5)
Extratreatment social support (support from practitioners after treatment)	16.2 (11.8, 20.6)
Other aversive smoking (negative consequence associated with smoking cigarette)	17.7 (11.2, 24.9)
Rapid smoking (i.e., smoke one cigarette, followed by another and another until sick)	19.9 (11.2, 29.0)

Source: Adapted from Surgeon General (2008).

Applying research in practice

A Randomized Controlled Trial of an Appearance-Related Smoking Intervention (Grogan et al., 2011). This paper investigated whether exposure to a smoke-related facial age progression technique impacted quit-smoking cognitions, nicotine dependence and self-reported and objectively assessed smoking in women aged between 18 and 34 years using a randomised control trial.

All the women were randomised to either an appearance-related intervention or a control group. Women completed questionnaires assessing attitudes, subjective norms, perceived behavioural control and intention to quit smoking immediately before, immediately after and 4 weeks after receiving the intervention or usual care.

Findings revealed that compared to the control group, the appearance-related intervention group had significantly more positive attitudes, subjective norms, perceived behavioural control and intention to quit smoking immediately after exposure.

It was concluded that an appearance-related smoking intervention may be useful with usual care for women who smoke.

As we can see from Table 8.9, there are several psychological approaches to smoking cessation. One of the earliest and most successful forms of psychological intervention is behavioural. According to behaviourists, all behaviour is learnt from the environment, can be reduced to simple stimulus-response associations and, regardless of its complexity, can be described and explained without reference to internal states (motivation, emotion, etc.) or mental events (e.g., perception, attention, memory or thinking). Thus, learning and experience are fundamental to the behaviourist approach.

Table 8.10 Why do you continue to smoke?

Antecedents (before the behaviour)	Behaviour (what did you do?)	Consequences (what happened after this)
• What were you doing? • What were you thinking? • What were you feeling? • Who were you with?	• Smoke!	• What happened after this? • How did you feel?

A
Example: I was stressed out because of the children
	B
	I had a cigarette
	  Or
	I went and sat down for 5 minutes to watch TV and relax
		C
		I felt guilty
		  Or
		I felt relaxed and ready to play with the children

Behavioural approaches

Behavioural approaches to smoking cessation are many and varied, yet are usually based on Marlatt and Gorden's (1985) relapse prevention model. This model suggests that common events (cognitive, behavioural or affective) lead to high-risk situations threatening abstinence, such as an argument with a partner or stress when driving to work. These situations can be identified with guided support by the individuals who smoke, although sometimes a table such as that presented in Table 8.10 may be useful to assist the person in identifying any triggers.

Consequently, it is suggested that individuals can prevent relapse by anticipating these events and learning to cope with them. This model has been taken up enthusiastically; however, the method's effectiveness has been questioned (Livingstone-Banks et al., 2019). At its simplest, any intervention based on the behavioural perspective would explore if there were any triggers for a person smoking and then either eradicate these triggers or teach the individual how to cope with them. For example, if every time a person sat down for a cup of coffee in the morning they had a cigarette, they would be taught to have the coffee in a place where they could not smoke or to take up some other activity during this time (e.g., reading the newspaper). Obviously, it would not be sensible to substitute one unhealthy behaviour for another, so replacing a cigarette with a cream cake would not be a good idea! Conversely, if the person reached for a cigarette every time they got stressed out with the children and wanted a '5-minute break with a smoke', different coping mechanisms for relaxation could be taught.

Applying this to Yuri

Yuri has several identified triggers—the pub and his friends. He needs to be taught coping mechanisms to deal with any potential triggers in these situations.

The transtheoretical model of change/stages of change

The most influential psychological model used in smoking cessation has been the transtheoretical model (TTM) of change or stages of change (DiClemente & Prochaska, 1982). The

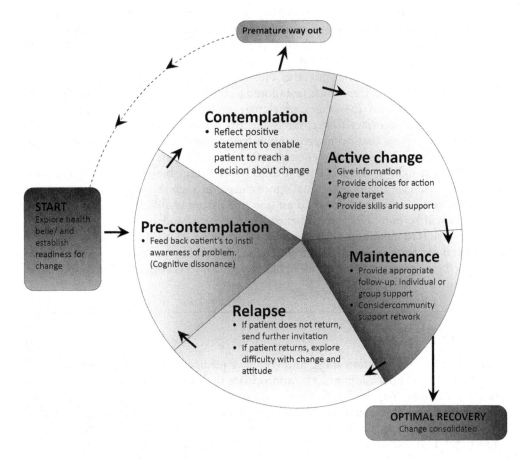

Figure 8.3 Stages of change model.

Source: Adapted from Silverman and Draper (2005).

model suggests that change proceeds through six stages, as summarised in Figure 8.3. Importantly, relapse can occur at any stage and can mean that the individual goes back to the very first stage—it is not a linear model of simple progression from one stage to another. Relapse means that you revert to a previous stage: you can revert to *any* previous stage.

Methods for assisting people to quit

The stages of change model has been used extensively to promote health and assist individuals in quitting smoking. This model is important because it allows professionals to identify where individuals are in their behaviour and then develop appropriate interventions (whether computer- or media-based, community- or individual-based, or pharmacologically or psychologically based). If, for example, an individual smokes and has no intention of giving up (i.e., the pre-contemplation stage), the intervention to be developed will be different from that of the individual who is preparing to give up (i.e., the contemplation stage) or has started the process (i.e., the action stage). In the first case, we should try to get quitting into the person's thought processes. We want to try to get the individual to consider quitting smoking—we want to shift them from the pre-contemplation stage to the contemplation stage. The most common method in this approach is a simple consciousness-raising exercise: increasing information about the problem and how it can affect the individual concerned. So, at this stage, it would simply be a case of getting them to realise that smoking is health-damaging and can affect them individually and then spelling out the individual health problems. This example demonstrates that interventions must be tailored to the individual's position in the cycle.

Interventions based on the stages of change model usually incorporate two key elements. First, it is necessary to accurately identify an individual's stage of change (or readiness to change) so that an appropriate intervention can be designed and applied. Second, the stage of change needs to be reassessed frequently, and the intervention needs to be modified in light of this assessment. In this way, stage-based interventions evolve and adapt in response to the individual's movement through the stages. It is suggested that such interventions are better than the 'one-size-fits-all' model and that the intervention will be more efficient and effective than such models.

The first task is to identify the stage at which the individual is. This is not as difficult as it sounds and can be completed using a simple 'readiness ruler', along with a 'confidence ruler', which can assist the practitioner in planning the intervention and the support that will be required.

Applying this to Yuri

Yuri is in the contemplation stage, and you have pushed him into the action stage. The methods you now adopt must be appropriate to this stage. Such methods could include providing Yuri with information on quitting, including preparing him for the physiological and psychological effects this may have. For example, Yuri will experience physiological withdrawal symptoms. In addition, now is also the perfect time to set Yuri some targets. Doing all of this will, in turn, provide Yuri with help and support during his attempt to quit.

The TTM has been primarily applied to smoking—West (2005) reported that a third of all TTM studies dealt with smoking, compared to only 13% for alcohol, cocaine, heroin, opiates and gambling—and has been *the* model for developing interventions. Indeed, surveys have suggested that the stages of change model and MI were the main topics covered in training courses and the primary theories used to explain behaviour change (West, 2005). The stages of change model has been popular with practitioners as a practical intervention guide for clinicians and as an example of applying complex theories of behaviour change in an approachable and understandable form. However, while the model and the concept of the stages of change are still widely used to design interventions, an increasing number of criticisms and limitations are being revealed. The main criticism is that the TTM is more useful in theory than practice.

Motivational interviewing

The concept of the TTM can be used clinically to work with people who smoke. One practical component that can be adopted from the model is MI, an innovative therapeutic approach for promoting behavioural change that is increasingly being applied to smoking cessation (Lindson et al., 2019). MI is 'a directive patient-centred style of counselling, designed to help people to explore and resolve ambivalence about behaviour change' (Lai et al., 2010).

The goal of MI reflects the simple expectation that increasing an individual's motivation to consider change—rather than showing them how to change—should be the key step. If a person is not motivated to change, whether or not they know how to do it is irrelevant. However, if a person is motivated to change, the interventions to change behaviour can begin.

MI is a technique based on cognitive behavioural therapy that aims to enhance an individual's motivation to change health behaviour. The whole process aims to help the patient understand their thought processes and identify how they help produce the inappropriate behaviour, which can be changed to develop alternative, health-promoting behaviours. MI differs from counselling because it is directive—the health care professional elicits and selectively reinforces change talk that resolves ambivalence and moves the individual towards change.

Motivational strategies include eight components designed to increase the person's motivation towards changing a specific behaviour. It is important to note that motivation is specific to one behaviour, so being motivated to quit smoking does not simply transfer to being motivated to reduce alcohol consumption. The eight components are:

- giving advice (about specific behaviours to be changed)
- removing barriers (often about access to particular help)
- providing choice (making it clear that if they choose not to change, that is their right and it is their choice; the therapist is there to encourage change but not insist on change)
- decreasing desirability (of the ambivalence towards change or the status quo)
- practising empathy
- providing feedback (from a variety of perspectives—family, friends, health professionals— to give the patient a full picture of their current situation)
- clarifying goals (feedback should be compared with a standard [an ideal], and clarification of the ideal can provide the pathway to the goal)
- active helping (such as expressing caring or facilitating a referral, both conveying a real interest in helping the person to change).

MI has been considered a successful technique in aiding long-term behaviour change concerning smoking (Lindson et al., 2019). Although the method sounds relatively simple and straightforward and, to a certain extent, it is, there are a number of key skills you need to employ to motivate people to quit smoking successfully. Some of these are presented in Table 8.11.

Applying this to Yuri

It is important that Yuri progresses from the action stage and can maintain his ability to quit for his health to benefit. In continuing to support Yuri, MI could be used and obstacles that impact his ability to maintain his quitting behaviour can be addressed.

Table 8.11 Key skills for motivational interviewing

Skill	Comment
Express empathy	There should be no criticism or blame as acceptance facilitates change
Develop discrepancy	Change is motivated by a perceived discrepancy between present behaviour and personal goal
Roll with resistance	Avoid arguing for change or providing change—see the smoker as the source of information
Support self-efficacy	The smoker's belief in the possibility of change is an important motivator for change
Use open-ended questions	Encourage the client to do most of the talking: 'What are your concerns about smoking?'
Use reflective listening	Reflect back change talk in a statement: 'I had real cravings this morning' to 'You are a little concerned about the cravings in the morning'
Use affirmation	Use to build rapport: 'You are right to be concerned about smoking in front of the children'
Summarise	Link together and reinforce what has been discussed: 'You are concerned that your smoking may cause lung cancer'
Reframe or agree with a twist	Address resistance by reinterpreting: 'My kids nag me about giving up smoking' to 'It sounds like they really care about your health'
Emphasise personal choice	Reinforce that is the client's choice to change their behaviour
Evocative questions	
Increasing confidence	Use open questions to evoke confidence talk: 'How might you go about making this change?'
Confidence ruler	Use the ruler to ask 'What would it take to score higher?'
Strengths and successes	Review obstacles and how the client has overcome them
Reframing	'I've tried three times to quit and failed' to 'You have had three good attempts already and are learning new skills'
Prompt coping strategies	Ask for potential obstacles and putative coping strategies

Sources: Adapted from Miller and Rollnick (2002).

With an estimated 67% of people who smoke reporting a desire to quit smoking (The Health and Social Care Information Centre, 2011), it is important to highlight some of the specific interventions available to all individuals. Examples of such programmes are discussed below.

The National Health Service Stop Smoking Service

The NHS provides a free stop-smoking service across England to anyone who is trying to quit. The service offers a combination of NRTs, counselling and support on a one-to-one or a group basis. Individuals who wish to quit start their support before any attempt to reduce smoking rates. The trained staff offer advice on quitting and recommend the best strategy for that individual. Once the individual decides to quit, carbon monoxide monitors are used to take biochemical measures of the carbon monoxide levels in the individual's breath. The higher the level of carbon monoxide, the more the individual is smoking. For example, a non-smoker should measure 0–10 on the reader as opposed to a heavy smoker, who will show a range of >20. This tool is used to motivate the individual to continue to quit as they will be able to see the benefits of their efforts. One evaluation concluded that over 250,000 people had quit smoking through the service (Dobbie et al., 2015).

Quit4life

Provided by the NHS, the service delivers smoking cessation support for individuals across Hampshire. The programme adopts a multifocused approach, including psychological and physiological support throughout the quitting process. Like the NHS Stop Smoking Service, smoking cessation support is offered through support groups from trained smoking cessation advisers. In addition, the service offers advice on tackling issues related to quitting and NRT. It is suggested that providing individuals with a combination of support mechanisms, such as those seen in Quit4life, can increase cessation rates (Fiore, 2009). Quit4life's most recent programme was an innovative vaping voucher scheme in 2018. The scheme offers people who smoke a choice regarding how they want to quit by offering a £25 voucher to people who smoke who want to quit tobacco by switching to an e-cigarette. Since the programme began, over 400 Quit4life participants have quit smoking. Overall, using e-cigarettes as a smoking cessation tool remains controversial, with concerns around safety, potential negative effects and regulation. In an upcoming section of this chapter, we will delve into the distinct perspectives and policies of the UK and Australia concerning e-cigarettes.

Stoptober

In October 2012, the NHS launched their first 'Stoptober' campaign. Backed by Cancer Research UK and the British Heart Foundation, the campaign encouraged people who smoke to stop smoking for 28 days, as those who do so are five times more likely to stay smoke-free (Department of Health, 2012). Participants could download the Stoptober app or access the Facebook page, where they were provided with tips, advice and encouragement. Between 2012 and 2021, 2.3 million people have made a quit attempt as part of the campaign.

Community-level interventions

Having considered individual-level interventions, it is also important to consider community-based interventions and policies. Such interventions aim to promote behaviour change in individuals who would not consider individual-level assistance. Tobacco-controlling interventions and policies have been found to be successful in reducing smoking prevalence (Wilson et al., 2012). Some examples of community-level interventions are outlined below.

Smokefree generation

The Department of Health has launched many advertising campaigns over the years to encourage people to quit smoking. One recently launched campaign was 'smoke-free generation'. Re-launched in November 2011, the campaign focused on the children of smokers and emphasised their worries regarding their parents' smoking habits. These were conveyed through short video clips using real children and their accounts instead of child actors. Within these campaigns, the children make stop-smoking appeals to make the parents realise that their smoking habits affect others around them.

Smoking cessation and technology

The delivery and effectiveness of advertising campaigns and interventions are now better than ever due to the popularity of social media. Social media has become one of the most influential platforms for smoking cessation techniques. A 2021 systematic review of the outcomes of 13 original studies concluded that social media is an effective, low-cost intervention, with the average 7-day point prevalence abstinence rate ranging from 7% to 75% (Luo et al., 2022). For social media interventions, cessation outcomes increased as the assessment time increased; this contrasts with in-person counselling, whereby outcomes decreased as the assessment time increased. It may be that the extra support received during and after intervention in social media-based programmes means that participants can maintain smoking cessation (Luo et al., 2022).

One feasible way smoking cessation programmes can be implemented through social media is via instant messaging platforms (such as Facebook Messenger, WhatsApp and WeChat). Luk et al. (2019) conducted a qualitative study into the perceptions of instant messaging platforms as a tool for smoking cessation among people who smoke in Hong Kong. The study supported instant messaging as a potential option for providing more personalised and adaptive support to people who quit smoking.

Another promising initiative that utilises current technology is the NHS Quit Smoking app. The free app allows quitters to track their progress, see how much money they are saving and receive daily support. The website promoting the app states that those who make it to 28 days without smoking are five times more likely to quit permanently.

Smoke-free legislation

The smoke-free legislation introduced in 2007 saw enclosed public spaces such as bars and restaurants become smoke-free environments. Its introduction has had many benefits. One benefit is reduced exposure to second-hand smoke for individuals who do not smoke (Henderson et al., 2021). More specifically, benefits have been seen in the air quality in pubs and bars (Brennan et al., 2010). Additionally, more recent legislation aims to protect children and young people by prohibiting smoking in cars when children under 18 are present. This legislation was approved and implemented in 2015. In addition to direct health benefits, it is thought that introducing smoke-free legislation can impact quit rates and intentions to quit. Research suggests that the perceived unacceptability of smoking due to the smoke-free legislation encouraged quit attempts by people who smoke (Brown et al., 2009). This highlights the attitudinal changes of individuals concerning smoking and social norms. This can have future implications on quitting and the uptake of the behaviour in the first place. Overall, the legislation has been effective at a health and behavioural level and at an attitudinal level. This level is considered an important factor in successful behaviour change as outlined in health theories and models such as the TPB (Ajzen, 1991; Middlestadt et al., 2012).

Second-hand smoke campaign

We have seen several interventions aimed directly at the impact of smoking on the people who smoke; however, attention also needs to be paid to the effects of cigarette smoke on individuals who do not smoke. For example, WHO China launched the #healthismyright social media campaign in 2018, empowering people to stand up for their right to be protected from second-hand smoke in public places. In 2017, the New Mexico

Department of Health launched the 'Kids for Smoke-free Air Challenge' in collaboration with the local Boys & Girls clubs. The campaign targeted parents, family and friends who may be exposing their children to tobacco smoke in cars and homes. The children collected signatures and pledges from parents and family members promising to keep their cars and homes smoke-free, with incentives of up to $1,000 to be won for local clubs. A national advertising campaign in the UK warning of the dangers of second-hand smoke was launched in 2012. This campaign aims to increase awareness of the dangers of second-hand smoke. In doing so, it aims to increase the number of quit attempts and reduce air pollution for non-smokers. The importance of raising awareness of second-hand smoke comes from the potentially dangerous chemicals that are thought to be affecting individuals who do not smoke. It is thought that alongside physiological symptoms, individuals such as children can be affected psychologically by second-hand smoke (Bandiera et al., 2011). This implies that second-hand smoke always has health implications (ASH, 2011b). Sadly, while brief counselling interventions in a health care setting may be effective in encouraging individuals to consider quitting smoking for their own health, the same technique does not appear to be effective in encouraging parents and carers to limit their children's exposure to second-hand smoke. A Cochrane database systematic review of parental smoking control programmes for reducing exposure to environmental tobacco smoke has demonstrated the limited efficacy of these kinds of interventions (Behbod et al., 2018). To date, researchers have been unable to determine the efficacy of any particular style of parent-level intervention because of the poor-quality research available. There is limited evidence to suggest MI and intensive counselling have some impact on getting parents to stop smoking around their children. Still, it has been suggested that population-based interventions are needed in this area (Baxi et al., 2014). Indeed, tobacco control programmes routinely involve an education component about the dangers of smoking in the home and in cars (Grace et al., 2022). Since legislation in many countries now prohibits smoking in cars in the presence of children, there is some evidence of emerging social change as a result, with some households voluntarily extending the restriction of smoking around children to smoking in the home as well, despite the lack of specific legislation around this.

Applying this to Yuri

Community-level campaigns, such as the second-hand smoke campaign, could be shown to Yuri as part of educating him about the potential health consequences of smoking. Yuri must realise how much his second-hand smoke can affect his grandchild, Dmitry. This factor could then impact his motivation to maintain his quitting behaviour.

Working effectively with others

In attempting to reduce smoking rates, providing individuals with the professional advice they will need is important. Below are examples of how health professionals can help with smoking cessation and contribute to successfully maintaining the behaviour to prevent relapse.

Nurses

Nurses have a wide patient base and, as such, provide a good basis for promoting smoking cessation to the general population (Rice et al., 2017). This, in turn, could help with the UK's government's aims to reduce smoking. More specifically, the NHS provides special training and resources to specific health care professionals such as midwives. Reducing and stopping pregnant women's smoking is important due to the detrimental health implications for both the mother and the child. The effects of smoking during pregnancy have been well documented. Alongside health implications, foetal development is also affected (Morales-Prieto et al., 2022). The National Institute for Health and Clinical Excellence (NICE) recognised the importance of midwives in this role and produced updated outlined guidance on the matter (NICE, n.d.). Recommendations for midwives include making the mother aware of the risks of smoking, supporting partners who also smoke and referring them to a stop-smoking service.

GPs

In addition to nurses having good access to the general population, GPs also have a wide client base and constitute a means of advice for smoking cessation. However, it has been noted that 11% of individuals who talk to their GP regarding smoking cessation are advised to stop but are not offered any support (Fidler et al., 2011). When the GP offered support and advice, positive associations were noted in attempted quit rates (Fidler, et al. 2011). This highlights the GPs' importance in promoting smoking cessation to their patients and providing a first point of call.

When looking to change behaviour permanently, a plan for change must be developed once the people who smoke are ready to quit. This can be used alongside any other methods when attempting to quit and comes from the person who smokes, though it is a process best shared with a health care professional. This plan involves setting goals, considering change options, arriving at a plan and eliciting commitment (see Table 8.12). It can be helpful for individuals to create a physical plan as this will provide reinforcement and something concrete to explore when challenges occur.

Maintaining the quit behaviour

Once the initial behaviour change is undertaken, it is important to work on maintaining it. Most quit attempts fail within the first week; hence, it is important to follow up with the individual on a frequent and regular basis—probably during the first 1, 2 and 3 weeks. Having follow-up text messages or phone calls during the first 10 days may also

Table 8.12 Developing a change plan

Aspect of change	Comment	Questions to ask
Setting goals	The smoker's goals are the ones that matter most	What do you want to achieve?
Considering change options	Useful to provide range of optional strategies	What do you think will work for you?
Arrive at a plan	Summarise the smoker's plan	How will you go about it?
Elicit commitment	Useful to agree some immediate steps to implement the plan	What date are you going to quit?

Table 8.13 Withdrawal symptoms commonly experienced

Withdrawal symptom	Duration	Proportion of smokers affected
Light-headedness	< 2 days	10%
Night-time awakenings	< 1 week	25%
Poor concentration	< 2 weeks	60%
Cravings	> 2 weeks	70%
Irritability or aggression	< 4 weeks	50%
Restlessness	< 4 weeks	60%
Depression	< 4 weeks	60%
Increased appetite and weight gain	> 10 weeks	80%

Source: Reproduced from *British Medical Journal*, 328, pp. 277–79 (Jarvis, Martin J. 2004), with permission from BMJ Publishing Group Ltd.

be useful. Following the withdrawal of nicotine, there may be unpleasant symptoms of nicotine withdrawal (see Table 8.13). These physical and mental symptoms occur because of the brain's adaptation to long-term nicotine administration. Withdrawal symptoms are normally temporary but can be very distressing for the first few weeks and may lead to relapse. It takes considerable willpower and support to deal with the withdrawal symptoms, and the cravings often prompt people to return to cigarettes immediately. Appropriate psychological support is necessary during this time, and this is where NRTs can be particularly effective (see previous discussion).

Relapse

Cigarette smoking is a behaviour that is relatively difficult to change. Despite the health risks associated with smoking, relatively few people who smoke succeed in their quit attempts (Pierce, 2022). Even with successful treatment, relapse can occur quickly, with most abandoning their quit attempts within 5–10 days. To explore relapse, researchers have explored psychological processes such as withdrawal, urge and craving and negative affect.

Applying this to Yuri

It is essential and important to maintain contact during the first 4 weeks to support Yuri through the initial changes he will experience as a result of quitting. After the initial 4 weeks, monitoring Yuri is still important, but this can be less frequent.

Factors associated with successful cessation

Although most people who smoke want to stop smoking, and 55.1% reported having attempted to quit smoking the previous year, the success rate is low, with only 7.5% of adults successfully managing to quit smoking (Centers for Disease Control and Prevention, 2022). Several studies have been undertaken exploring factors associated with successful quitting, which were often interrelated. For example, Zhou et al. (2009) found that individuals who experienced sleep disturbance, anxiety and depression were

Table 8.14 Factors associated with successful smoking cessation

Positive	Negative
Smoke-free home	Multiple previous attempts
No-smoking policy at work	Switching to low-tar products
Aged 35+	
Having university education	
Being married/cohabiting	
One previous attempt at quitting	
Social support	

Table 8.15 Potential coping strategies

Situation	Potential coping strategy
When stuck in the car in a traffic jam	Chew NRT gum or have a lozenge
In the pub	Let the smokers go outside by themselves
	Stop going to the pub!
After a meal	Move on to something else—cleaning table, etc.—rather than mulling over a cigarette
On waking	Use patch or gum, or clean teeth/shower immediately
When stressed	Relaxation techniques, exercise
When bored	Displacement
When anxious	Relaxation techniques
When relaxed	Displacement or avoidance
When angry	Relaxation techniques
Cravings	NRT
	Use support—either personal or professional
	Have a healthy snack (fruit, vegetables)
	Keep hands occupied
	Think positively about reasons for quitting

more likely to be unsuccessful in their quit attempts. Further, the environment was also found to be important—being in daily contact with other smokers, for example, is associated with less success, whether in the workplace or at home (see Table 8.14).

As an individual's confidence grows, some problem situations may arise with which he or she must cope. In these situations, the health care professional may have a key role in assisting the patient in reviewing the problem situations and suggesting potential coping strategies (see Table 8.15).

Applying this to Yuri

You need to ensure that the positive factors associated with quitting are in place in Yuri's life, such as social support from his friends and family and ensuring his home is smoke-free, so behavioural triggers are reduced.

Many who smoke who are willing and ready to quit struggle and often relapse at moments when some form of support would have seen them succeed. Support can make all the difference—whether from family, friends, a health care professional (e.g., nurse or health trainer), a support group, a helpline or social media and instant messaging services.

Conclusion

Smoking results in significant health problems, including an abbreviated life expectancy. Consequently, all health care professionals must explore how they can assist their clients and patients in stopping smoking. In those groups at risk for starting to smoke (e.g., adolescents or those with a family history of smoking), appropriate messages about the harm caused by smoking should be provided.

To assist those who smoke, a number of resources and pharmacological and psychological methods can be used to support smoking cessation. The stages of change model and MI are key methods that can be employed by the health care professional.

Key points

- Cigarette smoking remains the single most avoidable cause of death and disability in the UK and the Western world.
- There are differences in the prevalence rates of smoking in England, Wales, Scotland and Northern Ireland.
- The number of people smoking, including the young and older generations, has decreased considerably. Smoking has been linked to a whole host of diseases and chronic conditions, including heart disease, cancer, peripheral vascular disease, premature and low-weight babies, bronchitis, emphysema, sinusitis, peptic ulcers and dental hygiene problems and can worsen the effects of asthma and infections.
- Despite knowledge of the health risks associated with smoking, people continue to smoke and display unrealistic optimism regarding the impact of their smoking behaviour.
- The most influential model used in smoking cessation is the transtheoretical or stages of change model. This model suggests that people move between different stages of 'readiness' for change. People can move forwards or backwards, and relapse can occur at any time. However, there is limited evidence that smoking cessation programmes based on the TTM are effective.
- MI can be used to increase a person's motivation to quit.
- Individual-level smoking cessation interventions include (either alone or in combination) behavioural and pharmaceutical interventions ranging from brief advice and counselling to intensive support and administration of medications that contribute to reducing or overcoming dependence.
- Community-level interventions and legislation have been useful in raising awareness of the health consequences of smoking alongside impacting attitude change towards the behaviour.
- Society as a whole must continue to work together in an attempt to impact smoking rates. Working effectively with others and having a multi-angled approach is key in implementing behaviour change.
- Lapse and relapse rates are high in people who smoke and are attempting to quit. Contact with other people who smoke, gender and previous quit attempts can all impact the likelihood that a quit attempt will be successful.

Points for discussion

- Critically discuss the importance of attitudes regarding smoking cessation.
- Consider the current and future implications of smoke-free legislation from a psychological stance.
- Evaluate the importance of social support in quit attempts.

Further resources

Coleman, T. (2004a). Cessation interventions in routine health care. BMJ, *328*, 631–633.

Wilson, A., Agarwal, S., Bonas, S., Murtagh, G., Coleman, T., Taub, N., & Chernova, J. (2010). Management of smokers motivated to quit: A qualitative study of smokers and GPs. Family Practice, *27*(4), 404–409. 10.1093/fampra/cmq027

Useful web links

British Heart Foundation: 0800 169 1900. www.bhf.org.uk

NHS Stop Smoking Quitline: 0800 169 0169. www.givingupsmoking.co.uk

Quitline: 0800 002 200. www.quit.org.uk

Ash: 0207 739 5902. www.ash.org.uk

Smokefree—help to quit website: http://smokefree.nhs.uk/ways-to-quit/local-nhs-stop-smoking-service/

Smokefree helpline: 0800 022 4332

Quitting during pregnancy helpline: 0800 169 9169

Quit4life website: http://www.quit4life.nhs.uk/about_quit4life.html

References

Ahluwalia, I. B., Tripp, A. L., Dean, A. K., Mbulo, L., Arrazola, R. A., Twentyman, E., & King, B. A. (2021). Tobacco smoking cessation and Quitline use among adults aged ≥15 years in 31 countries: Findings from the global adult tobacco survey. American Journal of Preventive Medicine, *60*(3), 128–135. 10.1016/j.amepre.2020.04.029

Ajzen, I. (1991). The theory of planned behavior. Organizational Behavior & Human Decision Processes, *50*(2), 179.

Akanbi, M. O., Carroll, A. J., Achenbach, C., O'Dwyer, L. C., Jordan, N., Hitsman, B., Bilaver, L. A., McHugh, M. C., & Murphy, R. (2019). The efficacy of smoking cessation interventions in low- and middle-income countries: a systematic review and meta-analysis. Addiction (Abingdon, England), *114*(4), 620–635. 10.1111/add.14518

Armitage, C. J, & Conner, M. (2001). Efficacy of the theory of planned behaviour: A meta-analytic review. British Journal of Social Psychology, *40*(4), 471–499.

ASH. (2011a). Smoking statistics: Young people and smoking. London, UK: ASH.

ASH. (2011b). Research report: Second-hand smoke. London, UK: ASH.

ASH. (2017). Smoking and cancer. London, United Kingdom: ASH. https://ash.org.uk/resources/view/smoking-and-cancer

ASH. (2021). Smoking statistics. Retrieved from https://ash.org.uk/wp-content/uploads/2019/10/SmokingStatistics.pdf

Bandiera, F., Richardson, A., Lee, D., He, J. & Merikangas, K. (2011). Second-hand smoke exposure and mental health among children and adolescents. Archives of Paediatrics & Adolescent Medicine, *165*(4), 332–338.

Banks, E., Yazidjoglou, A., & Joshy, G. (2023). Electronic cigarettes and health outcomes: epidemiological and public health challenges. International Journal of Epidemiology, dyad059.

Baxi R, Sharma M, Roseby R, Polnay A, Priest N, Waters E, Spencer N, Webster P. (2014). Family and carer smoking control programmes for reducing children's exposure to environmental tobacco smoke. Cochrane Database of Systematic Reviews, Issue 3. Art. No.: CD001746. DOI: 10.1002/14651858.CD001746.pub3. Accessed 21 October 2023.

Beard, E. E., McNeill, A. A., Aveyard, P. P., Fidler, J. J., Michie, S. S., & West, R. R. (2011). Use of nicotine replacement therapy for smoking reduction and during enforced temporary abstinence: A national survey of English smokers. Addiction, *106*(1), 197–204.

Behbod, B., Sharma, M., Baxi, R., Roseby, R., & Webster, P. (2018). Family and carer smoking control programmes for reducing children's exposure to environmental tobacco smoke. The Cochrane Database of Systematic Reviews, *1*(1), CD001746. 10.1002/14651858.CD001746.pub4

Brady, K. T. (2020). Social determinants of health and smoking cessation: A challenge. The American Journal of Psychiatry, *177*(11), 1029–1030. 10.1176/appi.ajp.2020.20091374

Brennan, E., Cameron, M., Warne, C., Durkin, S., Borland, R., Travers, M. J., ...Wakefield, M. A. (2010). Second-hand smoke drift: Examining the influence of indoor smoking bans on indoor and outdoor air quality at pubs and bars. Nicotine & Tobacco Research, *12*(3), 271–277.

Bromley, C., Given, L. & The Scottish Government. (2011). The Scottish health survey 2010, volume 1: Main report. Edinburgh, United Kingdom: The Scottish Government. Retrieved from http://www.scotland.gov.uk/Publications/2011/09/27084018/91

Brown, A., Moodie, C. & Hastings, G. (2009). A longitudinal study of policy effect (smoke-free legislation) on smoking norms: ITC Scotland/United Kingdom. Nicotine & Tobacco Research, *11*(8), 924–932.

Bullen, C., Howe, C., Laugesen, M., McRobbie, H., Parag, V., Williman, J., & Walker, N. (2013). Electronic cigarettes for smoking cessation: A randomised controlled trial. Lancet (London, England), *382*(9905), 1629–1637. 10.1016/S0140-6736(13)61842-5

Centers for Disease Control and Prevention. (2022). Smoking and tobacco use: Electronic cigarettes. Retrieved from https://www.cdc.gov/tobacco/basic_information/e-cigarettes/index.htm

Chaffee, B. W., Watkins, S. L., & Glantz, S. A. (2018). Electronic cigarette use and progression from experimentation to established smoking. Pediatrics, *141*(4), e20173594. 10.1542/peds.2017-3594

Clift, A. K., von Ende, A., Tan, P. S., Sallis, H. M., Lindson, N., Coupland, C. A. C., ...Hopewell, J. C. (2022). Smoking and COVID-19 outcomes: An observational and Mendelian randomisation study using the UK Biobank cohort. Thorax, *77*(1), 65. 10.1136/thoraxjnl-2021-217080

Cofta-Woerpel, L., Wright, K. L., & Wetter, D. W. (2007). Smoking cessation 3: Multicomponent interventions. Behavioural Medicine, *32*, 135–149.

Department of Health, Social Services and Public Safety. (2011). Health survey Northern Ireland: First results from the 2010/11 Survey. Retrieved from http://www.dhsspsni.gov.uk/index/stats_research/stats-public-health.htm

Department of Health. (2011). Healthy lives, healthy people: A tobacco control plan for England. London, United Kingdom: Department of Health.

Department of Health. (2012). Stoptober campaign will encourage smokers to quit for 28 days. Retrieved from http://www.dh.gov.uk/health/2012/09/stoptober/

DiClemente, C. C., & Prochaska, J. O. (1982). Self-change and therapy change of smoking behaviour: A comparison of processes of change in cessation and maintenance. Addictive Behaviours, *7*, 133–142.

Dobbie, F., Hiscock, R., Leonardi-Bee, J., Murray, S., Shahab, L., Aveyard, P., ... & Bauld, L. (2015). Evaluating long-term outcomes of NHS stop smoking services (ELONS): A prospective cohort study. Health Technology Assessment (Winchester, England), *19*(95), 1.

Doll, R., & Hill, A. B. (1952). A study of the aetiology of carcinoma of the lung. British Medical Journal, *2*(4797), 1271–1286.

European Commission (2014). Tobacco product directive. https://health.ec.europa.eu/tobacco/product-regulation_en. Accessed 21st October 2023

Everest, G., Marshall, L., Fraser, C., & Briggs, A. (2022). Addressing the leading risk factors for ill health. The Health Foundation. Retrieved from 10.37829/HF-2022-P10

Faber, T., Been, J. V., Reiss, I. K., Mackenbach, J. P., & Sheikh, A. (2016). Smoke-free legislation and child health. NPJ Primary Care Respiratory Medicine, 26(1), 1–8.

Fadus, M. C., Smith, T. T., & Squeglia, L. M. (2019). The rise of e-cigarettes, pod mod devices, and JUUL among youth: Factors influencing use, health implications, and downstream effects. Drug and Alcohol Dependence, 201, 85–93. 10.1016/j.drugalcdep.2019.04.011

Fagerström K. O. (1978). Measuring degree of physical dependence to tobacco smoking with reference to individualization of treatment. Addictive Behaviors, 3(3-4), 235–241. 10.1016/03 06-4603(78)90024-2

Fidler, J. A., Shahab, L., West, O., Jarvis, M. J., McEwen, A., Stapleton, J. A., ... & West, R. (2011). 'The smoking toolkit study': A national study of smoking and smoking cessation in England. BMC Public Health, 11(1), 1–9.

Fiore, M. (2009). Treating tobacco use and dependence: 2008 update: clinical practice guideline. Diane Publishing.

Goniewicz, M. L., Smith, D. M., Edwards, K. C., Blount, B. C., Caldwell, K. L., Feng, J., Wang, L., Christensen, C., Ambrose, B., Borek, N., van Bemmel, D., Konkel, K., Erives, G., Stanton, C. A., Lambert, E., Kimmel, H. L., Hatsukami, D., Hecht, S. S., Niaura, R. S., Travers, M., ...Hyland, A. J. (2018). Comparison of Nicotine and Toxicant Exposure in Users of Electronic Cigarettes and Combustible Cigarettes. JAMA Network Open, 1(8), e185937. 10.1001/jamanetworkopen.2018.5937

Gorukanti, A., Delucchi, K., Ling, P., Fisher-Travis, R., & Halpern-Felsher, B. (2017). Adolescents' attitudes towards e-cigarette ingredients, safety, addictive properties, social norms, and regulation. Preventive Medicine, 94, 65–71.

Grace, C., Greenhalgh, E. M., & Tumini, V. (2022). Smoking bans in the home and car. In E. M. Greenhalgh, M. M. Scollo, & M. H. Winstanley (Eds.), Tobacco in Australia: Facts and issues. Melbourne, Australia: Cancer Council Victoria.

Grogan, S., Flett, K., Clark-Carter, D., Gough, B., Davey, R., Richardson, D., & Rajaratnam, G. (2011). Women smokers' experiences of an age-appearance anti-smoking intervention: a qualitative study. British Journal of Health Psychology, 16(4), 675–689. 10.1348/2044-8287. 002006

Hall, M. G., Mendel, J. R., Noar, S. M., & Brewer, N. T. (2018). Why smokers avoid cigarette pack risk messages: Two randomized clinical trials in the United States. Social Science & Medicine (1982), 213, 165–172. 10.1016/j.socscimed.2018.07.049

Hartmann-Boyce, J., McRobbie, H., Lindson, N., Bullen, C., Begh, R., Theodoulou, A., Notley, C., Rigotti, N. A., Turner, T., Butler, A. R., Fanshawe, T. R., & Hajek, P. (2021). Electronic cigarettes for smoking cessation. The Cochrane Database of Systematic Reviews, 4(4), CD010216. 10.1002/14651858.CD010216.pub5

Henderson, E., Continente, X., Fernández, E., Tigova, O., Cortés-Francisco, N., Gallus, S., ... López, M. J. (2021). Secondhand smoke exposure assessment in outdoor hospitality venues across 11 European countries. Environmental Research, 200, 111355. 10.1016/j.envres.2021. 111355

Himelfarb-Blyth, S., Vanderwater, C., & Hartwick, J. (2021). Implementing a 3As and 'opt-out'tobacco cessation framework in an outpatient oncology setting. Current Oncology, 28(2), 1197–1203.

Hollis, J. F., McAfee, T. A., Fellows, J. L., Zbikowski, S. M., Stark, M. & Riedlinger, K. (2007). The effectiveness and cost effectiveness of telephone counselling and the nicotine patch in a state tobacco quitline. Tobacco Control, 16(Suppl. 1), i53–i59. 10.1136/tc.2006.019794

Hrubá, D., & Zaloudíková, I. (2010). Why to smoke? Why not to smoke? Major reasons for children's decisions on whether or not to smoke. Central European Journal of Public Health, 18(4), 202.

Jackson, S. E., Kotz, D., West, R., & Brown, J. (2019). Moderators of real-world effectiveness of smoking cessation aids: A population study. Addiction (Abingdon, England), *114*(9), 1627–1638. 10.1111/add.14656

Jarvis, M. K. (2004). Why people smoke. British Medical Journal, *328*, 277–279.

Jassem J. (2019). Tobacco smoking after diagnosis of cancer: Clinical aspects. Translational Lung Cancer Research, *8*(Suppl 1), S50–S58. 10.21037/tlcr.2019.04.01

Kotz, D., Brown, J., & West, R. (2014). 'Real-world' effectiveness of smoking cessation treatments: A population study. Addiction, *109*(3), 491–499. 10.1111/add.12429

Kotz, D., Fidler, J., & West, R. (2009). Factors associated with the use of aids to cessation in English smokers. Addiction (Abingdon, England), *104*(8), 1403–1410. 10.1111/j.1360-0443. 2009.02639.x

Lai, D. T., Cahill, K., Qin, Y., & Tang, J. (2010). Motivational interviewing for smoking cessation. Cochrane Database of Systematic Reviews, *20*(1), CD006936. Retrieved from 10.1002/14651858. CD006936.pub2

Leslie F. M. (2020). Unique, long-term effects of nicotine on adolescent brain. Pharmacology, Biochemistry, and Behavior, *197*, 173010. 10.1016/j.pbb.2020.173010

Lindson, N., Thompson, T. P., Ferrey, A., Lambert, J. D., & Aveyard, P. (2019). Motivational interviewing for smoking cessation. Cochrane Database of Systematic Reviews, *7*, CD006936. 10.1002/14651858.CD006936.pub4

Livingstone-Banks, J., Norris, E., Hartmann-Boyce, J., West, R., Jarvis, M., Chubb, E., & Hajek, P. (2019). Relapse prevention interventions for smoking cessation. Cochrane Database of Systematic Reviews, *10*, CD003999. 10.1002/14651858.CD003999.pub6

Luk, T. T., Wong, S. W., Lee, J. J., Chan, S. S. C., Lam, T. H., & Wang, M. P. (2019). Exploring community smokers' perspectives for developing a chat-based smoking cessation intervention delivered through mobile instant messaging: Qualitative study. JMIR mHealth and uHealth, *7*(1), e11954.

Luo, Q., Steinberg, J., Yu, X. Q., Weber, M., Caruana, M., Yap, S., Grogan, P. B., Banks, E., O'Connell, D. L., & Canfell, K. (2022). Projections of smoking-related cancer mortality in Australia to 2044. Journal of Epidemiology and Community Health, *76*(9), 792–799. Advance online publication. 10.1136/jech-2021-218252

Marlatt, G. A., & Gorden, G. (Eds.). (1985). Relapse prevention: Maintenance strategies in addictive behavior change. New York, NY: Guilford Press.

McNeill, A., Brose, L., Robson, D., Calder, R., Simonavicius, E., East, K., … & Zuikova, E. (2022). Nicotine vaping in England: an evidence update including health risks and perceptions, 2022. King's College London: A report commissioned by the Office for Health Improvement and Disparities, available at: www.gov.uk/government/publications/nicotine-vaping-in-england-2022-evidence-update

Middlestadt, S. E., Seo, D., Kolbe, L. J., & Jay, S. J. (2012). Applying the theory of planned behavior to explore the relation between smoke-free air laws and quitting intentions. Health Education & Behavior, *39*(1), 27–34.

Miller, W. R., & Rollnick, S. (2002). Motivational interviewing: Preparing people for change (2nd ed.). New York, NY: Guilford Press.

Mohiuddin, S., Mooss, A., Hunter, C., Grollmes, T., Cloutier, D. & Hilleman, D. (2007). Intensive smoking cessation intervention reduces mortality in high-risk smokers with cardiovascular disease. Chest, *131*(2), 446–452.

Morales-Prieto, D. M., Fuentes-Zacarías, P., Murrieta-Coxca, J. M., Gutierrez-Samudio, R. N., Favaro, R. R., Fitzgerald, J. S. & Markert, U. R. (2022). Smoking for two—effects of tobacco consumption on placenta. Molecular Aspects of Medicine, *87*, 101023. 10.1016/j.mam.2021. 101023

Mullen, K. A., Manuel, D. G., Hawken, S. J., Pipe, A. L., Coyle, D., Hobler, L. A., Younger, J., Wells, G. A., & Reid, R. D. (2017). Effectiveness of a hospital-initiated smoking cessation programme: 2-year health and healthcare outcomes. Tobacco Control, *26*(3), 293–299. 10.1136/tobaccocontrol-2015-052728

Nabi-Burza, E., Drehmer, J. E., Walters, B. H., Willemsen, M. C., Zeegers, M. P. A., & Winickoff, J. P. (2021). Smoking cessation treatment for parents who dual use E-cigarettes and traditional cigarettes. Journal of Smoking Cessation, *2021*, 6639731. 10.1155/2021/6639731

Nargis, N., Yong, H.-H., Driezen, P., Mbulo, L., Zhao, L., Fong, G. T., ...Siahpush, M. (2019). Socioeconomic patterns of smoking cessation behavior in low and middle-income countries: Emerging evidence from the Global Adult Tobacco Surveys and International Tobacco Control Surveys. PLOS ONE, *14*(9), e0220223. 10.1371/journal.pone.0220223

NICE. (n.d.). Stopping smoking during pregnancy and after childbirth. Retrieved from https://pathways.nice.org.uk/pathways/tobacco-use#path=view%3A/pathways/tobacco-use/stopping-smoking-during-pregnancy-and-after-childbirth.xml&content=view-index

O'Connell, N., Burke, E., Dobbie, F., Dougall, N., Mockler , D., Darker, C., Vance, J., Bernstein, S., Gilbert, H., Bauld, L., & Hayes, C.B. (2022). The effectiveness of smoking cessation interventions for socio-economically disadvantaged women: a systematic review and meta-analysis. Systematic Reviews,*11*(1), 111. https://doi.org/10.1186/s13643-022-01922-7

Office for National Statistics. (2020). Adult smoking habits in the UK: 2019. Retrieved from https://www.ons.gov.uk/peoplepopulationandcommunity/healthandsocialcare/healthandlifeex-pectancies/bulletins/adultsmokinghabitsingreatbritain/2019

Okuyemi, K. S., Nollen, N. L., & Ahluwalia, J. S. (2006). Interventions to facilitate smoking cessation. American Family Physician, *74*, 262–271.

Papadakis, S., Anastasaki, M., Papadakaki, M., Antonopoulou, M., Chliveros, C., Daskalaki, C., Varthalis, D., Triantafyllou, S., Vasilaki, I., McEwen, A., & Lionis, C. (2020). 'Very brief advice' (VBA) on smoking in family practice: A qualitative evaluation of the tobacco user's perspective. BMC Family Practice, *21*(1), 121. 10.1186/s12875-020-01195-w

Pierce, J. P., Kealey, S., Leas, E. C., Pulvers, K., Stone, M. D., Oratowski, J., ... & Strong, D. R. (2022). Effect of graphic warning labels on cigarette pack–hiding behavior among smokers: The CASA Randomized Clinical Trial. JAMA Network Open, *5*(6), e2214242–e2214242.

Rice, V. H., Heath, L., Livingstone-Banks, J., & Hartmann-Boyce, J. (2017). Nursing interventions for smoking cessation. The Cochrane Database of Systematic Reviews, *2017*(12), CD001188. 10.1002/14651858.CD001188.pub5

Rigotti, N. A. (2022). Pharmacotherapy for smoking cessation in adults, UpToDate. Retrieved from https://www.uptodate.com/contents/pharmacotherapy-for-smoking-cessation-in-adults/print

Schachter, S., Silverstein, B., Kozlowski, L. T., Herman, C. P., & Liebling, B. (1977). Effects of stress on cigarette smoking and urinary pH. Journal of Experimental Psychology: General, *106*, 24–30.

Sheikh, M., Mukeriya, A., Shangina, O., Brennan, P., & Zaridze, D. (2021). Postdiagnosis smoking cessation and reduced risk for lung cancer progression and mortality: A prospective cohort study. Annals of Internal Medicine, *174*(9), 1232–1239. 10.7326/M21-0252

Silverman, J., & Draper, J. (2005). Skills for communicating with patients (2nd ed.). Oxford, United Kingdom: Radcliffe Publishing.

Smith, B., Bean, M., Mitchell, K., Speizer, I., & Fries, E. (2007). Psychosocial factors associated with non-smoking adolescents' intentions to smoke. Health Education Research, *22*(2), 238–247.

Sniehotta, F. F., Presseau, J., & Araújo-Soares, V. (2014). Time to retire the theory of planned behaviour. Health Psychology Review, *8*(1), 1–7. 10.1080/17437199.2013.869710

Soneji, S., Yang, J., Knutzen, K. E., Moran, M. B., Tan, A. S., Sargent, J., & Choi, K. (2018). Online tobacco marketing and subsequent tobacco use. Pediatrics, *141*(2).

Song, F., Elwell-Sutton, T., & Naughton, F. (2020). Impact of the NHS stop smoking services on smoking prevalence in England: A simulation modelling evaluation. Tobacco Control, *29*(2), 200–206.

Splete, H. (2022). E-cigarettes don't help smokers quit, suggests new research. Networks, *17*, 21.

Stead, L. F., Perera, R., Bullen, C., Mant, D., Hartmann-Boyce, J., Cahill, K., & Lancaster, T. (2012). Nicotine replacement therapy for smoking cessation. Cochrane Database of Systematic Reviews, *11*, CD000146.

Tate, C., Kumar, R., Murray, J. M., Sanchez-Franco, S., Montgomery, S. C., Montes, F., ... Hunter, R. F. (2021). Socio-environmental and psychosocial predictors of smoking susceptibility among adolescents with contrasting socio-cultural characteristics: A comparative analysis. BMC Public Health, *21*(1), 2240. 10.1186/s12889-021-12351-x

The Health and Social Care Information Centre. (2011). Statistics on smoking. London, United Kingdom.

Truth Initiative (2018). E-Cigarettes: Facts, Stats and Regulations. https://truthinitiative.org/ research-resources/emerging-tobacco-products/e-cigarettes-facts-stats-and-regulations Accessed October 21st 2023

UOHI (2023. Quit smoking program. https://www.ottawaheart.ca/clinic/quit-smoking-program Accessed October 21st 2023

US Surgeon General. (2008). Treating tobacco use and dependence (2008 update). Atlanta, GA: Department of Health and Human Services.

Ussher, M. H., Faulkner, G. E. J., Angus, K., Hartmann-Boyce, J., & Taylor, A. H. (2019). Exercise interventions for smoking cessation. The Cochrane Database of Systematic Reviews, *2019*(10), CD002295. 10.1002/14651858.CD002295.pub6

van Schayck, O.C.P., Bindels, L., Nijs, A. et al. (2020). The experience of general practitioners with very brief advice in the treatment of tobacco addiction. npj Primary Care Respiratory Medicine, *30*, 40. https://doi.org/10.1038/s41533-020-00200-0

Wardle, J., & Steptoe, A. (2003). Socioeconomic differences in attitudes and beliefs about healthy lifestyles. Journal of Epidemiology and Community Health, *57*(6), 440–443. 10.1136/jech.57. 6.440

Welsh Government. (2011). Welsh Health Survey 2010. Retrieved from http://www.wales.gov.uk/ statistics

West, R. (2004). ABC of smoking cessation: Assessment of dependence and motivation to stop smoking. British Medical Journal, *328*, 338–339.

West, R. (2005). Time for a change: Putting the transtheoretical (stages of change) model to rest. Addiction, *100*(8), 1036–1039.

WHO (2003). WHO Framework Convention on Tobacco Control https://fctc.who.int/who-fctc/ overview. Accessed October 21st 2023

WHO. (2021). Noncommunicable diseases. Retrieved from https://www.who.int/news-room/fact-sheets/detail/noncommunicable-diseases

Wilson, L., Avila Tang, E., Chandler, G., Hutton, H., Odelola, O., Elf, J., ...Apelberg, B. (2012). Impact of tobacco control interventions on smoking initiation, cessation, and prevalence: A systematic review. Journal of Environmental and Public Health, *2012*, 961724.

Zhou, X., Nonnemaker, J., Sherrill, B., Gilsenan, A., Coste, F., & West, R. (2009). Attempts to quit smoking and relapse: Factors associated with success or failure from the ATTEMPT cohort study. Addictive Behaviors, *34*(4), 365–373.

9 Sexual health

____

LEARNING OUTCOMES

At the end of this chapter, you will be able to:

- appreciate how 'sex', 'safe sex' and 'safer sex' have been defined by professionals and the lay public alike.
- understand the nature of sexually transmitted infections (STIs) and their health consequences, such as disease.
- be able to evaluate the psychological determinants of sexual behaviour and safe-sex practices.
- recognise and be able to review how psychological interventions can assist in promoting safer sex.
- understand how the Transtheoretical Model can be used to develop interventions to promote safer sex.
- understand how sexual health applies to LGBTQIA+ populations.

____

Case Study

Noah is a 21-year-old cisgender male currently working as a car mechanic and enjoying life to the fullest. He works hard in a local garage and earns a steady income. He has recently moved out of his parent's house to set up a home with his partner, Emma, in a rented flat. They previously had an on–off relationship where they agreed to see other people, but they have lived together as a couple for 3 months now. Noah has a varied sexual history and has sex with men and women. He has reported having more than 15 sexual partners since his introduction to sex in his early teens. Indeed, despite his determination to remain with Emma, Noah is having occasional sexual encounters with men he meets at the local pub or night club (although Noah claims that these encounters do not often result in 'full sex'—sexual intercourse). Noah's human immunodeficiency virus (HIV) status is unknown.

Emma is a 19-year-old cisgender woman and has estimated having 10 sexual partners, which have all been male; she considers herself heterosexual. Emma's only current sexual partner is Noah, but the couple are openly non-monogamous.

DOI: 10.4324/9781003471233-9

She does not want to get pregnant since she wants to complete her university degree; hence, she is using the contraceptive pill. Initially, when they got together, Noah and Emma did use condoms, but Noah felt it reduced sensation, so they decided that Emma should go on the pill despite her initial apprehension. Noah has recently experienced some pain 'down below' and has gone to a sexual health clinic to get it checked out. He feels that he may have contracted an STI from a recent unprotected sexual encounter with someone he met on a night out; however, it has been more than 12 months since he has been tested for any STIs. You have recommended both Noah and Emma be tested for STIs. He does not report any recent HIV exposure (in the last 72 hours) and, thus, does not qualify for post-exposure prophylaxis (antiviral medication that can prevent HIV if taken within 72 hours of exposure to the virus). You have recognised that both Noah and Emma may be at ongoing risk of contracting STIs and begin the process of promoting safer sex through the use of barrier protection methods and recommending STI check-ups at the clinic at least every 6 months. Since Noah is a man who has sex with men and Emma is a heterosexual woman with a male bisexual partner at risk of contracting HIV in the future, they may qualify for preexposure prophylaxis (Hammoud et al., 2019).

Applying This to Noah and Emma

Consider Emma and Noah's potential difficulties in their relationship and how their lifestyle may affect their sexual health. Evaluate how Noah could reduce the risk involved in his sexual behaviour.

Introduction

The first question we must ask, of course, is what is sexual behaviour? Although most people would not struggle when asked this question, further thought suggests that there are difficulties, which may implicate assessment by a health care professional and any planned intervention. A simplistic, biological definition of 'sexual behaviour' could refer to all actions and responses that make fertilisation possible. To achieve fertilisation, a male and female must perform a specific series of actions and experience specific physiological responses. However, this definition may be a little restrictive, and sexual behaviour is more than vaginal intercourse between a male and a female. A more pragmatic definition refers to any behaviour that involves a body's 'sexual response'. In this way, the physical actions associated with sexual behaviour do not have to result in fertilisation. This definition covers all types of human sexual activity (e.g., sexual self-stimulation, heterosexual and homosexual intercourse) but does not imply any hierarchical order. Moreover, it leaves each of these activities open to interpretation. In short, the above definition does not equate sex with reproduction or any other particular purpose. It merely calls attention to a certain physical response common to a variety of activities.

A final definition includes all actions and responses related to pleasure seeking. This modern, very wide definition can be traced to Sigmund Freud and his psychoanalytic theory. Thus, in this view, 'the sex drive' came to stand for pursuing pleasure in all its forms. 'Sex' was the underlying motive of every life-enhancing activity. As we can see, when used in this fashion, the term 'sexual behaviour' becomes quite inclusive. The only question in all of these cases is one of motivation. If the behaviour is somehow motivated by the wish for pleasure, if it is prompted by an individual's inner need for self-fulfilment, if it satisfies or gives the individual comfort, if it heightens the sense of being alive, then it is clearly sexual.

Most sexual researchers use the second of these definitions. The definition does not equate sex with reproduction or any other particular purpose. It merely highlights a certain physical response common to a variety of activities. Obviously, this definition is important for health researchers. When asking members of the population if they engage in 'sex', 'dangerous sexual behaviour' or 'safe sexual behaviour', it is important to define clearly what this covers.

Applying This to Noah

Sex can be defined as physical actions between two (or more) individuals that produce a physiological sexual response, which may or may not result in fertilisation. Noah would define sex as a pleasure-seeking act.

Most United Kingdom (UK) adults obtain their sexual health information from media such as television, newspapers and magazines (NICE, 2022). This means that individuals may not define sexual behaviour as professionals define it. Hence, when asking, 'Have you engaged in sex?' or 'When was the last time you had sexual behaviour?' you may not get a consistent response. For example, a study (Byers et al., 2009) of university students' views on what activities count as 'having sex' suggested that a small proportion (1.4%) regarded tongue kissing as having sex, while 8% regarded touching of the genitals without an orgasm, 20% regarded oral sex without an orgasm and 25% regarded oral sex with an orgasm as having sex. Over 70% thought that vaginal intercourse was sex, whereas around 80% thought anal intercourse was sex. This suggests that non-coital sex may not be defined as sex by certain key groups, particularly the younger respondents. Further, whether an act is considered 'sex' or not appears to differ depending on sexual orientation. For example, unidirectional and non-penetrative acts are more likely to be considered 'sex' by lesbian women and gay men than heterosexual males (Horowitz & Bedford, 2017). Accordingly, the definitions of 'sex', 'sexual activity' and 'risky sexual behaviour' must be extended and clearly defined for the health care professional and the individual.

In another study of undergraduate students by Hans et al. (2010), only around 20% of respondents regarded oral sex as 'sex'. This low value may result from some considering safe sex a form of sexual intercourse that does not result in pregnancy. Undergraduate students and sexual health care professionals' opinions differ regarding whether oral sex maintains virginity; 90.4% and 79.3%, respectively, believe oral sex maintains virginity (Hans & Kimberly, 2011). Of course, this only applies to hetero-normative/heterosexual couplings.

It is possible that individuals who engage in oral sex but do not consider it 'sex' may not associate the acts with their potential health risks (Chambers, 2007). In fact, evidence suggests that oral sex can contribute to the development of several STIs such as HIV; herpes simplex virus (HSV; types 1 and 2); syphilis, gonorrhoea and hepatitis (Saini et al., 2010); and the human papillomavirus virus, which is linked to various cancers (D'Souza et al., 2009). In support of this, research has also found that 16.1% of adolescents believe that participating in anal sex also maintains their virginity (Bersamin et al., 2007). More recently, what constitutes sex and virginity loss has undergone theoretical re-evaluation. Horowitz and Bedford (2017) proposed that what constitutes sexual behaviour be graded rather than dichotomous and moderated by sexual orientation. In their research, ratings of virginity loss were significantly greater for vaginal intercourse than anal intercourse for all groups except for gay males. The authors suggest that this graded approach allows research that predicts sexual behaviour rather than describes it, meaning such research could be used to provide targeted preventative and remedial sexual health intervention. It is by acknowledging this evidence that sexual health interventions should be implicated.

Having sex (however defined) with more than one partner in a lifetime may be a common experience. This means, of course, that calling on people to refrain from having sex does not work from a public health point of view, nor does it fit with the modern definition of sexual health (see next section). If we consider potential chains of sexual networking, as described in Figure 9.1, we can see that from being apparently monogamous, the number of potential partners from which STIs could have been contracted expands considerably. For example, in Figure 9.1, the male has had previous sexual contact with three women, who have each had three previous male partners. So, the first male has to consider the consequences not just of having sex with an individual woman but also with her partners. Hence, the female in the apparently monogamous relationship would have to deal with the consequences of 13 separate sexual couplings.

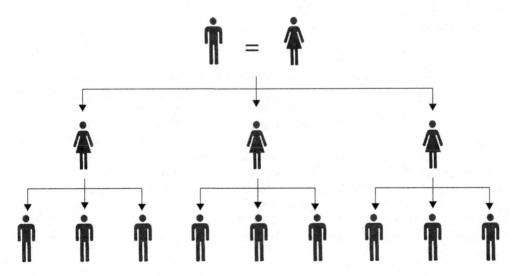

Figure 9.1 An example of a chain of sexual networking.

Applying This to Noah

Noah has had 15 previous sexual partners. If each of those individuals had had two other previous sexual partners, this would mean that Emma is being exposed to 45 separate couplings.

Government recommendations

The UK government has spent millions of pounds on promoting 'safe sex' and has promoted the use of condoms to prevent STIs. The concept of 'safe sex' was derived in response to the HIV/AIDS epidemic, and consequently, it originally focused on male homosexuals, the community where the outbreak originated, with the earliest reference to this term being in 1984 (Morin et al., 1984). A government definition of 'safe sex' involves taking precautions during sex that can keep you from getting an STI or giving one to your partner. In 1985, the Coalition for Sexual Responsibility drafted safe-sex guidelines to promote the distribution and use of condoms 'to eliminate the exchange of body fluids during anal intercourse or oral sex' (Lindsey, 1985). Subsequently, health-promotion officials extended the definition to hetero-sexual adolescents: 'judicious selection of sexual partners, the use of mechanical and chemical barriers during intercourse, and avoidance of sex practices such as those in which bodily fluids are exchanged' (Slevin & Marvin, 1987). The UK Government accepts a more recent definition of sexual health provided by the World Health Organization (WHO), which:

> Defines sexual health as a state of physical, emotional, mental and social wellbeing in relation to sexuality—it is not just the absence of disease, dysfunction or infirmity. Sexual health requires a positive and respectful approach to sexuality and sexual relationships, as well as the possibility of having pleasurable and safe sexual experiences, free of coercion, discrimination and violence. (Office for Health Improvement and Disparities, 2023)

These days, in addition to promoting condom use, key interventions involve education, testing/diagnosis and treatment for the prevention and control of STIs. More recently, the UK Government's guidance on sexual and reproductive health and HIV extends the definition of sexual health beyond the mere absence of disease, dysfunction or infirmity. That is, to be considered sexually healthy also means to be in a state of physical, emotional, mental and social wellbeing concerning one's sexuality. This means that a positive and respectful approach to sexuality and an awareness of the sexual rights of all persons are key to achieving and maintaining good sexual health (Department of Health, 2023). Specific sexual health recommendations also exist for certain communities; for example, gay or bisexual men are encouraged to have a sexual health check-up at least every 6 months (NHS Choices, n.d.). Meanwhile, the Australian STI guidelines recommend testing for STIs every 3 months for men who have sex with men (Ong et al., 2023).

Applying This to Noah and Emma

Noah thinks he is practising safer sex as he rarely has 'full sex' with the individuals with whom he has occasional sexual encounters. As a couple, Noah and Emma are predominantly concerned with preventing pregnancy and have not properly considered the health consequences of failing to practice safe sex.

Recently, the use of the term *safer sex* rather than *safe sex* has been used more frequently by health workers, with the realisation that the risk of transmitting STIs in various sexual activities is a continuum rather than a simple dichotomy between risky and safe. Additionally, the term safer sex is employed because condoms and other barrier methods are not 100% effective at preventing STIs (Grubb et al., 2020). However, the term *safe sex* is still commonly used by sex educators. Most STIs can be prevented by proper condom use; however, a 2009 survey indicated that individuals are less likely to use condoms for this preventative purpose, with 90% of men and 89% of women citing prevention of pregnancy as their reason for using condoms, and only 45% citing prevention of infection, most of whom cited pregnancy prevention as well (Lader, 2009). Interestingly, the percentage of men who used condoms to prevent infection declined with age, from 50% of men aged 25–34 to 33% among men aged 45 and over. This difference might indicate the belief that STIs only occur among the younger generations, which is worrying considering there has been a recent rise in STIs among those over 50. In 2006, for example, 10% of newly diagnosed HIV cases in the United States (US) were among the over 50 s (Minichiello et al., 2011). In the UK, more recently, in 2019, people over 50 accounted for 19% of new HIV diagnoses- a position still of concern in 2023 (Department of Health, 2023). The potential for STIs arising from this lack of knowledge and appropriate usage has to be stressed. For example, the use of condoms during oral sex rather than vaginal or anal intercourse is relatively low, below 20% (Stone et al., 2006), despite oral sex being a transmission route for many STIs. Further, in a national Spanish survey on sexuality and contraception among young people, many respondents stated that the main reason for not using a condom was linked to the number of instances oral sex was practised and that the use of condoms was reducing over time (Ballester-Arnal et al., 2022). According to Habel et al. (2018), as few as 7% of respondents reported using a condom during oral sex.

Most adults (over 50%) report making no changes to their behaviour due to what they hear regarding sexual health (NSOS, 2009). It is clear that information and awareness campaigns do not achieve their goal, and other strategies must be implemented.

Evidence suggests a reduction in STI transmission when consistent and correct use of condoms is employed (McKay, 2007). For example, the Cochrane review found that the consistent use of condoms reduces the risk of contracting HIV by 80% (Weller & Davis-Beaty, 2002). Similarly, Wald et al. (2005) found that participants reporting more frequent use of condoms were at a lower risk for acquiring HSV-2 than participants who used condoms less frequently. More recently, however, the protective power of condoms to reduce HSV-2 transmission has been found to differ significantly depending on the sex of the partner possessing versus contracting the virus. Magaret et al. (2016) found that external condom use reduced the risk of HSV-2 transmission from men to women by 96%. Female-to-male transmission, however, was less significantly reduced by condom use, by 65%.

Although abstinence seems to be an absolute answer to preventing STIs, abstinence is not always a practical or desirable option. Research has indicated that individuals' underlying attitudes concerning abstinence and sex drive the uptake of sexual intercourse in the teenage population (Masters et al., 2008). Therefore, attitudes must be addressed to make abstinence more popular among teenagers. Studies have found that a more comprehensive approach to educating adolescents about safe sex, including dispensing contraceptives and condoms, reduces risky sexual behaviour more than abstinence-only education (Underhill et al., 2008). Unfortunately, despite strong support for sexual education in schools, the delivery of such programs is declining in the US (Szucs et al., 2022). After abstinence, the next least risky approach is to have a monogamous sexual relationship with someone you know is free of any STI. Condoms can be used to avoid contact with semen, vaginal fluids or blood. Both male and female condoms dramatically reduce the chance of individuals getting or spreading an STI (McKay, 2007). WHO cite the male/external condom as the single most efficient available technology to reduce the sexual transmission of HIV and many other STIs, with the dual benefit of preventing unwanted pregnancy by up to 98% when used correctly (WHO, 2011). Some recent recommendations suggest the need for female-driven protective devices (Marfatia et al., 2015). The female/internal condom, though effective and safe, has not achieved its national potential due to its high costs, but both should be readily and consistently available to reduce the spread of STIs. However, it should be noted that condoms (internal or external) may not significantly reduce infections that are transferred via skin-to-skin contact (i.e., human papillomavirus virus) because of the possibility that not all affected areas are covered by the condom. This suggests that recommending condom use alone is likely insufficient for optimising the sexual health of all individuals. Thus, education, routine testing and early treatment are becoming increasingly important to staying sexually healthy.

However, although the 'official' and 'educational' definitions of 'sex' and 'safe sex' are well known and agreed upon, there is a paucity of literature on how the general public (and those at risk in particular) define 'safe sex' (Moskowitz et al., 2006). A Californian study reported that most defined safe sex in terms of condom use (with 26.3% suggesting that this alone was 'safe sex'). Condom use, in conjunction with other common methods (e.g., abstinence, safe partner or monogamy), was mentioned by two-thirds of respondents. Definitions of safe sex varied across sociodemographic groups. For example, males were more likely to mention monogamy and less likely to mention abstinence. Condom use was mentioned most often by adults aged 18–24 and tended to decrease with age. Adults aged 25–64 were most likely to mention monogamy, and those aged 45–64 were most likely to mention a safe partner (Moskowitz et al., 2006). In the study by Bourne and Robson (2009), participants offered an alternative view to 'safe sex' health-promotion campaigns and thought that sex could be safe in a loving relationship in which partners trusted each other whether condoms were used or not.

Applying This to Noah and Emma

Emma's definition of safe sex would be to take the pill, so she doesn't get pregnant.

The NHS Choices website, Livewell—Sexual Health and Sexwise (sexwise.org.ul) provides a wealth of information on various STIs, their symptoms and how they can be caught; oral sex and the use of sex toys; and 15 different forms of contraception and their availability (NHS Choices, n.d.). Additionally, Sexwise is a program commissioned by Public Health England to provide honest information and advice on sexual and reproductive health and pleasure. Both websites are interactive and easy to navigate, allowing people to gain information without the embarrassment of visiting their clinician.

The NATSAL-3 (The National Survey of Sexual Attitudes and Lifestyles) examined the sexual behaviour of over 15,162 adults across Britain and produced considerable data on factors such as age of first intercourse, sexual behaviour and contraception use. The report indicates that the most popular form of contraception for people aged 16–24 was condom use. It was rather worrying, however, that 10% of young adults in this age group reported using either no contraception or potentially unreliable methods such as withdrawal or the 'safe period'. In terms of safe sex, health care professionals should try to encourage condom use to prevent STIs along with potentially unwanted pregnancies. NATSAL-4 is underway and aims to survey 10,000 individuals between 16 and 59 between 2022 and 2023.

Other reports have investigated the views of both men and women. In general, men tend to report numerous negative attitudes towards condom use, including a reduction in behaviour spontaneity and reduced sexual pleasure. It has been found that men's perceptions of comfort while using a condom were a predictor of actual behaviour. The males who perceived condoms as uncomfortable were less likely to use them for the duration of intercourse (Hensel et al., 2011). According to Dalessandro et al. (2019), many young men prioritise their sexual pleasure by staying silent about condom use during sexual encounters and putting the responsibility for sexual health and contraception onto women. Some men believe they only need to protect themselves but not others (such as using the same condom to engage in group sex with multiple individuals; see Sousa et al., 2023). According to Campbell et al. (2016), rather than forgetfulness or physical discomfort, women mostly avoid condoms due to worries about negative reactions from their partners. They also tend to hold unrealistic perceptions of contracting an STI, this appearing to differ between men and women (Leval et al., 2011). That is, women tended to associate condom use with STI prevention, whereas men did not. However, STI risk perception, condom use and their association with relationship status and number of temporary partners did not differ between men and women.

Applying This to Noah and Emma

Noah and Emma, like some other young people, tend to underestimate their personal risk of STIs.

There are also several other negative attitudes held by women that can potentially hinder condom use, including:

- anticipated male objection to a female suggesting condom use (denial of their pleasure)
- difficulty/embarrassment in raising the issue of condom use with a male partner

- worry that suggesting use to a potential partner implies that either they or their partner is HIV+ or has another STI
- lack of self-efficacy or mastery in condom use.

As we will see, these negative attitudes or misconceptions must be addressed by the health care practitioner to promote condom use.

Applying This to Noah and Emma

Noah believes that wearing a condom reduces his sensation. Emma has not been able to discuss using condoms with Noah and has taken the simple route of 'going on the pill'.

Applying Research in Practice

Associations between sexually experienced adolescents' sources of information about sex and sexual risk outcomes (Secor-Turner et al., 2011). This study examined prevalent informal sources of information about sex and examined associations between informal sources of information about sex and sexual risk outcomes among sexually experienced adolescents. The sample included 22,828 sexually experienced adolescents aged between 13 and 20 years.

Findings revealed that peers and siblings were the most commonly reported informal, proximal source of information about sex. It was also reported that parents or parents plus peers and siblings as a source of information led to significantly lower odds of having multiple sex partners in the past year. Further, informal sources of information about sex had significantly lower odds of lifetime pregnancy involvement.

It was concluded that information about sex from people in adolescents' everyday lives can diminish the likelihood of involvement in sexual risk behaviours. Therefore, formal sex education programs should engage informal sources of information about sex to adolescents as having these informal, familiar sources of information about sex appears to serve as a protective factor against sexual risk outcomes, especially among younger adolescents.

Consequences of unsafe sex

Sex is, for the main part, a pleasurable activity and a normal and natural part of human behaviour. Sexual pleasure is both physical and psychological in nature and can result from a range of erotic interactions. However, it also comes with potential health consequences, such as STIs, which can lead to disease. Unprotected sex and having multiple sexual partners can lead to unwanted pregnancies and STIs, including HIV. At the end of 2020, approximately 38 million people were living with HIV worldwide (UNAIDS, 2020). The good news is that there has been a 35% reduction in new HIV cases in the UK since 2014. An estimated 94% of HIV-infected individuals have been diagnosed, 98% of those were receiving treatment, and 97% of those in treatment had an undetectable viral load, meaning they are unable to infect others with HIV. To achieve this and to attain the ultimate goal of ending HIV, the advice and motto of the UK Government has been to prevent, test, treat and retain. However, STIs are not only HIV (the virus that causes AIDS); there are numerous other infections that can result from unsafe sex (see Table 9.1).

Table 9.1 Symptoms of sexually transmitted diseases

STI	Comment
Chlamydia trachomatis	Can be transmitted in vaginal or seminal fluids. Although chlamydia is most often asymptomatic, untreated infections can progress to pelvic inflammatory disease, and approximately 40% of women later have decreased fertility
Gonorrhoea	Transmitted via seminal and vaginal fluids and easily transmitted through sexual activity. Gonococcal urethritis causes painful urination and discharge, although approximately 25% of men have no symptoms. Among women, gonorrhoea can cause cervicitis, with vaginal discharge, pain with intercourse, or painful urination; however, approximately half of infected women are asymptomatic
Nongonococcal urethritis (NGU)	NGU is the most common clinical sexually transmitted syndrome among men and is characterised by painful urination with or without discharge
Syphilis	Clinical manifestations of syphilis are varied, and its natural history is complex. It can be transmitted through sexual intercourse or direct contact with syphilitic sores or rash
Herpes	Genital herpes is the most common ulcerative STI in the UK, with diagnosis rates showing an increasing trend (HPA, 2011). There is no cure, and as with other STIs transmission of herpes simplex virus (HSV) can occur with unprotected sex or direct contact with genital ulcers. There is an especially high risk of transmission when those infected have an active genital sore or an active oral cold sore
Hepatitis B virus (HBV)	Can be passed via seminal and vaginal fluids and is approximately 100 times more transmissible than HIV. About a fifth of all new HBV infections occur among men having sex with men (MSM) and people are often unaware of their status. Vaccination is the most effective strategy against HBV (HPA, 2009)
Hepatitis C virus	The virus can be transmitted through seminal and vaginal fluids; however, the risk of sexual transmission is low. It is likely that if condoms are used consistently then sexual transmission of hepatitis C will be avoided
Human papillomavirus (HPV)	In total, 40 types of HPV can infect the genital tract. HPV-16 or -18 causes over 70% of cervical cancers worldwide, whereas HPV-6 or -11 causes over 90% of genital warts. HPV infection is extremely common. At

(*Continued*)

Table 9.1 (Continued)

STI	Comment
	least 50% of sexually active men and women acquire genital HPV infection at some point in their lives and may develop warts. The disease can be transmitted through unprotected sex or direct contact with genital warts
Human immunodeficiency virus (HIV)	An uninfected individual is most at risk of acquiring HIV from receptive anal or vaginal sex. Infection is initially asymptomatic. Signs of primary HIV include: fever, swollen glands, sore throat, rash on the body or face, painful muscles or joints, headache, feeling sick and vomiting, ulcers on the mouth, genitals and oesophagus. After the early symptoms, HIV may remain undetected for a number of years until the body's ability to fight infections is reduced. This leaves the body vulnerable to infections. If a person develops certain life-threatening illnesses it is known as AIDS (2007c)

Table 9.2 Rates per 100,000 of population of STI diagnoses by country (2011)

	Gonorrhoea	Syphilis	Chlamydia	Genital warts	Genital herpes
England	30.8	4.8	359.4	141.7	55.6
Wales	16	1.1	126	125	22
Northern Ireland	11	1.7	115	125	22
Scotland	17	3.7	170	135	27
UK	32	4.6	189	139	36

One common STI that can result from unprotected sex is chlamydia. Over 2 million chlamydia tests were conducted on individuals aged 15 to 24 in 2011; these resulted in over 140,000 new diagnoses (HPA, 2012). In 2018, Sexual Health Services England reported 447,694 new cases of STIs, a 5% increase since 2017. A large contribution to this rise in STI diagnoses was a 26% increase in gonorrhoea cases. Chlamydia, however, was the most common STI at 49% of all new cases (Department of Health, 2023). Chlamydia and gonorrhoea are the two most common STIs, and both are a key cause of preventable infertility amongst women and, along with other STIs, possibly make the acquisition and transmission of HIV more likely (Ward & Rönn, 2010), although there is some debate as to whether this is causal.

In the UK, the number of reported STI cases has risen considerably, particularly among young people (see Table 9.2). For instance, between 1995 and 2003, diagnoses of new episodes of gonorrhoea and chlamydia increased by 197% and 409%, respectively, among men aged 16–19 years (HPA, 2008). Table 9.3 (adapted from HPA, 2011) shows massive increases—a 135% increase in chlamydia, for example. Given the increase in STIs and unwanted pregnancies in adolescence, it is hard to disagree with the contention that the sexual health of England and Wales is in crisis and the worst in Europe (Evans & Tripp, 2006). The UK has the highest rates of teenage pregnancy in western Europe (WHO, 2011), and Scotland has recently introduced a new sexual health and blood-borne virus policy to tackle the level of STIs in the country, drawing parallels with other policy areas such as drugs and alcohol misuse (The Scottish Government, 2011).

Table 9.3 New STI diagnoses England: 2013–2022

New STI diagnoses	2013	2014	2015	2016	2017	2018	2019	2020	2021	2022	Change 2021 to 2022
Chlamydia	211,370	210,857	202,442	204,380	205,618	219,607	230,028	161,875	160,279	199,233	24%
Gonorrhoea	31,177	37,150	41,290	36,545	44,839	56,690	71,133	50,678	54,961	82,592	50%
Herpes: genital herpes (first episode)	34,294	34,132	33,922	33,005	32,911	33,737	34,464	20,693	21,892	24,910	14%
Mycoplasma genitalium	[x]	[x]	79	210	433	1,986	5,345	4,241	5,127	7,232	41%
Non-specific genital infection (NSGI)	49,628	47,246	42,253	36,800	33,491	31,199	28,091	15,302	14,512	16,655	15%
Pelvic inflammatory disease (PID) and epididymitis (non-specific)	22,484	22,120	21,098	19,975	18,702	17,747	16,223	10,573	10,500	10,796	3%
Syphilis: primary, secondary and early latent	3,345	4,445	5,313	5,932	7,036	7,405	8,040	6,941	7,543	8,692	15%
Warts: genital warts (first episode)	76,987	73,691	68,871	63,349	59,201	57,217	50,940	27,672	28,497	26,079	-8%
Other new STI diagnoses	25,756	25,417	24,090	22,905	22,909	23,167	23,996	13,505	13,711	16,264	19%
New STI diagnoses total	455,041	455,058	439,358	423,101	425,140	448,755	468,260	311,480	317,022	392,453	24%

Source: ONS (2022) Sexually transmitted infections (STIs): annual data tables.

Positively, however, the results of the NATSAL-3 revealed that unplanned pregnancy rates were lower than figures in other wealthy countries, such as the US. It has been suggested that this may reflect that contraception is provided to the public for free under the NHS in Britain. However, not surprisingly, most people who engage in sexual activity are less inclined to think about their risk of STI than they are with the pursuit of pleasure (Philpott, Knerr & Boydell, 2006). Further, those who do use contraception (in heterosexual couplings) may be primarily motivated by avoiding pregnancy rather than infection. Thus, the health care professional has to deal with a tricky dilemma—promoting safe sex without denying the pursuit of pleasure. Indeed, some have argued that denying the possibility of pleasure in sexual relations harms active negotiations for safer sex, especially among adolescents (Brown et al., 2008).

Applying This to Noah and Emma

Noah and Emma are both exposing themselves to several STIs. As Noah is already experiencing pain 'down below', he could have contracted gonorrhoea.

Why do people have safe/unsafe sex?

To combat the spread of STIs and deliver good sexual health outcomes, the government's current message is education, correct condom use, regular testing/diagnosis and treatment (Department of Health, 2023). Research evidence supports that consistent condom use is associated with a reduced risk of STIs (e.g., Gallo et al., 2007) and the use of condoms during risky sexual encounters is the only efficient way to prevent the spread of most STIs (Carey et al., 1992). However, in one US study, 82% of individuals attending a follow-up study conducted in a sexual health clinic reported using a condom at least once in the last year. However, 94% of individuals reported that they had participated in sex without using a condom. In addition, it also concluded that only 5% of this high-risk population reported using condoms consistently over the year of the study (Peterman et al., 2009). Not only does the condom have to be used, but it has to be used effectively (i.e., properly).

Hatherall et al., (2007) report that a sizeable minority (between 12% and 40%) applied a condom imperfectly. Given that using condoms imperfectly reduces their effectiveness as a method of STI prevention, it is important to address this through appropriate public health messages. For example, the UK public health initiative Sexwise provides some guidance on proper condom use, but more work is likely needed to motivate their use in the first place.

So, why do some people not use a condom? And if they do, why do they not use them correctly? Why is it that individuals still take the risk and have unsafe sex? There are, of course, several possible reasons why this might be, and many of these are psychological. Barriers to condom use may also include accessibility, lack of education or confidence surrounding condom use, presence of stigma and experiences of embarrassment around purchasing or obtaining condoms (Farrington et al., 2016).

There may be some external factors to consider as well. For example, young peoples' sexual encounters are often unplanned; sporadic; and sometimes the result of social pressure, coercion or alcohol. It is estimated that 11% of teenagers regret a sexual encounter they had while under the influence of alcohol (Hibell et al., 2009). One American study of close to 1,000 college students found that around 25% had had one or more alcohol-related regretted sex occurrence in the month before, a very short space of time (Orchowski et al., 2012). Early sexual activity is strongly associated with alcohol use, with both possibly relating to poor wellbeing at school (Philips-Howard et al., 2010). The two decisions (young age of first sex and non-use of condom) may be related, and it may be that younger teens are less able to negotiate condom use or that younger age at first sex is a marker for other underlying risk-taking propensities. However, alcohol plays a significant role in sexual behaviour for adolescents. For example, one study (Phillips-Howard et al., 2010) reported that alcohol increased the chances of children (11–14-year-olds) partaking in sexual activity and intercourse. The chances of individuals experiencing some sexual behaviour increased by up to 12-fold when the individual drank alcohol at least once a week. Therefore, inferring that alcohol contributed to them doing 'more' sexually than they would when sober is reasonable.

Buhi and Goodson (2007) reviewed the predictors of risky sexual behaviour in adolescents and classified these factors under common themes (see Table 9.4).

According to the International Society for Sexual Medicine, LGBTQIA+ youth are at a higher risk of STIs, with rates of chlamydia, gonorrhoea and HIV twice as high in gay, lesbian and bisexual youth compared to heterosexual males (Hubach et al., 2022). The reasons for higher transmission rates in this population may be due to several factors. For instance, it has been suggested that LGBTQIA+ youth may be more inclined to engage in risky sexual behaviour than their heterosexual peers. Research also suggests

Table 9.4 Summary of predictors of sexual behaviour

Theme	Element
Intention to have sex Environmental constraints	• Initiation of sexual behaviour (–); • Greater parental involvement (–/0); • High quality of relationship with parents (–/0); • Fewer rules/boundaries (–/0); • Increased parental support (–/0/–); • Greater parental monitoring/supervision (–/0); Increased peer support (0); • Increased time home alone (without a parent) (–);
Norms	• Perceptions of peer sex behaviours (believing most peers have had sex) (–/0); Perception of peer disapproval of sex or negative attitudes • towards sex (–/0); Perceived parental disapproval of engaging in sexual • intercourse (–); • Self-efficacy (–/0); • Pro abstinence self-standards (–); Negative emotions regarding sex/positive emotions • towards sexual abstinence (–/0); Positive attitudes toward abstinence/fewer sexually • permissive attitudes (/0);

Source: Buhi and Goodson (2007).
Note: (–) indicates that this element is a risk factor, (–) indicates a protective factor, (0) indicates a non-statistically significant finding.

there may be certain barriers to STI and HIV testing in gender-diverse populations. For example, according to Hibbert et al. (2020), 50% of trans people who reported having anal sex without a condom had never been tested for HIV and were far less inclined to seek sexual health services than their cisgender counterparts. Importantly, however, this is likely a by-product of having less targeted education on sexual health matters and less access to health care resources. The relationship between mental health and sexual wellbeing has also been highlighted. Unfortunately, people in the LGBTQIA+ community suffer discrimination, stigma and systemic inequalities in society and the health care system that ultimately lead to poorer health outcomes. On a positive note, LGBTQIA+ individuals with the protective factors of strong family and community support often report better health outcomes than those without support systems. Nevertheless, it is imperative that in addition to heterosexual information, sexual education addresses common LGBTQIA+ sexual activities and issues specifically so that the sexual health of all people is supported equally.

Several psychological variables may be important when discussing sexual behaviour. One of the most important of these may be self-efficacy. Studies (e.g., Buhi & Goodson, 2007) have indicated a protective effect of self-efficacy. For example, intention was found to be a predictive factor for adolescents' sexual behaviour, alongside perceived norms and time spent at home alone (Buhi & Goodson, 2007). A different approach was adopted by Reissing et al. (2012), who reported on the relationship between individuals' first sexual experiences and their future sexual attitudes. They suggested that an individual's first sexual experience can influence psychological factors in several ways. For example, it was concluded that women who were older at the time of their first sexual experience had less sexual self-efficacy. That is, they had less belief in their capabilities to enact certain behaviours and responses in a sexual context. Conversely, a higher degree of sexual self-efficacy has been shown to relate to better sexual adjustment. A study by Sprecher (2014) spanning 23 years and over 5,000 university students in the US found gender differences in pleasure, guilt and anxiety in response to first intercourse. For example, while men reported more anxiety than women, they also reported more pleasure but less guilt. This again highlights the importance of psychology and attitudes concerning sexual behaviour.

Applying This to Noah and Emma

Noah is not as likely to practice safe sex as he reports sensation loss when using a condom. Emma may worry about Noah's reaction to wanting to use a condom.

Concerning the impact of psychological variables on safe sex, it is thought that moral norms impact condom use and safe-sex practices (Sarkar, 2008). This variable represents personal feelings of moral obligation or responsibility for adopting a given behaviour. This is perceived as a variable of growing importance in the health-related domain and affects the development of appropriate interventions and media campaigns.

Another reason unprotected sex may occur is that there may be other goals besides health. For example, sharing intimacy, experiencing belongingness and increasing one's self-esteem are goals that may override thoughts of health in an immediate situation (e.g.,

Gebhardt et al., 2006). These psychological functions of sexual behaviour may impact safe-sex behaviour. For example, heterosexual men's accounts of sexual pleasure while using a condom can be found to correlate with negative perceptions of psychological factors such as perceived penis size (Hensel et al., 2012). Investigations into condom use and sexual pleasure concluded that sexual pleasure and age were correlated: the older the male is, the higher the sexual pleasure that is experienced while using a condom (Hensel et al., 2012). In particular, men who believe condoms reduce sexual pleasure are less likely to engage in safe sex and use condoms (Randolph et al., 2007).

Finally, psychological research on the determinants of unsafe sexual practice usually employed the social cognition models outlined in Chapter 3, including theories such as the Health Belief Model (Rosenstock, 1990), the Protection Motivation Theory (Rogers, 1975), the Theory of Reasoned Action (Fishbein & Ajzen, 1975) and the Theory of Planned Behaviour (TPB) (Ajzen, 1985). Within this type of conceptualisation, it is assumed that individuals are motivated to use a condom if the benefits of doing so outweigh the costs and they can perform the behaviour.

Health care professionals must consider these factors when attempting to devise intervention strategies.

Applying This to Noah and Emma

Environmental factors should be considered when designing an intervention to assist Noah and Emma due to their non-monogamous relationship.

Interventions to promote safer sex

Individual-level interventions

Shrier et al. (2001) explored whether an individual intervention based on various psychological models, including the Stages of Change (SoC) (Prochaska & DiClemente, 2002), and implemented through motivational interviewing (Miller & Rollnick, 2002) could improve condom use. The intervention they suggested began with a 7-minute video in which popular entertainers and sports figures discussed and dramatised condom names, buying condoms and negotiating condom use, and two female adolescents demonstrated condom use to their peers. Condom use was portrayed as normative behaviour.

In addition, female health educators were employed and trained in various theories and taught to use a standardised intervention manual that outlined key points to cover, activities to perform and motivational strategies to employ. At the outset, participants were asked how much they needed and wanted to change their sexual risk behaviour (on a so-called 'wheel of change'). The intervention ensured that the same information was provided to all participants, but the educator tried to individualise the session based on the stage of change. Based on this intervention, condom use improved; that is, more of the participants used condoms during sex than before. However, this is one specific example, and there are many others based on the SoC model.

Support for the SoC model can also be found in a recent meta-analysis (Noar et al., 2009), which considered 12 randomised control trials of computer-based HIV prevention interventions. Interventions that adopted the SoC model were found to be more effective. This is thought to be due to the intervention's tailoring to an individual and its personalised approach.

Applying This to Noah and Emma

Health care professionals could work with Noah and Emma to encourage the use of condoms. The SoC model could be a starting point for health professionals to tailor interventions to Noah and Emma. The couple will be able to identify the stage they are currently at and gradually complete activities and strategies using motivational interviewing. This will allow Noah and Emma to explore the underlying reasons for Noah's negative views of condoms and endeavour to change his behaviour in the longer term.

Other psychological models can contribute to promoting safer sex and can be incorporated into any intervention based on the SoC model. One example would be from the TPB (Fishbein & Ajzen, 1975), which suggests that subjective norms, including peer norms, are important factors related to the SoC. For example, adolescents who perceive greater support for safer sex are more likely to improve and maintain their sexual behaviour (e.g., Sieving et al., 2006).

The SoC model has been described extensively elsewhere in this book; see, for example, how it can be applied to smoking cessation in Chapter 8. However, it serves as a useful model for developing and implementing intervention strategies for a range of lifestyle behaviours, and safe sex is one of them. The SoC model (Prochaska & DiClemente, 1983) has been used as a foundation for intervention design, and its benefit is that it allows an intervention to be tailored to an individual's needs and their specific stage. A further strength of the model is that the individual's current stage can be used to indicate success. If we examine the SoC model when applied to condom use, we can explore how we can place individuals within each of the stages (see Figure 9.2).

In this model, women who reported using condoms consistently (i.e., every time they had sex) for at least 6 months with their main partners were in 'maintenance', those using condoms consistently but for less than 6 months were in 'action', those who intended to use condoms consistently in the next month were in 'preparation', those who intended to use condoms consistently sometime within the next 6 months were in 'contemplation' and those who did not intend to use condoms consistently were in 'pre-contemplation'.

Applying This to Noah and Emma

Noah is in the pre-contemplation stage of change when considering condom use.

There are other, more sophisticated models. Level of motivation to practise safer sex can be reported in numerous ways. For example, asking individuals a set of questions allows them to be categorised into each of the stages (see Table 9.5).

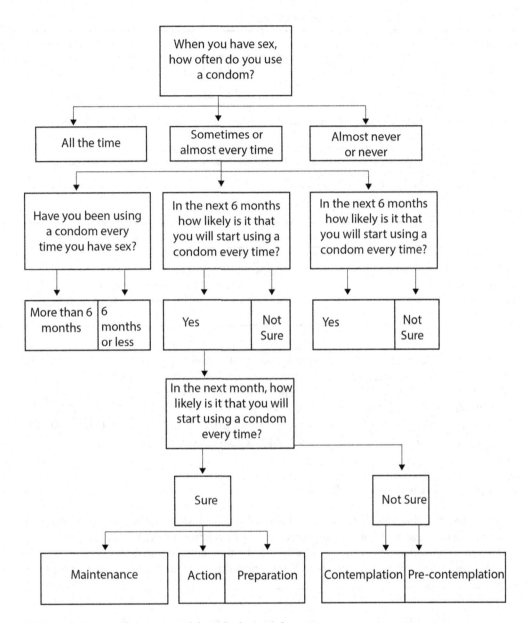

Figure 9.2 Stages of change model applied to condom use.

Alternatively, (in a less formal manner), the health care professional could simply ask the individual what their sexual behaviour was and whether they intended to change it.

According to the SoC model, there are two important factors for predicting the adoption of safer behaviour: self-efficacy and decisional balance. An individual's self-efficacy for performing the behaviour has been shown to have a linear relationship with more movement to safer behaviour. As individuals progress towards maintaining positive health behaviour, their confidence in their ability to carry out the behaviour

Table 9.5 Allocating individuals to stage of change

Question	Stage of change
Are you basically satisfied with your sexual behaviours and don't want to change them?	Pre-contemplators
Are you thinking about making changes to your sexual behaviour soon (i.e., in the next month)?	Contemplators
Are you going to make changes to your sexual behaviour in the next month?	Preparation
Have you made changes to your sexual behaviour in the past 6 months?	Action
Have you made changes to your sexual behaviour in the past 6 months and not returned to the previous pattern?	Maintenance

Table 9.6 Pros and cons of condom use

Pros	Cons
Protects from STIs	Sensation reduced
Prevents unwanted pregnancy	Interrupts the moment
Reduces mess	Added expense/inconvenience to obtain
Increases female pleasure	Embarrassment when communicating with partner
Lengthens time for intercourse	

increases (see Chapter 4 for a fuller discussion of self-efficacy). Decisional balance is simply weighing the perceived pros and cons of behaviour change and how these cognitions about health behaviour relate to the SoC. Typically, people in the pre-contemplation stage identify more cons associated with the behaviour, whereas those in the action or maintenance stages perceive more pros. Some of the most frequently reported pros and cons of condom use are presented in Table 9.6.

Applying This to Noah and Emma

Presented in Table 9.6 are the pros and cons of condom use. Another way of looking at this is the pros and cons of unprotected sex. In relation to Noah, a con of Noah having unprotected sex is the possibility that he may contract an STI. A pro of this behaviour (according to Noah) is that sensation during sexual activity is increased.

Studies have indicated that, not surprisingly, the pros and cons of condom use are consistently the best predictor of progression to and maintenance of consistent condom use. Hence, the message for the health care professional is clear: deal with the pros and cons of condom use at the outset. One of the major tasks may be dealing with the negative aspects of condom wear and correcting misconceptions.

Community-level interventions

Within the UK, the Department of Health suggested several actions needed to be implemented. The first of these was to develop a national campaign aimed at younger men and women to ensure that they understand the real risk of unprotected sex and persuade them of the benefits of using condoms to avoid the risk of STIs or unplanned pregnancies (see, for example, www.nhs.uk/Livewell and www.sexwise.org.uk). Further, there was a longer-term strategy to ensure that children and young people were on the right path towards improving their sexual health by reducing teenage pregnancy and the consumption of alcohol and illicit drugs. Developments of new resources for the health service (e.g., a confidential email service and websites such as www.teenagehealthfreak. org and www.nhs.uk/Livewell/Sexandyoungpeople/Pages/Sex-and-young-people-hub. aspxr) are all part of this approach.

Over the last few years, considerable efforts have been made to recognise how sexual health needs affect individuals differently depending on their gender and sexuality and whether they are gender diverse. Several community-level interventions are aimed at targeting the most vulnerable groups. For example, the National Chlamydia Screening Programme, which, in 2021, changed its focus to reducing harm from untreated chlamydia infections. Since the harmful effects of chlamydia reside mainly in women, opportunistic screening outside of sexual health clinics will now chiefly be offered to women, even if they are asymptomatic. This strategy means that testing, treatment and partner notification can begin early to reduce the spread of chlamydia and the adverse reproductive health outcomes of the infection.

Regarding HIV, gay and bisexual men are statistically at the highest risk. The HIV education portal 'It Starts with Me'—provided by HIV Prevention England, the national program commissioned by Public Health England—has information and quizzes on the people who should be tested for HIV and when, the method to get tested or obtain self-testing kits for HIV and the assessment of eligibility for preexposure prophylaxis and post-exposure prophylaxis.

In an Australian context, the AIDS Council of NSW (ACON) was established in 1985 in response to the AIDS crisis, and is a health-promotion leader specialising in HIV prevention and support, in addition to LGBTQIA+ health. ACON offer a range of education programs and services aimed at understanding health issues that uniquely affect sexually and gender-diverse communities. For example, trans and gender-diverse people often face barriers to health care that is gender affirmative, which may compound their already high risk of STIs in numerous ways. Thus, part of community-level sexual health intervention more broadly involves coordinating a comprehensive plan to deliver strategies to improve the health outcomes of gender-diverse populations, which many have suggested is currently at a crisis level. One such plan from ACON is *A Blueprint for Improving the Health and Wellbeing of the Trans and Gender Diverse Community in NSW*. Such interventional programs promoting condom use and STI testing have used various strategies and media, including lectures, leaflets, interactive games and websites, films, role-modelling and posters. Public health campaigns have employed poster campaigns, TV, newspaper and cinema advertising, interactive computer and web programs and health-promotion leaflets (e.g., https://www.nhs.uk/live-well/sexual-health/).

Theoretically derived interventions have mostly used social cognition models to address safer sexual behaviour. These models suggested that knowledge about STIs and beliefs about infection, risk and symptom severity are weaker predictors of condom use than action-specific cognitions, such as attitudes towards condom use, perceived self-efficacy concerning condom use, the social acceptability of condom use and condom use intentions. The TPB has been widely used as a basis for understanding condom use behaviour and developing interventions. In addition, it has been shown to be a useful model for varying subsamples of the population, including drug addicts, concerning safe-sex practices (Mausbach et al., 2009).

Research by Abraham et al. (2011) investigated the predictive ability of the TPB on condom use while accounting for social structure. It was recognised that accounting for social structure while using this theory enabled it to predict condom use behaviour more reliably. The study identified key messages and recommendations about applying cognitive theory and condom use. Some of these are:

- Cognition models do not successfully account for social structure, such as socio-economic status, on behaviour.
- Mothers' socioeconomic status accounted for 5% of the variance.
- Condom use was correlated with condom-use cognitions.
- Individuals from areas with greater levels of deprivation reported using a condom less frequently.
- Positive attitudes towards condom use were associated with greater educational aspirations, lower parental aspirations and being female.
- College aspirations explained 4% of the variance in consistent condom use, which highlights the importance of social structures in predicting behaviour.

Overall, it was suggested that more research should be conducted into the effects of the social structure, including socioeconomic status, aspirations, gender and deprivation, alongside cognitions when considering teenagers' behaviours concerning condoms. In addition, the research highlighted the potential underlying factors that influence condom-related behaviour in this sample of teenagers. It can be suggested that by considering social structural factors, health behaviour concerning condoms could be better understood. Other research has demonstrated similar conclusions, acknowledging the need for the TPB to be used with other variables to predict condom use better (Turchik & Gidycz, 2012).

Investigations into the effectiveness of leaflet-based interventions derived from the TPB highlight interesting findings and implications for using this model in health promotion regarding condom use. Krahé et al. (2005) performed an experiment on the effectiveness of a leaflet promotion aimed to impact safe-sex practices. The leaflet was developed based on research into cognitive correlates with condom use (Sheeran et al., 1999). However, mixed results on the effectiveness of the leaflet alone were seen. The experimental conditions tested by this research suggested that the leaflet alone provided similar results to the no-leaflet condition. The research highlighted the importance of motivation regarding getting the individual to spend time and read the leaflet. Thus, the experimental group, which received an intrinsic reward for reading and processing the leaflet, experienced lasting behavioural effects at 1-month follow-up. Consequently, it is important to note that interventions specifically tailored for individuals must attempt to increase motivation for actual engagement with the material and develop appropriate materials appropriately.

Research has shown that abstinence programs can successfully prevent adolescent sexual involvement (Jemmott et al., 2010). There is a growth of abstinence movements in the US (e.g., The Silver Ring Thing); however, similar trends have not been seen in the UK. This may be because health educators fear their audience will be unwilling to contemplate delaying sexual intercourse. The other problem with this approach, as discussed above, is defining what abstinence is. Does it mean only 'not having sexual

Table 9.7 Misconceptions around condom wear

Cons	How
Sensation reduced	Add additional lube which can enhance the experience for both partners
Interrupts the moment	Can add to the moment, as it can signify to the partner that they are ready for sex
Added expense/inconvenience to obtain	Can be obtained free from a number of sources
Embarrassment when communicating with partner	Should be able to embrace the moment and actually can add to the pleasure for both parties

intercourse'? Or does it also mean not kissing or touching? Further, most adolescents experience some form of sexual desire. As Berer (2006) suggests: 'The prescription of abstinence is a potential death sentence for anyone who wants to have sex if the means to make it safe, at whatever age, are withheld' (p. 7).

A potential strategy to attempt to change individuals' condom-use behaviour is to attempt to reinterpret the use of condoms, for example, moving from the condom as 'safety wear' to condoms as 'pleasure promoters' or eroticising the condom. One project, the Pleasure Project (Philpott et al., 2006), aims to promote condoms as sexy and pleasurable and lists several 'quick and dirty ways' to illustrate the benefits of condoms. So, for example, opening a male condom packet can be a sign that a person is ready for sex. Carrying condoms in a pocket or handbag when going out and showing them to a potential partner can illustrate how interested the person is in sex while also encouraging condom use (Philpott et al., 2006, p. 25). A Turkish condom company saw a considerable boost in sales through the use of social networking sites by reinventing the condom using slogans like 'safe and fun sex is your right' and aiming to market condoms as playful and fun through colourful packaging and a range of flavours, shapes and textures (Purdy, 2011). For example, Table 9.7 outlines the previously highlighted disadvantages associated with condom wear and suggests how these can be corrected or addressed.

A second key element derived from the studies exploring the SoC is that interventions need to be tailored to the SoC. The model suggests that different processes in behaviour change, such as raising consciousness and self-reinforcement, are necessary at different stages. Thus, interventions focusing on cognitive and emotional factors will be the most influential in the early stages, whereas action-orientated approaches are effective in later stages.

For example, for inconsistent condom users, interventions should first target increasing the advantages of using condoms (e.g., lengthening the duration of sexual intercourse, decreasing messiness and increasing female pleasure) and then promoting and modelling skills for communication with partners about condoms. Maintaining consistent condom use is a challenge, and interventions will need to focus on novel ways to sustain interest in the effectiveness and positive aspects of condoms. For individuals who use condoms consistently, interventions might adhere to relapse-prevention models whereby the goals are to preserve the positive attitude towards condoms, maintain consistent communication with partners about condoms and reinforce perceptions of vulnerability to STIs.

There is a difference between some of the other behaviours discussed in this book and safer sex: for example, with smoking, diet and exercise, behaviour change is largely an individual choice. The adoption of condom use, however, is a behaviour that often demands communication and agreement between partners. It may necessitate an assessment of one's own risk and the risk of one's partner(s). Therefore, communication with partners about condom use and perceived personal vulnerability to STIs and HIV must be considered. Further, we must return to our original point: sex is a pleasurable activity that must be encouraged with partners and individuals. The fear message will not work.

Applying This to Noah and Emma

Noah and Emma need to talk about using condoms within their relationship, reconcile their differences regarding their use and, in turn, use contraception that they are both 100% happy with.

Working effectively with others

Given that attempting to provide safer sex education can be problematic, it is essential that some broad-based messages are promoted. These are provided in Table 9.8. As can be noted, the emphasis is on pleasure rather than fear. It is about safely promoting the activity rather than attempting to scare people into changing.

Table 9.8 Tips for sexual health educators

Tip	Comment
Have a realistic attitude	Appreciate that different sexual practices and attitudes are evident
Get advice from the target audience	Pleasure and sexiness are often culturally specific, so tailor the message appropriately
Remain comfortable about talking about sex and pleasure	Trainers and health educators need to be able to talk about sex and pleasure seeking in appropriate language
Focus on pleasure and sex rather than disease	It is important to strike a balance between promoting pleasure and promoting health
Promote positive messages rather than messages of fear or shame	If people are fearful or shamed then they are less likely to request assistance
Focus on the individual issues	Ensure that any counselling/intervention is tailored to deal with the individual concerns and not a predetermined agenda
Be realistic in an assessment of risk	Ensure the individual client assesses their own risks and acceptable measures of risk reduction
Support positive changes	Small steps are positive, and moving from one stage to another can be seen as positive
Clarify misconceptions	Clarify rather than deal with general discussions
Use appropriate language	Ensure that over-technical language is avoided and that the individual feels comfortable when discussing sex

School nurses and sexual education

School nurses provide students with a wide variety of services during school hours, one of which is free, confidential advice on sexual health and contraception. Using school nurses to provide this service enables the young population to gain accurate advice and information relating to sexual health. Although using school nurses could potentially positively impact teenagers' sexual health, it is suggested that such staff are not used to their full advantage when considering sexual health (Westwood & Mullan, 2009).

Research into children's experiences of sex education in schools has provided some insightful findings. Children were found to want the most advice on STIs, and wide variation between preferred delivery methods was seen throughout the sample (Newby et al., 2012). This challenges schools trying to effectively deliver messages in the sex education sessions to all, especially when society is becoming increasingly diverse. Therefore, better thought-out recourses should be implemented; this will not only address worries regarding the transmission of STIs but also impact teenage pregnancy concerns. Working with the school nurse, schools could potentially develop a more successful sex education program.

Sexual health and family-planning clinics

Sexual health clinics or genitourinary medicine clinics provide a vast range of services to the general population. The services include treatment for STIs, contraception advice, sexual health advice, free condoms and counselling services for individuals who have suffered sexual attacks or been diagnosed with an STI. Trained health professionals from various backgrounds, such as doctors, nurses and counsellors, are all available to offer free, confidential advice offered in a non-judgemental way. The non-judgemental attitude of staff is a crucial element of the service, and younger people especially consider the staff's attitudes to be important in reducing barriers to sexual health advice (Baxter et al., 2011).

In addition, research has identified that using psychological behaviour change techniques within this setting and family-planning clinics can positively affect emergency contraception consultation rates (Martin et al., 2011). It is suggested that by using techniques that specifically outline behaviours, such as the 'if-then' technique, implications can be seen concerning effective contraception behaviour. Again, in turn, this technique could be applicable to reducing STIs and unwanted pregnancy rates.

Applying This to Noah and Emma

Noah and Emma could both visit their local sexual health clinic to get tested for STIs. In addition, they could also get some advice on safe sex and using condoms correctly, so they don't 'reduce sensation' for Noah.

Conclusion

Sexual behaviour is a natural behaviour that has at its root, a fundamental physiological purpose. However, it serves a range of other cultural, emotional, psychological and social purposes that must be considered when attempting to promote safe sexual behaviour. Promoting a safe-sex message is important given the rise in sexually transmitted diseases nationally and worldwide. Psychological factors contribute to whether people engage in safe sex, and social cognitive models have successfully predicted condom use. Several key elements from the SoC model can be used to promote safe sex.

Key points

- Researchers generally define sexual behaviour as any behaviour that involves a sexual response of the body; however, individuals will define it differently, depending on, for example, age, experience and sexual orientation.
- Safe sex is hard to define but involves taking steps to reduce the chance of contracting or transmitting STIs. Most people associate this with condom use and/or monogamy, but advancements in antiviral medications such as post-exposure prophylaxis and preexposure prophylaxis to prevent HIV are changing the landscape of 'safer sex', particularly in the gay community.
- The UK has seen the largest rise in the number of HIV cases since 2000 and cases of other STIs, such as chlamydia and herpes, are also increasing.
- Evidence suggests that consistent and correct condom use is associated with reduced STI transmission. Despite this, many people in the UK are not consistently practising safe sex.
- Alcohol is associated with risky sexual behaviours.
- Social cognition models have been shown to predict some safe-sex practices.
- Self-efficacy is a key variable in promoting safe sex.
- Interventions to reduce unsafe sex include providing sex education in schools and mass-media campaigns.
- Interventions have been shown to be more effective when they are targeted to specific audiences and are based on psychological theory.
- Individuals can be classified according to their SoC, and this information can be used to promote condom use.
- Misconceptions about condom use must be addressed, and these can be redefined positively.
- Sexual behaviour change is more effective if promoted within a positive pleasure framework.

Points for discussion

- Consider how attitudes towards condom use have changed and discuss the potential reasons underlying the attitude changes. In doing so, identify any subgroups where attitudes are less positive.
- Critically evaluate psychological theory concerning the promotion of safe sex.
- Consider Noah and Emma:
  - What sort of problems are Emma and Noah potentially facing?
  - Develop an action plan for Noah (and discuss how to involve Emma).

Further resources

Sexual health: https://www.nhs.uk/live-well/sexual-health/
Teenage Health Freak: https://www.healthforteens.co.uk/sexual-health/
Brook—Free and confidential information for under 25 s—Ask Brook 0808 802 1234 or http://www.brook.org.uk/

References

Abraham, C., Sheeran, P. & Henderson, M. (2011). Extending social cognition models of health behaviour. Health Education Research, *26*(4), 624–637.

Ajzen, I. (1985). From intention to actions: A theory of planned behaviour. In J. Kuhl, & J. Beckman (Eds.), Action-control: From cognition to behaviour (pp. 11–39). Heidelberg, Germany: Springer. Retrieved from http://www.people.umass.edu/aizen/publications.html

Ballester-Arnal, R., Giménez-García, C., Ruiz-Palomino, E., Castro-Calvo, J., & Gil-Llario, M. D. (2022). A trend analysis of condom use in Spanish young people over the two past decades, 1999–2020. AIDS and Behavior, *26*(7), 2299–2313. 10.1007/s10461-021-03573-6

Baxter, S., Blank, L., Guillaume, L., Squires, H., & Payne, N. (2011). Views of contraceptive service delivery to young people in the UK: A systematic review and thematic synthesis. Journal of Family Planning & Reproductive Health Care, *37*(2), 71–84.

Berer, M. (2006). Dual protection: More needed than practised or understood. Reproductive Health Matters, *14*(28), 162–170.

Bersamin, M., Fisher, D., Walker, S., Hill, D., & Grube, J. (2007). Defining virginity and abstinence: Adolescents' interpretations of sexual behaviors. Journal of Adolescent Health, *41*(2), 182–188.

Brown, L., DiClemente, R., Crosby, R., Fernandez, M., Pugatch, D., Cohn, S., ...Schlenger, W. (2008). Condom use among high-risk adolescents: Anticipation of partner disapproval and less pleasure associated with not using condoms. Public Health Reports, *123*(5), 601–607.

Bourne, A. H., & Robson, M. A. (2009). Perceiving risk and (re)constructing safety: The lived experience of having 'safe' sex. Health, Risk & Society, *11*(3), 283–295.

Buhi. E. R. & Goodson, P. (2007). Predictors of adolescent and sexual behaviour and intention: A theory-guided systematic review. Journal of Adolescent Health, *40*(1), 4–21.

Byers, E., Henderson, J. & Hobson, K. M. (2009). University students' definitions of sexual abstinence and having sex. Archives of Sexual Behaviour, *38*(5), 665–674.

Campbell, A. N., Brooks, A. J., Pavlicova, M., Hu, M. C., Hatch-Maillette, M. A., Calsyn, D. A., & Tross, S. (2016). Barriers to condom use: Results for men and women enrolled in HIV risk reduction trials in outpatient drug treatment. Journal of HIV/AIDS & Social Services, *15*(2), 130–146. 10.1080/15381501.2016.1166090

Carey, R. F., Herman, W. A., Retta, S. M., Rinaldi, J. E. R., German, B. A. & Athey, T. W. (1992). Effectiveness of latex condoms as a barrier to human immunodeficiency virus-sized particles under conditions of simulated use. Sexually Transmitted Disease, *19*, 230–234.

Chambers, W. C. (2007). Oral sex: Varied behaviours and perceptions in a college population. Journal of Sex Research, *44*(1), 28–42.

Dalessandro, C., James-Hawkins, L., & Sennott, C. (2019). Strategic silence: College men and hegemonic masculinity in contraceptive decision making. Gender & Society, *33*(5), 772–794.

Department of Health (2023). A framework for sexual health improvement in England. London: UK Government.

D'Souza, G., Agrawal, Y., Halpern, J., Bodison, S., & Gillison, M. (2009). Oral sexual behaviors associated with prevalent oral human papillomavirus infection. Journal of Infectious Diseases, *199*(9), 1263–1269.

Evans, D. L., & Tripp, J. H. (2006). Sex education: The case for primary prevention and peer education. Current Paediatrics, *16*, 95–99.

Farrington, E. M., Bell, D. C., & DiBacco, A. E. (2016). Reasons people give for using (or not using) condoms. AIDS and Behavior, *20*(12), 2850–2862. 10.1007/s10461-016-1352-7

Fishbein, M., & Ajzen, I. (1975). Belief, attitude, intention and behaviour: An introduction to theory and research. London, United Kingdom: Addison-Wesley.

Gallo, M. F., Steiner, M. J., Warner, L., Hylton-Kong, T., Figueroa, J. P., Hobbs, M. M. & Behets, F. M. (2007). Self-reported condom use is associated with reduced risk of chlamydia, gonorrhoea, and trichomoniasis. Sexually Transmitted Diseases, *34*(10), 829–833.

Gebhardt, W. A., Kuyper, L. & Dusseldorp, E. (2006). Condom use at first intercourse with a new partner in female adolescents and young adults: The role of cognitive planning and motives for having sex. Archives of Sexual Behaviour, *35*(2), 217–223.

Grubb, L. K., Alderman, E. M., Chung, R. J., Lee, J., Powers, M. E., Rahmandar, M. H., ... & Wallace, S. B. (2020). Barrier protection use by adolescents during sexual activity. Pediatrics, *146* (2), 130–133.

Habel, M. A., Leichliter, J. S., Dittus, P. J., Spicknall, I. H., & Aral, S. O. (2018). Heterosexual anal and oral sex in adolescents and adults in the United States, 2011–2015. Sexually Transmitted Diseases, *45*(12), 775–782. 10.1097/OLQ.0000000000000889

Hammoud, M. A., Vaccher, S., Jin, F., Bourne, A., Maher, L., Holt, M., ... & Prestage, G. P. (2019). HIV pre-exposure prophylaxis (PrEP) uptake among gay and bisexual men in Australia and factors associated with the nonuse of PrEP among eligible men: Results from a prospective cohort study. JAIDS Journal of Acquired Immune Deficiency Syndromes, *81*(3), e73–e84.

Hans, J. D., Gillen, M., & Akande, K. (2010). Sex redefined: The reclassification of oral-genital contact. Perspectives on Sexual and Reproductive Health, *42*(2), 74–78.

Hans, J. D., & Kimberly, C. (2011). Abstinence, sex, and virginity: Do they mean what we think they mean? American Journal of Sexuality Education, *6*(4), 329–342.

Hatherall, B., Ingham, R., Stone, N., & McEachran, J. (2007). How, not just if, condoms are used: The timing of condom application and removal during vaginal sex among young people in England. Sexually Transmitted Infections, *83*, 68–70.

Hensel, D. J., Stupiansky, N. W., Herbenick, D., Dodge, B., & Reece, M. (2011). When condom use is not condom use: An event-level analysis of condom use behaviors during vaginal intercourse. Journal of Sexual Medicine, *8*(1), 28–34. 10.1111/j.1743-6109.2010.02031.x

Hensel, D. J., Stupiansky, N. W., Herbenick, D., Dodge, B., & Reece, M. (2012). Sexual pleasure during condom-protected vaginal sex among heterosexual men. Journal of Sexual Medicine, *9*(5), 1272–1276. 10.1111/j.1743-6109.2012.02700.x

Hibell, B., Guttormsson, U., Ahlström, S., Balakireva, O., Bjarnason, T., Kokkevi, A., & Kraus, L. (2009). The 2007 ESPAD report. Substance use among students in 35 European countries. Stockholm, Sweden: The Swedish Council for Information on Alcohol and Other Drugs.

Hibbert, M. P., Wolton, A., Weeks, H., Ross, M., Brett, C. E., Porcellato, L. A., & Hope, V. D. (2020). Psychosocial and sexual factors associated with recent sexual health clinic attendance and HIV testing among trans people in the UK. BMJ Sexual & Reproductive Health, *46*(2), 116–125. 10.1136/bmjsrh-2019-200375

Horowitz, A. D., & Bedford, E. (2017). Graded structure in sexual definitions: Categorizations of having "had sex" and virginity loss among homosexual and heterosexual men and women. Archives of Sexual Behavior, *46*(6), 1653–1665. 10.1007/s10508-016-0905-1

HPA. (2008). All new episodes seen at GUM clinics: 1998–2007. United Kingdom and country specific tables. London, United Kingdom: HPA.

HPA. (2009). Health Protection Agency. Hepatitis B—General information. Retrieved from http://www.hpa.org.uk/Topics/InfectiousDiseases/InfectionsAZ/HepatitisB/GeneralInformationHepatitisB/hepbGeneralInfo/

HPA. (2011). Number and rates of new STI diagnoses in England, 2002–2011. London, United Kingdom: Public Health England. Retrieved from http://www.hpa.org.uk/webc/HPAwebFile/HPAweb_C/1215589015024

HPA (2012). HIV in the United Kingdom: 2012 report. London, United Kingdom: Health Protection Services, Colindale. Retrieved from http://www.hpa.org.uk/webc/HPAwebFile/HPAweb_C/1317137200016

Hubach, R. D., Zipfel, R., Muñoz, F. A., Brongiel, I., Narvarte, A., & Servin, A. E. (2022). Barriers to sexual and reproductive care among cisgender, heterosexual and LGBTQIA+ adolescents in the border region: Provider and adolescent perspectives. Reproductive Health, *19*(1), 1–11.

Jemmott III, J. B., Jemmott, L. S., & Fong, G. T. (2010). Efficacy of a theory-based abstinence-only intervention over 24 months: A randomized controlled trial with young adolescents. Archives of Paediatrics and Adolescent Medicine, *164*(2), 152–159.

Krahé, B., Abraham, C. & Scheinberger-Olwig, R. (2005). Can safer-sex promotion leaflets change cognitive antecedents of condom use? An experimental evaluation. British Journal of Health Psychology, *10*(2), 203–220.

Lader, D. (2009). *Contraception and sexual heath, 2008/09.* London: ONS.

Leval, A., Sundström, K., Ploner, A., Dahlström, L., Widmark, C., & Sparén, P. (2011). Assessing perceived risk and STI prevention behaviour: A national population-based study with special reference to HPV. Plos ONE, *6*(6), 1–10.

Lindsey, R. (1985, 24 October). Bathhouse curbs called help in coast AIDS fight. New York Times, p. A19.

Martin, J., Slade, P., Sheeran, P., Wright, A. & Dibble, T. (2011). 'If-then' planning in one-to-one behaviour change counselling is effective in promoting contraceptive adherence in teenagers. Journal of Family Planning & Reproductive Health Care, *37*(2), 85–88.

Marfatia, Y. S., Pandya, I., & Mehta, K. (2015). Condoms: Past, present, and future. Indian Journal of Sexually Transmitted Diseases and AIDS, *36*(2), 133–139. 10.4103/0253-7184.167135

Magaret, A. S., Mujugira, A., Hughes, J. P., Lingappa, J., Bukusi, E. A., DeBruyn, G., Delany-Moretlwe, S., Fife, K. H., Gray, G. E., Kapiga, S., Karita, E., Mugo, N. R., Rees, H., Ronald, A., Vwalika, B., Were, E., Celum, C., Wald, A., & Partners in Prevention HSV/HIV Transmission Study Team (2016). Effect of condom use on per-act HSV-2 Transmission Risk in HIV-1, HSV-2-discordant couples. Clinical Infectious Diseases: An Official Publication of the Infectious Diseases Society of America, *62*(4), 456–461. 10.1093/cid/civ908

Masters, N., Beadnell, B., Morrison, D., Hoppe, M., & Gillmore, M. (2008). The opposite of sex? Adolescents' thoughts about abstinence and sex, and their sexual behaviour. Perspectives on Sexual & Reproductive Health, *40*(2), 87–93.

Mausbach, B., Semple, S., Strathdee, S., & Patterson, T. (2009). Predictors of safer sex intentions and protected sex among heterosexual HIV-negative methamphetamine users: An expanded model of the theory of planned behaviour. AIDS Care, *21*(1), 17–24.

McKay, A. (2007). The effectiveness of latex condoms for prevention of STI/HIV. Canadian Journal of Human Sexuality, *16*(1–2), 57–61.

Minichiello, V., Hawkes, G., & Pitts, M. (2011). HIV, sexually transmitted infections, and sexuality in later life. Current Infectious Disease Reports, *13*(2), 182–187.

Miller, W. R., & Rollnick, S. (2002). Motivational interviewing: Preparing people for change (2nd ed.). New York, NY: Guilford Press.

Morin, S. F., Charles, K. A., & Malyon, A. K. (1984). The psychological impact of AIDS on gay men. American Psychologist, *39*, 1288–1293.

Moskowitz, J. M., Assunta Ritieni, A., Tholandi, M., & Xia, M. (2006). How do Californians define safe sex? Californian Journal of Health Promotion, *4*(1), 109–118.

Newby, K., Wallace, L. M., Dunn, O., & Brown, K. E. (2012). A survey of English teenagers' sexual experience and preferences for school-based sex education. Sex Education, *12*(2), 231–251.

NHS Choices. (n.d.). Retrieved from www.nhs.uk/Livewell/STIs

NICE (2022) Reducing sexually transmitted infections. https://www.nice.org.uk/guidance/ng221 Accessed: 3rd February 2024.

Noar, S. M., Black, H. G., & Pierce, L. B. (2009). Efficacy of computer technology-based HIV prevention interventions: A meta-analysis. Aids, *23*(1), 107–115.

Office for Health Improvement and Disparities. (2023). Sexual and reproductive health and HIV: Applying all our health. Retrieved from https://www.gov.uk/government/publications/sexual-and-reproductive-health-and-hiv-applying-all-our-health/sexual-and-reproductive-health-and-hiv-applying-all-our-health

Orchowski, L. M., Mastroleo, N. R., & Borsari, B. (2012). Correlates of alcohol-related regretted sex among college students. Psychology of Addictive Behaviors, 26(4), 782–790.

Ong, J. J., Bourne, C., Dean, J. A., Ryder, N., Cornelisse, V. J., Murray, S., Kenchington, P., Moten, A., Gibbs, C., Maunsell, S., Davis, T., Michaels, J., & Medland, N. A. (2023). Australian sexually transmitted infection (STI) management guidelines for use in primary care 2022 update. Sexual Health, 20(1), 1–8. https://doi.org/10.1071/SH22134

Peterman, T., Tian, L., Warner, L., Satterwhite, C., Metcalf, C., Malotte, K., ...Douglas, J. (2009). Condom use in the year following a sexually transmitted disease clinic visit. International Journal of STD & AIDS, 20(1), 9–13. 10.1258/ijsa.2008.008177

Phillips-Howard, P., Bellis, M., Briant, L., Jones, H., Downing, J., Kelly, I., ...Cook, P. (2010). Wellbeing, alcohol use and sexual activity in young teenagers: Findings from a cross-sectional survey in school children in North West England. Substance Abuse Treatment, Prevention, and Policy, 5, 27.

Philpott, A., Knerr, W., & Boydell, V. (2006). Pleasure and prevention: When good sex is safer sex. Reproductive Health Matters, 14, 23–31.

Prochaska, J. O., & DiClemente, C. C. (1983). Stages and processes of self-change smoking: Towards an integrative model of change. Journal of Consulting and Clinical Psychology, 51, 390–395.

Prochaska, J. O., & DiClemente, C. C. (2002). Transtheoretical therapy: Toward a more integrative model of change. Psychotherapy: Theory, Research and Practice, 19, 276–288.

Purdy, C. H. (2011). Using the internet and social media to promote condom use in Turkey. Reproductive Health Matters, 19(37), 157–165.

Randolph, M. E., Pinkerton, S. D., Bogart, L. M., Cecil, H., & Abramson, P. R. (2007). Sexual pleasure and condom use. Archives of Sexual Behaviour, 36(6), 844–848. 10.1007/s10508-007-9213-0

Reissing, E. D., Andruff, H. L., & Wentland, J. J. (2012). Looking back: The experience of first sexual intercourse and current sexual adjustment in young heterosexual adults. Journal of Sex Research, 49(1), 27–35.

Rogers, R. W. (1975). A protection motivation theory of fear appeals and attitude change. Journal of Psychology, 91, 93–114.

Rosenstock, I. (1990). The health belief model: Explaining health behaviour through expectancies. In K. Glanz, F. M. Lewis, & B. K. Rimmer (Eds.), Health behaviour and health education: Theory, research and practice. San Francisco, CA: Jossey-Bass.

Saini, R., Saini, S., & Sharma, S. (2010). Oral sex, oral health and orogenital infections. Journal of Global Infectious Diseases, 2(1), 57–62.

Sarkar, N. N. (2008). Barriers to condom use. European Journal of Contraception & Reproductive Health Care, 13(2), 114–122.

Sheeran, P., Abraham, C., & Orvell, S. (1999). Psychosocial correlates of heterosexual condom use: A meta-analysis. Psychological Bulletin, 125, 90–132.

Shrier, L. A., Ancheta, R., Goodman, E., Chiou, V. M., Lyden, M. R., & Emans, S. J. (2001). Randomized controlled trials of safer sex intervention for high-risk adolescent girls. Archives of Paediatrics and Adolescent Medicine, 155, 73–79.

Sieving, R., Eisenberg, M., Pettingell, S., & Skay, C. (2006). Friends' influence on adolescents' first sexual intercourse. Perspectives on Sexual and Reproductive Health, 38, 13–19.

Sousa, A. F. L. D., Lima, S. V. M. A., Ribeiro, C. J. N., de Sousa, A. R., Barreto, N. M. P. V., Camargo, E. L. S., ... & Mendes, I. A. C. (2023). Adherence to pre-exposure prophylaxis (PrEP) among men who have sex with men (MSM) in Portuguese-speaking Countries. International Journal of Environmental Research and Public Health, 20(6), 4881.

Sprecher, S. (2014). Evidence of change in men's versus women's emotional reactions to first sexual intercourse: A 23-year study in a human sexuality course at a midwestern university. The Journal of Sex Research, 51(4), 466–472.

Slevin, A. P., & Marvin, C. L. (1987). Safe sex and pregnancy prevention: A guide for health practitioners working with adolescents. Journal of Community Health Nursing, *4*, 235–241.

Stock, M. L., Peterson, L. M., Houlihan, A. E., & Walsh, L. A. (2013). Influence of oral sex and oral cancer information on young adults' oral sexual-risk cognitions and likelihood of HPV vaccination. Journal of Sex Research, *50*(1), 95–102.

Stone, N., Hatherall, B., Ingham, R., & McEachran, J. (2006). Oral sex and condom use among young people in the United Kingdom. Perspectives on Sexual and Reproductive Health, *38*, 6–12.

Secor-Turner, M., Sieving, R. E., Eisenberg, M. E., & Skay, C. (2011). Associations between sexually experienced adolescents' sources of information about sex and sexual risk outcomes. Sex Education, *11*(4), 489–500.

Szucs, L. E., Harper, C. R., Andrzejewski, J., Barrios, L. C., Robin, L., & Hunt, P. (2022). Overwhelming support for sexual health education in US Schools: A meta-analysis of 23 surveys conducted between 2000 and 2016. Journal of Adolescent Health, *70*(4), 598–606.

The Scottish Government. (2011). The sexual health and blood borne virus framework 2011–15. Retrieved from http://www.scotland.gov.uk/Resource/Doc/356286/0120395.pdf

Turchik, J. A., & Gidycz, C. A. (2012). Prediction of sexual risk behaviors in college students using the theory of planned behaviour: A prospective analysis. Journal of Social & Clinical Psychology, *31*(1), 1–27.

UNAIDS. (2020). UNAIDS Report on the global AIDS epidemic 2020. Retrieved from https://www.unaids.org/sites/default/files/media_asset/2020_aids-data-book_en.pdf

Underhill, K., Montgomery, P., & Operario, D. (2008). Abstinence-plus programs for HIV infection prevention in high-income countries. Cochrane Database of Systematic Reviews (Online), *23*(1), CD007006.

Wald, A., Langenberg, A. G. M., Krantz, E., Douglas, J. M., Handsfield, H. H., DiCarlo, R. P., … Corey, C. (2005). The relationship between condom use and herpes simplex virus acquisition. Annals of Internal Medicine, *143*, 707–713.

Ward, H., & Rönn, M. (2010). The contribution of STIs to the sexual transmission of HIV. Current Opinion in HIV and AIDS, *5*(4), 305–310.

Weller, S. C., & Davis-Beaty, K. (2002). Condom effectiveness in reducing heterosexual HIV transmission. Cochrane Database of Systematic Reviews, *1*, CD003255. 10.1002/14651858.CD003255

Westwood, J, & Mullan, B. (2009). Teachers' and pupils' perceptions of the school nurse in relation to sexual health education. Sex Education, *9*(3), 293–306.

WHO. (2011). Sexual health: A public health challenge in Europe. Entre Nous, The European Magazine for Sexual and Reproductive Health. Retrieved from http://www.euro.who.int/__data/assets/pdf_file/0019/142570/en72.pdf

10 Specific conditions

LEARNING OBJECTIVES

At the end of this chapter you will:

- Appreciate the impact that lifestyle can have on the onset and progression of specific diseases.
- Understand the importance of health promotion in their management.
- Have explored available interventions to promote the health of people with specific disorders.
- Understand how psychology can influence behaviour change in different client groups.
- Identify the role that health and allied professionals play in promoting health for each condition.

Introduction

The burden of lifestyle-related ill health for individuals, families and communities in the UK cannot be ignored. Modifiable risk factors such as physical inactivity, diet-related factors, smoking and alcohol use have been closely linked to the rising prevalence of many common chronic diseases, including coronary heart disease (CHD), Type 2 diabetes, liver disease and chronic obstructive pulmonary disease (COPD). Behavioural choices can not only increase a person's risk of developing health problems over time, but they can also hasten disease progression and contribute to greater morbidity and early mortality for those already diagnosed with a condition (Buck & Frosini, 2012). There are differential influences of lifestyle behaviours on development and trajectory of specific conditions. It is well known that smoking cessation significantly improves outcomes for people with COPD and the influence of increased physical activity in the prevention and management of Type 2 diabetes is well recognised. Understanding the impact of these behaviours on health and well-being for different medical conditions can help with the management of the conditions.

Behaviour change has a critical role to play in reducing and managing the burden of preventable and treatable diseases (NHS, accessed 2023). Consequently, there is a pressing need for effective lifestyle interventions and improved management of these conditions. However, changing lifestyle behaviour is challenging and requires time, effort

DOI: 10.4324/9781003471233-10

and motivation from both health professional and client (Noordman et al., 2012). Insight into effective behaviour change techniques can facilitate health care providers to better understand and support clients to adapt their lifestyle to manage their condition/s more effectively.

Health consequences of behaviour

Developing a chronic condition can be influenced by an unhealthy lifestyle and this is particularly true for multi-factorial disorders such as Type 2 diabetes, CHD, common mental health problems and COPD. Lifestyle factors play an important role not only in the onset but also in the progression of these conditions, so an important aspect of their management is the promotion of healthful behaviours and the modification of risky behaviours.

Type 2 diabetes

> ### Case study
>
> Paulette is a 48-year-old woman who works as an accounts clerk. Following the birth of her second daughter 10 years ago Paulette's weight has steadily increased, and she is now overweight for her height. Over the past 6 months Paulette has often complained of feeling tired and has less energy to do everyday activities which she has put down to 'her age'. Compensating for this tiredness, Paulette has found herself snacking frequently between meals for an energy boost.
>
> Recent symptoms of increased thirst during the day and at night have prompted Paulette to see her GP because her nights are becoming increasingly disturbed. Following tests, Paulette has been diagnosed with Type 2 diabetes. She is not entirely shocked by the diagnosis because her father similarly has Type 2 diabetes and has lived with the condition since his 50s. Having been told by her GP that Type 2 diabetes can 'run in the family' Paulette is unsure how changes in her current lifestyle will help to control and manage the progression of the condition. Although Paulette had previously enjoyed attending aerobics classes in her early 20s, her increasing family and work commitments have prevented her from sustaining a physically active lifestyle.

Introduction

Type 2 diabetes is a chronic and progressive disorder which, owing to its rapidly increasing prevalence, has reached epidemic proportions. Globally, more than 1 in 10 adults are living with Diabetes. In 2000, it was estimated that there were 151 million adults living with Diabetes, in 2021 it was estimated to be 537 million people worldwide and it has been predicted this will rise to 643 million by 2030 (International Diabetes Federation, 2021). Characterised by defects in both insulin secretion and insulin action, Type 2 diabetes accounts for around 90% of all diagnosed cases of diabetes (Nolan et al., 2011; International Diabetes Federation, 2021). It is the leading cause of kidney failure, blindness in adults, and amputation in the UK and is an independent risk factor for heart disease and stroke, reducing life expectancy on average by 10 years (Diabetes UK, accessed 2023). The macro-vascular and micro-vascular complications and associated organ damage resulting from poorly managed diabetes represent an enormous cost, both economically in terms of the financial cost of diabetes care and in terms of its impact on quality of life for the individual (Bommer et al., 2018). Although there is a genetic component to its aetiology, the environment also plays an important role in the onset of Type 2 diabetes (Kyrou et al., 2020). With levels of obesity rising and western lifestyles accepting sedentary behaviour as the norm, the rising prevalence of this condition is only set to continue (International Diabetes Federation, 2021; Jarvis et al., 2010; Ogurtsova et al., 2017). However, it is well established that lifestyle interventions that increase physical activity, improve diet, and prevent weight gain can prevent or delay the onset of diabetes and prevent or delay secondary conditions developing (Alouki et al., 2016).

Type 2 diabetes is a complex condition to manage. The need for continuous regulation of blood glucose means that a person living with Type 2 diabetes must manage their own condition outside of the clinical setting. Daily choices about diet, physical activity, taking medication and blood glucose monitoring are made by individuals with a diagnosis of diabetes and the consequences of these choices can affect health and progression of the disease (Jarvis et al., 2010; Carpenter et al., 2018). Monitoring and regulating blood glucose levels requires considerable effort on the part of the individual and these activities may be perceived as onerous and unnecessary if the individual generally feels well and the complications of the condition have yet to manifest (Carpenter et al., 2018). There is however promising evidence that behavioural interventions can improve diabetes control and health outcomes for people diagnosed with Type 2 diabetes (Galaviz et al., 2018).

Interventions to promote the health of people with Type 2 diabetes

Given its multi-factorial aetiology, people's lifestyle choices clearly play an important role in the onset and progression of Type 2 diabetes. Traditional approaches to its treatment focused on drug interventions to stabilise blood glucose levels and manage cardiovascular risk factors. However, long-term data from the UK Prospective Diabetes Study demonstrated that despite initial improvements, drug therapy was not effective in maintaining blood glucose control over time (UKPDS, 1998). These findings raise questions about the effectiveness of drug interventions alone for the long-term management of Type 2 diabetes (Jarvis et al., 2010).

It is important to recognise that effective diabetes management lies mainly in the hands of the person with the condition (Department of Health, 2001a). However, it is one of the most challenging chronic illnesses to manage and the demands of complex self-management can cause people considerable distress (Carpenter et al., 2018). High level self-management skills are required for people to manage their diabetes successfully and evidence suggests structured educational courses based on established standards for diabetes self-management education successfully improve clinical outcomes and quality of life (Steinsbekk et al., 2012; Carpenter et al., 2018). Unlike patient education within the medical model, where health professionals are considered to be the experts and patients the recipients of care (Brennan & Strombom, 1998), structured educational programmes are patient-centred and aim to empower patients to become active self-managers of their condition.

Individual level interventions

SELF-MANAGEMENT EDUCATION

Structured educational programmes have been recommended by NICE (2015, updated 2022) and championed by Diabetes UK who argue that all people newly diagnosed with Type 2 diabetes should attend a programme as these have been recognised to result in better self-management and clinical outcomes (Deakin et al., 2006; Wheatley et al., 2021). Based on theories of patient empowerment (Anderson & Funnell, 2000) and problem-based learning (Barrows, 1996), these programmes aim to provide individuals with the confidence, tools and techniques that will enable them to manage their condition more effectively (Loveman et al., 2008; Wheatley et al., 2021). The diabetes education and self-management for ongoing and newly diagnosed (DESMOND) intervention (Davies et al., 2008) and the Diabetes X-PERT programme (Deakin et al., 2006; Wheatley et al., 2021) are two examples of structured education programmes that are available nationally for people with Type 2 diabetes. In particular the X-PERT programme, which runs over 6 weeks, has been shown to be effective in improving clinical, lifestyle and psychosocial indicators in people with newly diagnosed and existing Type 2 diabetes (Deakin et al., 2006; Wheatley et al., 2021).

Structured educational programmes utilise behavioural strategies such as problem solving, goal setting and social support to facilitate dietary and physical activity behaviour change and self-monitoring among people with Type 2 diabetes. Self-directed behavioural goal setting is a strategy often used in structured programmes to increase self-efficacy and empowerment. It refers to the process of creating an action plan whereby individuals can accomplish behaviours necessary for the self-management of their condition. This process allows the individual to develop concrete, usually short-term goals, to facilitate lifestyle change (Funnell, 2010). Behavioural goals to improve diabetes self-management may include:

- Avoidance of foods with high sugar content in order to regulate blood glucose levels
- Reduction of daily calorie intake to achieve weight loss and reduce BMI
- Avoidance of foods high in fat to achieve weight loss and reduce BMI
- Increasing daily physical activity levels.

Diabetes self-management education can be delivered in many forms. A systematic review by Steinsbekk et al. (2012) concluded that group-based training for diabetes self-management improves diabetes control and knowledge of the condition in the short and longer term. The Diabetes X-PERT programme, which is a group-baschemes, which promote cyclingsed intervention, has proven to be particularly effective in improving blood glucose control (Wheatley et al., 2021). However, evidence shows that uptake of structured education programmes is extremely low; only 3.8% of people newly diagnosed with Type 2 diabetes attend a programme (Wenzel, 2016). Consequently, Diabetes UK has adopted a broad framework to consider patient education on three levels:

Level 1: The provision of information and advice on diabetes management on a one-to-one basis. This is typically provided by a health care professional at the time of diagnosis.

Level 2: These are less formal initiatives than level 3 structured and quality assured programmes. They are not targeted at the newly diagnosed and are often focused on a particular aspect of self-management, for example physical activity or aimed at a particular group, for example older adults. Their defining characteristic is that they offer people the opportunity to learn about self-management in a flexible and informal way. They can be led by health professionals or can be peer-led. For example: Living with Diabetes Days (Diabetes UK), CarbAware, a 3-hour carbohydrate counting course.

Level 3: Structured Education programmes that meet a set of nationally agreed criteria set out in NICE guidelines. For example DESMOND & X-PERT.

Wenzel (2016) reviewed the evidence of effectiveness of informal and flexible level 2 self-management initiatives. Given the low uptake of the level 3 structured education programmes it is important to understand the effectiveness of level 2 initiatives (Wheatley et al., 2021). Wenzel (2016) concluded that the situation is very ad hoc and robust evidence of positive outcomes limited. However, it is likely that people with diabetes are best served by having a menu of education options to choose from. This enables individuals to select the initiative that best suits their needs, lifestyle and learning style.

Opportunities clearly exist for individuals to establish social support when structured education is delivered within a group setting. As discussed in Chapter 4 of this book, specific social support can work at the individual level by providing positive feedback about successful behaviour change thereby improving self-efficacy (Wheatley et al., 2021). It can also provide instrumental and emotional support whereby members can draw on and learn from the experiences of others in the group (Jarvis et al., 2010).

TELEMEDICINE TECHNOLOGIES

Various telemedicine technologies such as text messages and computer and web-based interventions have been proven to be effective. Diabetes mobile phone applications are also promising tools for self-care. There are a great many lifestyle apps available and diabetes apps have been defined as software that accepts data (transmitted or manual) and provides feedback to patients on improved management (automated or by a health care professional). A review of ten studies looking at the impact of the use of diabetes apps for people with Type 2 diabetes indicated a consistent reduction in blood glucose of 0.5%. There was some evidence that they were more effective in younger people. Feedback options varied from automated and therefore dynamic, timely feedback and more individualised feedback from a health professional. It is postulated that the feedback triggered lifestyle choices which lowered blood glucose (Hou et al., 2016).

Applying this to Paulette

Referring Paulette to the X-PERT programme would enable her to develop knowledge and self-management skills to optimise her diabetes management. However, should Paulette not be able to attend, encouraging her to engage in other local initiatives or online courses could also be encouraged. Paulette's self-efficacy for dietary and physical activity behaviour change may be enhanced through developing good coping skills and setting achievable goals. The social support she receives from any group membership may facilitate her to adapt to her condition and make the necessary lifestyle changes to control its progression.

PROMOTING HEALTH THROUGH PHYSICAL ACTIVITY

Low cardio-respiratory fitness, an independent marker of long-term mortality in individuals with diabetes, is a modifiable risk factor that can lead to poor health outcomes for people with Type 2 diabetes (Balducci et al., 2019). Increasingly, it is recognised that interventions need to address both physical activity and time spent sedentary and that although these behaviours are related; greater time spent sedentary is associated with being metabolically unhealthy independent of other levels of physical activity (Bowden Davies et al., 2019; Balducci et al., 2019). Frequently described as the cornerstone of Type 2 diabetes management, regular physical activity has a positive effect on glycaemic control and has been associated with decreases in cardiovascular risk by lowering blood pressure and BMI and improving lipid profiles (Chudyk & Petrella, 2011; Kirk et al., 2009; Yates et al., 2009; Marwick et al., 2009). Despite its many health benefits, physical activity is underutilised by people with the condition who, according to Morrato et al. (2007), are less likely to meet physical activity guidelines compared to the general population. Reducing sedentary time can also have benefits for self-management of diabetes (Balducci et al., 2019). Challenges clearly exist for the successful promotion of physical activity in individuals with Type 2 diabetes and it is increasingly recognised that daily physical activity that isn't moderate or vigorous physical activity can still be beneficial for people with Type 2 diabetes (Hamasaki, 2016).

STRUCTURED EXERCISE PROGRAMMES

Simply advising people to become more physically active is generally ineffective when promoting lifestyle change (Upton & Thirlaway, 2010). A recent systematic review and meta-analysis of randomised controlled clinical trials supports this view by concluding that physical activity advice alone for people with diabetes was ineffective in reducing blood glucose concentrations over time (Umpierre et al., 2011). By contrast, structured exercise training that consisted of aerobic exercise, resistance training or a combination of the two was associated with reductions in blood glucose levels, the effects of which were similar across the three exercise modalities. This effect was greater again for people who engaged in structured exercise of moderate intensity for at least 150 minutes per week (Chudyk & Petrella, 2011; Umpierre et al., 2011), giving support to the argument that 150 minutes of physical activity a week is a minimum and more is better (Department of Health and Social Care, Welsh Government, Department of Health Northern Ireland, and the Scottish Government, 2019; WHO, 2020).

Despite structured exercise regimes of moderate intensity exhibiting a more significant impact on diabetes-related outcomes (Umpierre et al., 2011; Chudyk & Petrella, 2011), it is important to appreciate that higher intensity exercise may not be tolerated or may even be hazardous for individuals who have previously been sedentary and/or present with co-existing complications. It is generally accepted that physical activity at any level is better than no exercise at all (Kavookjian et al., 2007; Balducci et al., 2019), and emerging evidence also suggests that breaks in sedentary behaviour, such as non-exercise standing activity, and light intensity exercise are independently associated with improved blood glucose regulation for people with Type 2 diabetes (Healy et al., 2008; Healy et al., 2008; Department of Health, 2011; Balducci et al., 2019; Hamasaki, 2016). For individuals who are already exercising at a moderate level of intensity, health professionals may wish to consider encouraging exercise of a higher intensity and sustained duration because of the potential additional benefits on metabolic regulation and cardio-respiratory fitness (Kavookjian et al., 2007). It is vital therefore that interventions promoting physical activity for people with Type 2 diabetes are tailored to the specific health needs of the individual. An assessment of previous activity levels, cardiovascular risk factors and co-existing complications is therefore recommended (Box 10.1).

Applying this to Paulette

An assessment of Paulette's current health status, to include baseline measures of blood pressure, pulse, and current activity level, is recommended before she decides which form of physical activity is acceptable and appropriate for the self-management of her diabetes.

Her previous enjoyment of aerobics classes may allow Paulette to consider improving her cardio-respiratory fitness through this more structured form of exercise.

EXERCISE REFERRAL SCHEMES

Exercise referral schemes have been discussed in detail in Chapter 6. It is worth mentioning that these schemes are available through the NHS to patients with Type 2 diabetes; however their efficacy in promoting sustained behaviour change has not been demonstrated.

Box 10.1   Applying Research in Practice

Type 2 diabetes and dog walking: patients' longitudinal perspectives about implementing and sustaining physical activity (Peel et al., 2010)

This study explores the ways in which people with Type 2 diabetes talk about implementing and sustaining physical activity in their everyday lives.

Interviews were conducted with 40 patients newly diagnosed with Type 2 diabetes living in the Lothian region of Scotland. Participants were interviewed at baseline, 6 and 12 months. Twenty-one of the original sample not lost to follow-up were interviewed again after 4 years.

Regular physical activity was considered unsustainable by most participants and information and guidance about physical activity from health professionals was considered to be vague and non-specific. Walking, especially with a dog, was considered an achievable and sustainable form of exercise for people with Type 2 diabetes. Participants' accounts revealed how dog walking provided regular routine activity for the self-management of Type 2 diabetes which was maintained over the 4-year study period.

In conclusion, ascertaining patients' preferences and constraints on physical activity would facilitate the setting of individualised achievable goals. The potential for physical activity maintenance through dog walking is noteworthy in this client group.

Community level interventions

Many of the community level interventions promoting physical activity and healthy eating are of value for people with Type 2 diabetes. The influence of obesity, overweight and physical inactivity in the onset and progression of Type 2 diabetes is well documented (Diabetes UK, accessed 2023), so community-wide promotional activities that target important modifiable risk factors such as diet and exercise could greatly help the treatment of this condition (Bailey, 2011). One such example is the Better Health campaign which has been described in Chapter 2 (Better Health, accessed 2023). Although this intervention aims to tackle obesity in people of all ages through changes in dietary and exercise habits, these lifestyle measures are equally important for the management of Type 2 diabetes. Similarly, the Traffic Light System devised by the Food Standards Agency facilitates people to make healthy dietary choices by indicating the nutritional values in food. This informational intervention is particularly relevant to people with Type 2 diabetes because they are required to closely monitor and regulate their daily sugar intake in order to stabilise their blood glucose levels. Song et al. (2021) reviewed the impact of colour-coded and warning nutritional labelling and concluded that there was comprehensive evidence that colour-coded labels nudged consumers purchasing behaviours towards healthy products.

Public health campaigns addressing physical activity are as equally important for people with Type 2 diabetes. Active transport schemes, which promote cycling and walking, and green activities such as allotment gardening as part of a community group, have the potential to increase daily activity levels in people with diabetes. These community approaches may be particularly effective in promoting an active lifestyle because they enable people with the condition to incorporate physical activity into their daily lives more flexibly (These interventions are discussed in detail in Chapter 4).

Applying this to Paulette

Paulette could use the Traffic light system on food packaging to ensure that she successfully regulates her blood sugar by avoiding foods with high sugar content.

Environmental schemes encouraging active transport could enable Paulette to schedule physical activity into her otherwise busy work and home life. This could be achieved through either walking or cycling to work.

Working effectively with others

Multi-disciplinary team support is available to all people with Type 2 diabetes from diagnosis. GPs, practice nurses, dieticians, podiatrists, and other allied health professionals all have an important role to play in the provision of diabetes care. Traditionally, diabetes education was delivered in a didactic setting whereby health professionals were assumed to be the experts. However, the emphasis is shifting, and patients are now encouraged to have autonomy by working in alliance with professionals to identify successful strategies for diabetes self-management (Deakin et al., 2006).

PEER SUPPORT

Peer support is a promising approach for diabetes care. It harnesses the ability and experience of patients with diabetes to support others with the condition (Qi et al., 2015). However, the efficacy of these peer-led interventions is mixed with some studies indicating that 'expert' patients are as effective as specialist health professionals in imparting diabetes self-management knowledge (Baksi et al., 2008) and others saying there is no effect of group-based peer support interventions on diabetes control or psychosocial measures (Cade et al., 2009; Smith et al., 2011). However, a meta-review by Qi et al. (2015) concluded that peer support improved glycaemic control compared to usual care. Most studies were peer-led self-management education following a formal model suggesting that trained peer leaders may be critical for success. Peer support may offer the kind of emotional, social, and practical support that is necessary to achieve and sustain complex behaviour change necessary for the self-management of diabetes (Boothroyd & Fisher, 2010).

Applying this to Paulette

Paulette will work closely with members of the primary care team in order to establish self-directed goals to manage her diabetes autonomously.

Joining a peer support group may enable Paulette to meet and gain support from other people with Type 2 diabetes.

Coronary heart disease (CHD)

Case study

Matt has recently been discharged from hospital following a sudden heart attack at the age of 58. He had collapsed early one morning with pains in his neck, jaw and chest whilst collecting papers for his news agency business, which he has run for the past 30 years. Living in a rural location, Matt relies on his car to deliver papers to his clients. Starting work at 5 am most mornings to collect paper deliveries and working through until early evening when the shop closes means that Matt works long, often unsociable hours to meet the needs of the business. Weekends are similarly as busy in the shop, and he has limited leisure time activities as a consequence. These demands have taken a toll on Matt's mood and stress levels over the years, and he admits that he has used smoking as a coping strategy. Matt and his wife are keen to make changes to his current lifestyle because he is overweight for his height and has been for many years. However, they are fearful that by becoming more physically active he will increase his risk of having another heart attack.

Introduction

Coronary heart disease (CHD) is the term used to describe the build-up of fatty deposits in the coronary arteries and it affects the heart by restricting the flow of blood to the heart muscle. This can lead to a feeling of tightness or pain in the chest, known as angina, or to a myocardial infarction (heart attack). The condition is caused by a combination of genetic, environmental and lifestyle factors with long-term modification of behavioural-risk factors the most accessible route to reducing the risk of future health problems. CHD is a preventable disease, but cardiovascular diseases are the leading cause of death globally. Of the estimated 17.9 million people who died from Cardiovascular Diseases in 2019, 85% were due to Heart Attacks and Stroke (WHO, 2021). Despite decreasing trends in incidence and mortality, CHD continues to be the leading cause of premature death in the UK, accounting for 1 in 8 deaths in men and 1 in 14 deaths in women in 2021 (British Heart Foundation, 2022). These figures demonstrate a reduction in deaths from CHD since 2021 when 1 in 4 deaths in men and 1 in 6 deaths in women were recorded as due to CHD (British Heart Foundation, 2010). It is heartening that the treatment and lifestyle interventions provided in the UK have improved outcomes significantly but there are still 7.6 million people in the UK living with heart and circulatory diseases and as survival rates from acute events improve these numbers could rise. It becomes more important than ever that we support people to prevent CHD and limit the progression of disease (British Heart Foundation, 2022).

Having an acute cardiac event is a frightening and often life changing experience (British Heart Foundation, 2007). Indeed, many people with CHD experience reduced quality of life, often suffering from anxiety, depression, and emotional and social disturbances all of which can affect the development and progression of the condition (Richards et al., 2018). Even if the physical implications of an acute coronary event are minimised by prompt medical interventions such as angioplasty and antithrombotic drugs, many individuals find the long-term modification of lifestyle behaviours daunting and difficult to sustain (British Heart Foundation, 2007). The importance of pharmacological treatments to combat the associated risk factors of CHD is indisputable, however, Li et al. (2021) suggest that treatment of depression and anxiety in people with CHD is imperative because these factors reduce people's ability to make and sustain positive changes to their lifestyle. They also suggest they lead to reduced compliance with medication. Smoking, poor diet, and lack of exercise are important modifiable risk factors for CHD and even modest changes in these lifestyle behaviours can substantially improve outcomes for people with the condition (Artinian et al., 2010).

Individual level interventions

Cardiac rehabilitation

Cardiac rehabilitation is a complex intervention comprised of five core components: exercise training, nutritional counselling, risk factor modification, psychosocial management, and patient education (Mehra et al., 2020). The National Service Framework for Coronary Heart Disease (Department of Health, 2000) recommended that 85% of post myocardial infarction and re-vascularisation (angioplasty and bypass) patients should be offered cardiac rehabilitation. However, according to the latest figures from the 2017 National Audit for cardiac rehabilitation just 50% of heart patients in England participated in the programme (Doherty et al., 2018). Opportunities to promote health and reduce cardiac risk factors in the period immediately following a cardiac event are clearly being missed for patients who do not attend Cardiac Rehabilitation (CR).

Group-based educational classes are the preferred method for delivering behaviour change in CR at the individual level (British Heart Foundation, accessed 2023). However, NICE (2021) recognise that although pre-pandemic most rehabilitation was group based there has been an increase in the use of self-managed options such as REACH-HF. Programmes aim to support patients to become active self-managers in their health through participation in the four phases of Cardiac Rehabilitation:

- **Phase I:** pre-discharge care which includes medical risk factor assessment, education, correction of cardiac misconceptions and reassurance.
- **Phase II:** the immediate post-discharge period which includes home visits, telephone contact and supervised use of the Heart Manual (a self-help programme for patients recovering from a heart attack).
- **Phase III:** a 6 to 14-week multi-disciplinary behaviour change and rehabilitation programme, consisting of group sessions once or twice a week
- **Phase IV:** maintenance of lifestyle changes made in the preceding phases, including exercise opportunities accessed through local sports and leisure centres. This phase is not currently part of the NHS pathway.

Applying this to Matt

In order to reduce the risk of a recurrent heart attack, Matt would benefit from Cardiac Rehabilitation. His participation in the four phases of CR is essential to optimise early behaviour change that will support self-management of the condition.

BEHAVIOUR CHANGE IN CARDIAC REHABILITATION

Lifestyle modification is a central feature of cardiac rehabilitation. Patients are encouraged to develop skills in self-management and this often means making positive changes to their lifestyle in order to reduce behavioural-risk factors and promote cardiovascular health. Chow et al. (2010) highlighted the early benefits of lifestyle modification after acute coronary events. They found that adherence to diet, exercise, and smoking recommendations just 30 days following an MI was associated with a substantially lower risk of recurrent cardiovascular events and mortality at 6 months. Patient collaboration is essential to the behaviour change process, with health professionals taking on a facilitative role by assisting patients to identify patterns of helpful and unhelpful health behaviour in order to self-generate solutions for behaviour change. This partnership allows the patient to decide which health behaviour, if any; he/she would like or is ready to change (Tierney et al., 2011). NICE (2007a, accessed 2023) have developed guidelines relating to behaviour change in the health care context and these guidelines can be used by health professionals to facilitate patients receiving CR to effectively change their health behaviour (Table 10.1).

Table 10.1 NICE guidelines: Generic principles for effective health behaviour change at the individual level

---

Select interventions that motivate and support people to

- Understand the short, medium and long-term consequences of their health-related behaviours, for themselves and others
- Feel positive about the benefits of health-enhancing behaviours and changing their behaviour
- Plan their changes in terms of easy steps over time
- Recognise how their social contexts and relationships may affect their behaviour, and identify and plan situations that might undermine the changes they are trying to make
- Plan explicit 'if-then' coping strategies to prevent relapse
- Make a personal commitment to adopt health-enhancing behaviours by setting)and recording) goals to undertake clearly defined behaviours, in particular context, over a specified time
- Share their behaviour with others

National Institute for Health and Clinical Excellence (2007a).

STRATEGIES SUPPORTING BEHAVIOUR CHANGE IN CARDIAC REHABILITATION

Cognitive-behavioural strategies are an integral component of any behaviour change intervention (Artinian et al., 2010; Li et al., 2021). Chapter 4 provides a detailed discussion of the psychological interventions that are available to help people make changes to their lifestyle; these include CBT, goal setting and motivational interviewing. In terms of cardiac rehabilitation, these strategies enable individuals with CHD to:

1 Modify their lifestyle
2 Develop adaptive coping strategies
3 Change maladaptive illness beliefs
4 Improve physical and psychosocial outcomes

In their review, Janssen et al. (2012) found that lifestyle interventions that incorporated four self-regulation strategies: goal setting, self-monitoring, planning and feedback resulted in greater improvements in dietary and exercise behaviour for patients with CHD than interventions that included none of these techniques.

Goal setting Goal setting is an effective technique to achieve desired behaviour change within clinical groups. This technique is generally more successful when goals are specific in outcome, short term and realistic in terms of the patients' current capabilities and health status (Artinian et al., 2010). Behavioural goals to facilitate CHD self-management may include:

- Avoidance of foods high in saturated fats in order to improve cholesterol levels
- Reduction of daily calorie intake to achieve weight loss and reduce BMI
- Reduction of daily/weekly alcohol consumption in line with current government guidelines
- Increasing physical activity levels to improve cardiovascular fitness
- Smoking cessation/reduction of tobacco use

Self-monitoring Self-monitoring is an important self-regulatory strategy and refers to the process of observing one's behaviour and evaluating it in relation to identified goals.

Simple diaries can be used for self-monitoring of behaviours; individuals can chart their physical activity/dietary intake by logging number of steps taken, distance walked, calories consumed, or amount of weight lost (Burke et al., 2008). This strategy provides the individual with direct feedback on progress thus enhancing self-efficacy for behaviour change and facilitating the adoption of self-management behaviours for CHD management.

Action planning　Action planning has been described as a simple yet promising strategy to increase the uptake of phase IV CR (Sniehotta et al., 2010). As previously outlined, phase IV cardiac rehabilitation groups are usually community-based and provide patients with the opportunity to make sustained lifestyle changes generally through participation in physical activity programmes (British Heart Foundation, accessed 2023). A study by Sniehotta et al. (2010) demonstrated that among participants who planned where and when to attend phase IV CR in the third phase of this programme, 65.9% subsequently went on to attend a phase IV program compared to 18.5% of those who did not make a plan. These findings suggest that both intention and action planning are good predictors of phase IV CR attendance and give support to the utility of an extended Theory of Planned Behaviour to explain cardiac rehabilitation behaviour.

Feedback　Feedback is frequently included in successful behaviour change interventions and, when delivered by a health professional, it can act as a gauge upon which the individual can assess their progress (Artinian et al., 2010). Feedback about behavioural performance can motivate an individual to sustain changes made to their lifestyle, or it can facilitate them to adjust their behaviour in order to reach their goal/s for CR self-management. Increasingly, evidence suggests that feedback can be provided electronically by text, apps or other internet-based interventions (Pfaeffli Dale et al., 2015), However, NICE (2020) recommend commissioning digital and mobile interventions as a supplement to existing services not as a replacement and advise that evidence-based behaviour techniques should underpin any intervention.

Social support　Phase III of CR is particularly well placed to provide individuals with social support for a successful adaptive psychological coping response following an acute cardiac event (Barth et al., 2010). The group-based approach incorporates scheduled follow-up sessions for ongoing contact with multi-disciplinary team members and social support from the peer group. The frequency and duration of this group-based intervention may have the advantage of enhancing perceived social support for lifestyle change among patients referred to CR. In their review, Barth et al. (2010) distinguish between different dimensions of social support and their impact on CHD prognosis. They concluded that functional social support (e.g., perceived social support) was more important than structural support (e.g., living alone) for reducing cardiac mortality. Loneliness and social isolation are associated with an increased risk of developing CHD and stroke and hence this group may be particularly in need of the social support they can access through group-based rehabilitation (Valtorta et al., 2016) Social support through group participation is an important intervention strategy that may improve risk factors and related health behaviours for individuals with CHD.

> **Applying this to Matt**
>
> Encouraging Matt to attend the group-based CR programmes could provide him with additional social support to make changes to his current lifestyle and reduce the risk factors associated with poor cardiovascular outcomes.

THE ROLE OF PHYSICAL ACTIVITY IN CARDIAC REHABILITATION

Despite overwhelming evidence promoting an active lifestyle, many of people in the UK fail to meet government guidelines for being active (Department of Health and Social Care, Welsh Government, Department of Health Northern Ireland, and the Scottish Government, 2019; WHO, 2020). This is problematic because cardiorespiratory fitness is closely associated with overall risk of CHD (Lavie et al., 2009). The beneficial effects of increased physical activity in people with CHD are well documented (Artinian et al., 2010; Held et al., 2012; Stewart et al., 2017) and when delivered as a component part of Cardiac Rehabilitation favourable cardiovascular and psychosocial outcomes are observed (Lavie et al., 2009; Heran et al., 2011; NICE, 2021). Held et al. (2012) importantly identify that even minimal amounts of either mild or moderate intensity physical activity (e.g., from 0 to 30 minutes/week) can have a protective effect on the heart.

A common anxiety for people with heart disease is the belief that physical activity may further damage their heart or indeed increase their risk of sustaining another heart attack (Riegel, 1993; Farris et al., 2019). Evidence suggests that faulty illness beliefs in people with CHD can lead to maladaptive health behaviours such as abstaining from even low levels of physical activity. This inappropriate behavioural response can lead to low cardiorespiratory fitness, exacerbating the symptoms of CHD and making recurrence of an acute event more likely. NICE (2020) suggest that health professionals should endeavour to understand illness beliefs in order to encourage positive coping strategies and adaptive health behaviours. They conclude that cognitive behavioural interventions are particularly effective in both challenging cardiac misconceptions and creating positive belief change in people with CHD.

A substantial body of evidence demonstrates a strong link between depression and CHD (Goldston & Baillie, 2008; Wellenius et al., 2008; Whooley, 2006; Vaccarino et al., 2020). Interventions promoting physical activity have a clear role to play in the management of these co-existing conditions because physical exercise is known to improve both depressive symptoms and markers of cardiovascular risk (Blumenthal et al., 2007; Vaccarino et al., 2020). The underlying mechanisms linking depression and worse CHD outcomes are complex and undoubtedly multi-factorial. Pharmacologic and Non-pharmacologic interventions (such as psychotherapy and exercise) should be considered for CHD patients (Vaccarino et al., 2020).

> **Applying this to Matt**
>
> Tailoring physical activity advice to Matt's specific health needs will benefit from a pre-exercise assessment by a health professional or exercise specialist. This will establish how exercise can be incorporated into Matt's daily life to help him achieve improvements in cardio-respiratory fitness and mood.

Working with both Matt and his wife to explore their illness beliefs that exercise could further damage his heart is essential if he is to make an adaptive response to engage in physical activity for cardiac rehabilitation.

Community level interventions

Many of the community level interventions that target specific lifestyle behaviours such as smoking, eating healthily, and being physically active are important to people with CHD because these health behaviours are also important modifiable risk factors for the development and progression of the disease. Public health smoking campaigns are particularly relevant to people with CHD who smoke because smoking cessation or any reduction in cigarette use can have considerable benefits for coronary health. The Smokefree legislation introduced by the Department of Health in 2007 has been particularly successful in changing attitudes to smoking in public places, making this behaviour less socially acceptable. Smoke-free policies seek to encourage smoke-free environments to benefit the health of smokers and non-smokers alike, therefore this intervention can both directly and indirectly influence the health of people with CHD.

Public health campaigns to improve dietary habits and increase physical activity are equally important to people with CHD. The Better Health campaign (Better Health, accessed 2023) is one such example that targets these important risk factors for heart disease and aims to encourage a healthier lifestyle to reduce obesity. Similarly, the Traffic Light System can assist individuals with heart disease to make healthier food choices (Kunz et al., 2020). The colour coded labelling system can guide people to select foods that are low in saturated fats, salt, and sugar in order to facilitate weight loss and/or lower dietary fat intake to improve cholesterol levels.

A number of community interventions aim to increase physical activity and there has been much debate around the obesogenic environment. Active transport has emerged as an important intervention that could yield many benefits including improvements of public health by increasing physical activity and reducing air pollution and traffic congestion (Jarrett et al., 2012; Hirst, 2020). Increased walking and cycling and reduced use of private cars all have a positive effect on many health outcomes, and environments that support these activities are particularly important for coronary health.

Applying this to Matt

The opportunity for Matt to smoke in public places will be restricted by the enforcement of smoke-free policies. These smoke-free campaigns may alter Matt's attitude towards smoking through the alteration of social norms which makes smoking less socially acceptable.

Matt could use the Traffic Light System on food packaging to ensure that he reduces his intake of foods which are high in saturated fats. This food labelling system would enable him to make healthier food choices and monitor his overall calorie intake in order to reduce his weight and BMI.

Active transport is a strategy that Matt could use to increase his physical activity levels, either to get back and forth to work or to make deliveries to clients who are within easy reach of the business. Reducing his reliance on the car will ensure that he reduces time spent in sedentary activities.

Working effectively with others

Clinical guidelines emphasise the importance of a multi-disciplinary approach to CR (BHF, accessed 2023). Nurses, physiotherapists, dieticians, exercise specialists, occupational therapists and psychologists all have a role to play in supporting individuals with CHD to become active self-managers in the control of their condition.

Psychologists importantly address the psychological aspects of CHD management. Cognitive-behavioural therapy (CBT) is one such approach that clinical psychologists may use to enable patients to change any negative patterns of thinking or behaviour that may be impacting on their ability to manage their condition. A randomised controlled trial that compared cognitive behavioural therapy based on stress management and standard treatment for people with CHD found that group-based CBT delivered over a year was significantly more effective in lowering the rate of fatal and non-fatal recurrent coronary events (Gulliksson et al., 2011). Similarly, Li et al. (2021) concluded that CBT-based interventions are effective treatments for CHD patients significantly improving their symptoms of depression, anxiety, stress, body mass index and health-related quality of life. Having access to these psychological therapies is clearly fundamental because psychosocial factors such as work-related stress, depression, anxiety, and hostility, have been shown to account for approximately 30% of the attributable risk of acute heart attacks (Yusuf et al., 2004). Depression is two to three times more common in patients with CHD than in the general population (Vaccarino et al., 2020).

Applying this to Matt

In order to manage his current stress and low mood, Matt would benefit from assessment by a psychologist who can recommend an appropriate intervention. Attending a group-based stress or management intervention run by a psychologist as part of a Cardiac Rehabilitation programme may enable Matt to improve his mood and physical activity could also be of benefit.

Mental health

Introduction

Case study

Eve is a 22-year-old undergraduate student in the final year of her sociology degree. The past 6 months have been particularly difficult for Eve because she has been feeling very anxious and low and has been unable to get any enjoyment out of life.

Eve has actively avoided any social activities at college and when asked how she is feeling she will often become tearful and upset. Eve is particularly concerned because her sleep pattern has changed, and she is constantly over-tired because she wakes very early most mornings and is unable to get back to sleep. Her college work is suffering as a consequence, and this is adding to Eve's anxiety and feelings of hopelessness. Her recent weight loss due to her decreased appetite prompted Eve to visit her GP and having discussed her symptoms, Emily has been diagnosed with anxiety and depression. Although Eve has been prescribed anti-depressant medication, she is also keen to understand how changes to her lifestyle may help her to cope with her symptoms of anxiety and depression.

Common mental disorders

One in six adults in the UK will be experiencing a common mental disorder (such as anxiety or depression) in any snapshot week of 2022 (Flinders, 2022; McManus et al., 2016; World Federation for Mental Health, 2018). Common mental disorders (CMD), which comprise of different types of anxiety and depression, cause emotional distress for the individual, and interfere with physical and social functioning if left untreated (McManus et al., 2016). Overall prevalence of common mental health problems in the UK has gradually increased between 1993 and 2014 (McManus et al., 2016). Data from the 2014 Adults Psychiatric Morbidity Survey (AMPS) (McManus et al., 2016) also indicates that prevalence of common mental disorders continues to be higher for women than men: overall, 1 in 5 women had a common mental health disorder compared to 1 in 8 men. Reports of self-harming doubled in men and women between 2007 and 2014. This may be due to changes in reporting behaviour, perhaps people felt more able to disclose self-harm. However, it is possible that increased reporting of self-harm reflects a real increase in the behaviour.

Depression is characterised by the absence of a positive affect (a loss of interest and enjoyment in ordinary things and experiences), low mood and a range of associated emotional, cognitive, physical and behavioural symptoms (NICE, 2022). The ICD-10 uses a list of 10 depressive symptoms to categorise depression according to its severity (WHO, 2010). In terms of treatment and management, the common form of major depressive episode is divided into four distance groups based on the number of depressive symptoms experienced in the list.

ICD-10 DIAGNOSTIC CRITERIA FOR DEPRESSION: AN AGREED LIST OF 10 DEPRESSIVE SYMPTOMS

Key symptoms
 1 persistent sadness or low mood; and/or
 2 loss of interests or pleasure
 3 fatigue or low energy
 4 disturbed sleep
 5 poor concentration or indecisiveness
 6 low self-confidence
 7 poor or increased appetite
 8 suicidal thoughts or acts
 9 agitation or slowing of movements
10 guilt or self-blame   The 10 symptoms then define the degree of depression, and management is based on the particular degree

- **not depressed** (fewer than four symptoms)
- **mild depression** (four symptoms)
- **moderate depression** (five to six symptoms)
- **severe depression** (seven or more symptoms, with or without psychotic symptoms)

Symptoms should be present for a month or more and every symptom should be present for most of every day (NICE, 2017).

Commonly, people with depression remain low throughout the course of the day, although for some, mood may gradually improve during the day only to return to low mood upon waking (NICE, 2004). The symptoms of depression are often extremely distressing for the affected individual and for those close to them (McManus et al. (eds) 2016). Apart from the personal suffering experienced by individuals who are depressed, the impact of the condition on social and occupational functioning, physical health and mortality is substantial (Mental Health Foundation, accessed 2023).

Interventions to improve the health of people with common mental health disorders

Mental health disorders increase the risk of communicable and non-communicable diseases, and strong associations between depression and coronary heart disease have been found (Tylee et al., 2012). Treatment is critical to minimise the physical and psychosocial consequences of common mental disorders. Traditionally, depression and anxiety have been treated with medication and psychological interventions. However, lifestyle interventions also have an important role to play in the treatment of these conditions (Forsyth et al., 2009; Kandola et al., 2019). Smoking (Malone et al., 2018), physical inactivity (Rosenbaum et al., 2016), poor diet (Firth et al., 2019) and obesity (Sarwer & Polonsky, 2016) have all been associated with poor mental health and are risk factors for the development of depression and anxiety. Physical activity is probably the one lifestyle behaviour that is most closely associated with improved outcomes for people with depression and/or anxiety. The recurrent nature of these disorders suggests that interventions promoting sustained lifestyle changes are necessary for both symptom control and/or relapse prevention (Rebar et al., 2015).

Individual level interventions

PHYSICAL ACTIVITY IN THE TREATMENT OF DEPRESSION AND ANXIETY

There is a general belief that physical activity and exercise have positive effects on mood and anxiety. Indeed, the effect of exercise on depression has been scrutinised over many years and some have advocated its use as an adjunct or alternative treatment for the condition. The National Institute for Health and Clinical Excellence (NICE) guideline for depression recommends structured, supervised exercise programmes 2–3 times a week, for 45 minutes to 1 hour, over 10 to 14 weeks for the treatment of mild to moderate depression (NICE, 2009). Across the UK, exercise referral schemes are also available for people with depression through primary care (NICE, 2014).

It is now well accepted that physical activity is an effective treatment for both mild and more severe depression (Nystrom et al., 2015; NICE, 2017). It has been more challenging to determine the appropriate type and duration of physical activity. Research in the field has attempted to establish the optimal dose (frequency, duration and intensity) of physical activity necessary to improve mental health outcomes for people with depression and anxiety. A review by Teychenne et al. (2008) found that the greatest benefits of physical activity on mental health were achieved when higher doses of activity were achieved. This higher dose was comparable to current public health guidelines of 150 minutes of moderate-intensity physical activity over a week (UK Chief Medical Officers, 2019). However, support was also obtained for much lower doses of physical activity with evidence suggesting that as little as 20–60 minutes of exercise per week can be protective against depression. It has also been suggested that it is the practice of regular physical activity that is associated with improvements in mental health (Azevedo Da Silva et al., 2012). It is therefore important to initially reinforce frequency so that physical activity becomes habitual.

Generally, people with depression and anxiety are at greater risk of being physically inactive than non-depressed individuals (Roshanaei-Moghaddam et al., 2009). The relationship between physical activity and depression/anxiety is likely to be bidirectional: regular physical activity improves symptoms for individuals with these conditions, although having symptoms of depression/anxiety increases the probability of not meeting recommended levels of activity (Azevedo Da Silva et al., 2012). Cognitive-behavioural strategies such as goal setting, self-monitoring, activity assignments and supportive follow-up are effective techniques that may help depressed individuals adopt and maintain a more physically active lifestyle. Activity diaries are a particularly useful self-monitoring tool that may promote physical activity in people with common mental health conditions. Diaries that include measures for mood or anxiety can provide individuals with direct feedback of the effect of exercise on subjective well-being. Focusing on short-term mood changes associated with physical activity has been found to be more motivating and tangible to patients than changes in physical fitness because the results are more immediate (Forsyth et al., 2009).

Applying this to Eve

To enhance her mood, Eve would benefit from regular physical activity. Assessing her current activity level and supporting Eve to set realistic yet progressive goals would enable her to gradually increase her exercise to meet the recommended guideline of 150 minutes a week. An activity diary would reinforce the mood enhancing effects of exercise for behaviour change.

DIET IN THE TREATMENT OF DEPRESSION

Dietary habits have only recently been recognised as having an impact on mental health and a growing body of epidemiological studies has demonstrated an association between depression and unhealthy eating patterns and poor food choices (Jacka & Berk, 2012). It is generally accepted that overall dietary pattern may be more important for the prevention and management of depression than the effect of any single nutrient. Research has suggested that individuals adhering to a Mediterranean style diet reduced their risk of developing depression over time (Sanchez-Villegas et al., 2009; Firth et al., 2019). The Mediterranean dietary pattern includes foods which may be protective against depressive symptoms, for example:

- high ratio of monounsaturated fats to saturated fats
- high intake of vegetable
- high intake of fruit and nuts
- moderate alcohol intake
- low intake of meat or meat products
- high intake of cereal
- high fish intake

By contrast, a Westernised dietary pattern, which is typically characterised by the consumption of calorie-dense foods which are high in saturated fats and sugars and low in essential micro-nutrients, has been linked to poorer mental health measures in adolescents and to increased anxiety in men and women (Oddy et al., 2009; Jacka et al., 2011). Indeed, depression itself can have an effect on appetite (decreased or increased) and this may also result in the decline of essential nutrients for physical and mental health (Mikolajczyk et al., 2009). Adherence to national dietary guidelines is an important recommendation for people with depression, particularly when studies examining dietary improvements as a treatment strategy in depression are lacking (Jacka & Berk, 2012). In 2018, Tolkien, Bradburn and Murgatroyd concluded that an anti-inflammatory diet maybe an effective intervention or preventative means of reducing depression risk and symptoms.

A number of cognitive-behavioural techniques may be used to strengthen healthy eating patterns in individuals with depression. Forsyth et al. (2009) found that a goal-based approach to lifestyle change was well received by patients with depression and/or anxiety in a primary care setting. Activity scheduling is a behavioural treatment which enables individuals with depression to monitor their mood in response to daily activities in order to establish connections between the two.

Applying this to Eve

Maintaining a balanced diet through the increased consumption of fruit and vegetables and the avoidance of high fat and sugary foods may help Eve to regulate her mood.

Community level interventions

INTERVENTIONS TARGETING PHYSICAL ACTIVITY IN THE COMMUNITY

Being physically active has clear benefits for people with common mental disorders and community level interventions promoting an active lifestyle are particularly important for these individuals. Active transport is one such strategy that promotes active living at the community level, however, a recent meta-analysis by Barton and Pretty (2010) has also explored the impact of green exercise on mental health outcomes with promising results. They concluded that green space provides communities with a unique opportunity to improve mental health because physical activity in the presence of nature is associated with improvements in self-esteem and mood. Even short-duration and light-intensity physical activity in green space, such as walking in parks, resulted in immediate mental health benefits. The potential for green exercise as a therapeutic intervention for people with a mental health problem is great however access to green space, particularly within urban settings, requires planning and investment at a strategic level.

Applying this to Eve

Regular physical activity in green space has important mood enhancing benefits that may improve Eve's depression. Eve could try to self-regulate her mood by simply walking, jogging or cycling in local parks.

INTERVENTIONS TARGETING SMOKING CESSATION IN THE COMMUNITY

Smoking is a known risk factor for depression and some anxiety disorders and smokers who are nicotine dependent tend to have poorer mental health outcomes than non-dependent smokers (Pedersen & von Soest, 2009; Richardson et al., 2019). Policies promoting smoking cessation have a clear role to play in the physical and mental health of people who smoke. Smoke-free legislation in particular has the potential to reduce smoking prevalence at a population level by limiting people's opportunities to smoke in public places. The added advantage of this approach is that people's exposure to second-hand smoke is also reduced. The effects of this legislation are therefore two-fold because any reduction in smoke exposure, either directly through smoking behaviour or indirectly through second-hand smoke, has the potential to improve mental health outcomes.

Working effectively with others

People with common mental disorders are usually treated within primary care (NICE, 2009) with GPs playing a pivotal role because they are usually the first person that patients see regarding their symptoms. This puts them in an ideal position to identify unhealthy lifestyle behaviours that may be impacting on patients' mental health. A multi-disciplinary approach to mental health care means that the skill and expertise of health and other allied professionals are often called upon to support and treat people with mental health disorders in primary care. Community mental health nurses, dieticians, psychologists and exercise specialists may all be involved in the care of people with a mental health diagnosis, and the reinforcement of national guidelines for diet and physical activity should be standard practice for all patients with depression and anxiety.

Chronic obstructive pulmonary disease: COPD

Case study

Rob is 58 and has smoked for most of his life, having started as a young teenager. His early retirement from the steelworks 6 months ago was because Rob has been suffering with breathing problems which steadily worsened over time. Having suffered from a persistent productive cough and breathlessness on exertion for the past year, Rob reluctantly visited his GP for help. Tests revealed that Rob has moderate COPD. His family are particularly concerned because Rob has also lost a significant amount of weight and his breathing problems are beginning to limit his daily activities. Rob and his family are keen to make changes to his lifestyle in order to improve his breathing and overall health.

Introduction

Chronic Obstructive Pulmonary Disease (COPD) is a long-term irreversible disease of the lungs in which the flow of air into the lungs is restricted by inflammation and damage to the lung tissue (NICE, 2010). COPD is the third leading cause of death in the world (Terzikhan et al., 2016; WHO, 2023). Characteristic symptoms of COPD include a cough, sputum production and breathlessness on exertion and a diagnosis is made when airflow obstruction is detected on spirometry (Gruffydd-Jones & Loveridge, 2011). Bronchitis and emphysema are the two main types of COPD and an important causative factor for their development is smoking. It is estimated that 20% of smokers will develop COPD (Terzikhan et al., 2016). Other risk factors such as air pollution, respiratory infections, poor nutritional status, chronic asthma, impaired lung growth, poor socio-economic status and genetic factors are also important. The condition is described as being progressive because it gradually gets worse over time, and this deterioration is often associated with poorly managed exacerbations. Exacerbations are particularly debilitating for individuals because they accelerate loss of lung function and reduce physical activity in daily life (Bourbeau, 2009). This downward spiral can lead to physical de-conditioning and ultimately death. Early treatment is essential to manage acute exacerbations and slow any decline in lung function in order to lengthen the time in which the individual can maintain an active life (Polsky & Moraveji, 2021).

In the UK, annual deaths from COPD have been fairly consistent over the past 25 years, ranging between 25,000 and 30,000 deaths each year (Health and Safety Executive, 2012; British Lung Foundation, accessed 2023). It is the fifth biggest killer nationally, with death rates much higher in the 75+ age range for both men and women (this group accounts for two-thirds of all deaths from the disease). Mortality rates from COPD as a contributory cause have been rising since 2006 and increased significantly from 54 per 100,000 in 2019 to 68.8 per 100,000 in 2020 (Office for Health Improvement and Disparities, 2021). Accurately estimating prevalence rates for the disease is fraught with difficulties because levels of underdiagnosis and misdiagnosis in the early stages are high. However, any delay in diagnosis can result in patients needlessly suffering symptoms and limitations that could otherwise be alleviated by appropriate management (Price et al., 2011). According to the

National Institute for Health and Clinical Excellence, the mean delay from onset to diagnosis is 20 years (NICE, 2010; NICE, 2018). Opportunities to prevent its progression in the early stages are therefore being missed.

Interventions to improve the health of people with COPD

Although not curable, COPD can be treated at any stage of the disease: mild, moderate or severe (O'Donnell et al., 2008; NICE, 2011; NICE, 2018). Key to the successful management of the disease is the need for people to modify or change their health behaviour/s in order to preserve lung function and optimise their general health. In its early stages, opportunities exist to prevent disease progression through lifestyle modification. Smoking cessation and physical activity are the two important lifestyle behaviours that impact on the health of people living with COPD (NICE, 2010; NICE, 2011; NICE, 2018).

Individual level interventions

PULMONARY REHABILITATION

Available through the NHS for patients with a confirmed diagnosis of COPD, Pulmonary Rehabilitation seeks to restore individuals to the fullest possible physical, social and mental health. This is achieved through individually tailored physical exercise training, self-management advice and multi-disciplinary education (IMPRESS, 2008). Fundamentally, the programme aims to improve patients' exercise tolerance in order to support a more physically active lifestyle and it has been suggested the greatest positive effect of any current therapy is on exercise capacity in COPD (Spruit et al., 2015). This is particularly important for people with COPD because the negative impact of prolonged inactivity has far-reaching consequences, with research demonstrating that impaired exercise capacity is a significant determinant of disease burden (van Wetering et al., 2008; Spruit et al., 2015). Improving exercise tolerance to support an active lifestyle is therefore an important treatment goal for people attending Pulmonary Rehabilitation.

The effectiveness of Pulmonary Rehabilitation programmes to improve exercise tolerance, dyspnoea (breathlessness) and health-related quality of life is well established (Maltais et al., 2008; van Wetering et al., 2010; Spruit et al., 2015). Although the benefits do tend to wane over time (Guell et al., 2017). Its approach is similar to that of Cardiac Rehabilitation and Structured Education for Type 2 diabetes because it is underpinned by training in self-management and empowerment for behaviour change (Spruit et al., 2015). Exercise training is a central focus of the programme, and a combination of aerobic and strength training is advocated to concurrently increase exercise tolerance and improve muscle function. Indeed, low muscle mass due to skeletal muscle dysfunction is a strong predictor of mortality in COPD (Man et al., 2009). In contrast to the irreversible abnormalities of the lungs, the skeletal muscle abnormalities in COPD can be improved or reversed by exercise training. In turn, exercise training through Pulmonary Rehabilitation can restore the patient to the highest level of functional capacity possible relative to their breathing impairment (Rochester, 2003).

Pulmonary Rehabilitation typically consists of twice-weekly supervised sessions for a minimum of 6 weeks, although 12-week programmes produce greater sustained benefits (Guell et al., 2017). Best practice guidance outlined by the NHS England (2012) recommends the use of training diaries to log incremental progress through the setting of individualised goals for aerobic and strength (resistance) exercise training. As previously discussed, self-monitoring through diary keeping and goal setting are effective self-regulatory strategies for behaviour change. A review observed that Pulmonary Rehabilitation increases motivation, self-efficacy for physical activity and functional capacity to support an active lifestyle in people with the condition (ZuWallack, 2009). Gysels and Higginson (2009) found that patients who were most successful at self-management were all involved in Pulmonary Rehabilitation. In addition, Pulmonary Rehabilitation has been described as being instrumental in enhancing patients' participation in physical activity by improving their confidence to manage symptoms of breathlessness and by reducing their fear of exertional activity (Hogg et al., 2012) (Box 10.2).

Box 10.2 Applying research in practice

People with COPD perceive ongoing, structured and socially supportive exercise opportunities to be important for maintaining an active lifestyle following Pulmonary Rehabilitation: a qualitative study (Hogg et al., 2012)

This study explored the perceptions of people with COPD regarding maintaining an active lifestyle following participation in a Pulmonary Rehabilitation programme.

Focus groups were conducted with individuals with a diagnosis of COPD who had completed an 8-week Pulmonary Rehabilitation programme as an outpatient.

Ongoing peer and professional exercise-support was perceived as fundamental for maintaining an active lifestyle after Pulmonary Rehabilitation. Participants valued the peer support found within Pulmonary Rehabilitation and expressed that this was an important factor for their continued participation in physical activity following a rehabilitation programme. Pulmonary Rehabilitation was seen as a vehicle to facilitate greater participation in daily activities by improving self-confidence to manage breathlessness.

Applying this to Rob

Rob's capacity to become more physically active will be enhanced through participation in a Pulmonary Rehabilitation programme. The individualised exercise training component of rehabilitation will improve and strengthen Rob's muscle function and enable him to self-manage acute episodes of breathlessness. The support gained from peers and professionals during the programme may help Rob to increase his daily activity level.

INTERVENTIONS PROMOTING SMOKING CESSATION

Quitting smoking is the most effective way to slow decline in lung function for people with COPD (ZuWallack, 2007; van Eerd et al., 2016). It is also the most cost-effective intervention and smokers with COPD should therefore be offered smoking cessation support as treatment for their disease (Hoogendoorn et al., 2010). Health messages constructed around the concepts of lung health and lung age provide a positive way of expressing behaviour change messages and have demonstrated positive effects on smoking cessation in people with COPD (DoH, 2011). Sigurgeirsdottir et al. (2022) have suggested that shame patients felt in relation to their self-inflicted disease may make stopping smoking more difficult. Shame, or self-stigma rather than preventing the negative behaviour can trigger embedded habitual behaviours that function as coping strategies. Van Eerd et al. (2016) in their Cochrane review of the literature conclude that a combination of behavioural and pharmacological treatment is effective in helping smokers to quit with no convincing evidence for any particular form of behavioural or pharmacological treatment.

Applying this to Rob

Supporting Rob to give up smoking without triggering feelings of self-stigma will require non-judgemental behavioural therapy alongside pharmacological treatments.

Community level interventions

COPD is largely caused by smoking so interventions promoting smoking cessation at the community level have clear benefits to people with the condition. Policies that raise awareness of the dangers of second-hand smoke and legislation that restricts smoking in enclosed public spaces have been effective in altering peoples' attitudes towards the social acceptability of smoking. This shift in attitude may support the efforts of people with COPD who are attempting to quit because opportunities to smoke in public are reduced.

Physical activity is recognised as an important health behaviour in terms of benefits to quality of life and survival in people with COPD (Bourbeau, 2009; Guell et al., 2017). Public health campaigns that promote participation in physical activity at the community level are therefore important for this client group. Active Transport schemes are a good example of how physical activity can be promoted within the community through engagement in walking and cycling initiatives. Integrating physical activity flexibly into daily routine in this way may be an appealing alternative to other structured forms of exercise, particularly for people with physical limitations associated with this complex health condition.

Applying this to Rob

The opportunity for Rob to smoke when he socialises locally with friends is now restricted by smoking legislation. These restrictions will support his attempts to quit smoking.

Rob can increase his daily activity by walking to and from the local shops rather than relying on his car as a mode of transport. Incorporating regular physical activity into his daily routine will gradually increase his exercise capacity in order to prevent further decline in lung function.

Working effectively with others

COPD care is delivered by a multi-disciplinary team and may include input from respiratory nurse specialists, physiotherapists, occupational therapists and dieticians (NICE, 2010; Spruit et al., 2015). Although patients are generally cared for within primary care, acute exacerbations often require hospitalisation so a collaborative approach to disease management across the primary and secondary care sector is essential. Referral to a dietician is common for patients with moderate to severe COPD because this stage of the condition is associated with being underweight and having reduced muscle mass. Rawal and Yadav (2015) reported that 'pulmonary cachexia syndrome' which is characterised by loss of fat-free body mass and causes muscle wasting occurs in 25% to 40% of COPD patients.

Nutritional management is an important aspect of care in this client group because weight loss is associated with decreased lung capacity, health status and increased morbidity (Houghton, 2008). Nutritional supplements may be considered for individuals with a low BMI alongside regular exercise to increase muscle mass. Patients eating high-fat, low-carbohydrate diets have demonstrated improvements in pulmonary function compared to traditional high carbohydrate diets (Rawal & Yadav, 2015). As COPD progresses, breathlessness when eating may also restrict the amount a person can eat at one time so patients should be encouraged to adopt eating strategies to optimise their nutritional intake, such as eating frequent, small meals over the course of a day (Houghton, 2008).

Peer support is vital in motivating individuals to initiate and make sustained changes to their lifestyle (Matheson et al., 2010; Spruit et al., 2015). The efficacy of peer support to help people with COPD to stop smoking has been demonstrated by a buddy-led smoking cessation intervention (Cox, 2011). The Hope 2 Quit intervention harnessed the support of 'buddies' or expert patients with COPD who worked collaboratively with the multi-disciplinary team to design and deliver the smoking cessation intervention. The intervention was successful in supporting short and long-term quit rates for those receiving buddy support. With a 4-week quit rate of 81% and a 1-year quit rate of 50% it is hard to ignore the impact that social support from buddies can achieve in this client group.

Applying this to Rob

Rob would benefit from dietetic advice and support because of his ongoing weight loss. This may include advice about eating strategies and dietary supplementation to optimise his nutritional status and increase his body weight and muscle mass.

Conclusion

It is clear that the lifestyle choices we make can have a profound effect on our health over time. Rising prevalence rates for many of the chronic conditions that we see in UK today suggests that lifestyle behaviours are significantly impacting on the health of the nation. These conditions tend to be progressive and long-term, and when poorly managed can lead to further health problems and a reduced quality of life. Lifestyle interventions can be used effectively to manage conditions such as Type 2 diabetes, CHD, COPD, and depression. Health professionals must endeavour to work collaboratively with clients to promote health through behaviour change. There is evidence of a shift towards greater client autonomy whereby individuals are now encouraged to be active self-managers of their condition. This self-management often requires individuals to make and sustain multiple changes to their lifestyle. Behaviour change is never easy and challenges clearly exist for people with health limitations due to chronic illness. Nevertheless, psychological techniques for health behaviour change have been shown to be effective in improving health outcomes for people with specific conditions.

Key points

- Unhealthy lifestyles contribute to the high prevalence of chronic disorders in the UK
- Positive and sustained changes to lifestyle can help manage these long-term health conditions
- Self-regulatory techniques such as self-monitoring and goal setting are particularly effective in promoting behaviour change in clinical groups
- Individuals are encouraged to be active self-managers of their condition
- Multi-disciplinary teams are often involved in the care of people with ongoing health conditions

Points for discussion

- How would you support an individual who is newly diagnosed with Type 2 diabetes to self-manage their condition?
- Identify which self-regulatory strategies are important to support behaviour change in people with a long-term health condition. What are the relative benefits and limitations for each strategy you have identified?
- What factors do you need to consider when promoting a physically active lifestyle for individuals following a cardiac event?

Further resources

British Heart Foundation. www.bhf.org.uk
British Lung Foundation. www.blf.org.uk
Diabetes UK. www.diabetes.org.uk
Mental Health Foundation. www.mentalhealth.org.uk
Mind, the Mental Health Charity. www.mind.org.uk

References

Introduction

Buck D., & Frosini F. (2012). Clustering of unhealthy behaviours over time. *Implications for policy and practice*. London: The King's Fund.
Department of Health, Physical Activity, Health Improvement and Protection. (2011). *Start active, stay active*. London: Department of Health.
NHS. (Accessed 2023). NHS long term plan. www.longtermplan.nhs.uk
Noordman, J., van der Weijden, T., & van Dulmen, S. (2012). Communication-related behavior change techniques used in face-to-face lifestyle interventions in primary care: A systematic review of the literature. *Patient Education and Counseling, 89*(2), 227–244.

Type 2 diabetes

Alouki, K., Delisle, H., Bermudez-Tamayo, C., & Johri, M. (2016). Lifestyle interventions to prevent Type 2 diabetes: A systematic review of economic evaluation studies. *Journal of Diabetes Research*. 10.1155/2016/2159890. PMC4738686.

Anderson, R. M., & Funnell, M. M. (2000). *The Art of Empowerment: Stories and Strategies for Diabetes Educators*. In T Deakin (2012) X-PERT structured education programmes improve control in diabetes. *Journal of Diabetes Nursing, 16*(7), 266–272.

Bailey, C. J. (2011). The challenge of managing coexistent Type 2 diabetes and obesity. *BMJ, 342.* 10/1136/bmj.d1996

Baksi, A. K., Al-Mrayat, M., Hogan, D., Whittingstall, E., Wilson, P., & Wex, J. (2008). Peer advisers compared with specialist health professionals in delivering a training programme on self-management to people with diabetes: A randomized controlled trial. *Diabetic Medicine, 25*(9), 1076–1082.

Balducci, S., D'Errico, V., Haxhi, J., Sacchetti, M., Orlando, G., Cardelli, P., Vitale, M., Bollanti, L., Conti, F., Zanuso, S., Lucisano, G., Nicolucci, A., Pugliese, G., for the Italian Diabetes & Exercise study 2 (IDES_2) Investigators. (2019). Effect of a bheavioural intervention strategy on sustained change in physical activity and sedentary behavior in patients with Type 2 diabetes. *JAMA, 321*(9), 880–890. 10.1001/jM.2019.0922

Barrows H. S. (1996). Problem-based learning in medicine and beyond. In T Deakin (2012) X-PERT structured education programmes improve control in diabetes. *Journal of Diabetes Nursing, 16*(7), 266–272.

Better Health. (Accessed 2023). www.nhs.uk

Bommer, C., Sagalova, V., Heesemann, E., Manne-Goehler, J., Atun, R., Barnighausen, T., Davies, J., & Vollmer, S. (2018). Global economic burden of diabetes in adults: Projections from 2015 to 2030. *Diabetes Care, 41*(5), 963–970. 10.2337/dc17-1962

Boothroyd, R. I., & Fisher, E. B. (2010). Peers for progress: Promoting peer support for health around the world. *Family Practice, 27*(suppl 1), i62–i68.

Bowden Davies, K. A., Sprung, V. S., Norman, J. A., Thompson, A., Mitchell, K. L., Harrold, J. A., Finlayson, G., Gibbons, C., Wilding, J. P. H., Kemp, G. J., Hamer, M., & Cuthbertson, D. J. (2019). Physical Activity and Sedentary Time: Association with Metabolic Health and Liver Fat. *Medicine and Science in Sports and Exercise, 51*(6), 1169–1177.

Brennan, P.F., & Strombom, I. (1998). Improving health care by understanding patient preferences: the role of computer technology. *Journal of the American Medical Information Association, 5*(3), 257–262.

Cade, J. E., Kirk, S. F. L., Nelson, P., Hollins, L., Deakin, T., Greenwood, D. C., & Harvey, E. L. (2009). Can peer educators influence healthy eating in people with diabetes? Results of a randomized controlled trial. *Diabetic Medicine, 26*(10), 1048–1054.

Carpenter, R., DiChiacchio, T., & Barker, K. (2018). Interventions for self-management of Type 2 diabetes: An integrative review. *International Journal of Nursing Studies 6*, 70–91. 10.1016/j.ijns.2018.12.02

Casey, D., De Civita, M., & Dasgupta, K. (2010). Understanding physical activity facilitators and barriers during and following a supervised exercise programme in Type 2 diabetes: A qualitative study. *Diabetic Medicine, 27*(1), 79–84.

Chudyk, A., & Petrella, R. J. (2011). Effects of exercise on cardiovascular risk factors in Type 2 diabetes a meta-analysis. *Diabetes Care, 34*(5), 1228–1237.

Davies, M. J., Heller, S., Skinner, T. C., Campbell, M. J., Carey, M. E., Cradock, S., ...& Khunti, K. (2008). Effectiveness of the diabetes education and self management for ongoing and newly diagnosed (DESMOND) programme for people with newly diagnosed Type 2 diabetes: Cluster randomised controlled trial. *BMJ, 336*(7642), 491–495.

Deakin, T. A., Cade, J. E., Williams, R., & Greenwood, D. C. (2006). Structured patient education: The Diabetes X-PERT Programme makes a difference. *Diabetic Medicine, 23*(9), 944–954.

Department of Health. (2001a). *National Service Framework for Diabetes*. London: Department of Health. Available at: http://www.doh.gov.uk/nsf/diabetes/index.htm. Accessed 1 September 2012.

Department of Health. (2001b). *The Expert Patient*. London: Department of Health. Available at: http://www.doh.gov.uk/cmo/ep-report.pdf. Accessed 10 September 2012.

Department of Health. (2009). *Change4Life*. London: Department of Health. Available at: www.dh.gov.uk/en/MediaCentre/Currentcampaigns/Change4Life/index.htm

Department of Health and Social Care, Llwodraeth Cymru Welsh Government, Department of Health Northern Ireland and the Scottish Government. (2019). UK Chief Medical Officers Physical Activity Guidelines. www.gov.uk/dhsc

Department of Health, Physical Activity, Health Improvement and Protection. (2011b). *Start active, stay active*. London: Department of Health.

Diabetes UK. (accessed 2023). Diabetes UK: Complications of diabetes. www.diabetes.org.uk

Duke, S. A., Colagiuri, S., & Colagiuri, R. (2009). Individual patient education for people with Type 2 diabetes mellitus. *Cochrane Database of Systematic Reviews*, 1(1). 10.1002/14651858. CD005268.pub2. PMC6486318

Funnell, M. M. (2010). Peer-based behavioural strategies to improve chronic disease self-management and clinical outcomes: Evidence, logistics, evaluation considerations and needs for future research. *Family Practice*, 27(suppl 1), i17–i22.

Gruber, K. J. (2008). Social support for exercise and dietary habits among college students. *Adolescence (San Diego): An International Quarterly Devoted to the Physiological, Psychological, Psychiatric, Sociological, and Educational Aspects of the Second Decade of Human Life*, 43(171), 557.

Gysels, M. H., & Higginson, I. J. (2009). Self-management for breathlessness in COPD: the role of pulmonary rehabilitation. *Chronic Respiratory Disease*, 6(3), 133–140.

Hamasaki, H. (2016). Daily physical activity and Type 2 diabetes: A review. *World Journal of Diabetes*, 7(12), 243–251. 10/4239/wjd.v7.i12.243

Healy, G. N., Dunstan, D. W., Salmon, J., Cerin, E., Shaw, J. E., Zimmet, P. Z., & Owen, N. (2008). Breaks in sedentary time beneficial associations with metabolic risk. *Diabetes Care*, 31(4), 661–666.

Healy, G. N., Wijndaele, K., Dunstan, D. W., Shaw, J. E., Salmon, J., Zimmet, P. Z., & Owen, N. (2008). Objectively measured sedentary time, physical activity, and metabolic risk the Australian Diabetes, Obesity and Lifestyle Study (AusDiab). *DiabetesCare*, 31(2), 369–371.

Hou, C., Carter, B., Hewitt, J., Francisa, T., & Mayor, S. (2016). Do Mobile Phone Applications Improve Glycemic control (HbA1c) in the self-management of diabetes? A systematic review, meta-analysis, and GRADE of 14 randomised trails. *Diabetes Care*, 39(11), 2089–2095. 10.2337/dc-0346

International Diabetes Federation. (2021). IDF Diabetes Atlas 2021. 10th edition. www.diabetesatlas.org

Jarvis, J., Skinner, T. C., Carey, M. E., & Davies, M. J. (2010). How can structured self-management patient education improve outcomes in people with Type 2 diabetes? *Diabetes, Obesity and Metabolism*, 12(1), 12–19.

Kavookjian, J., Elswick, B. M., & Whetsel, T. (2007). Interventions for being active among individuals with diabetes a systematic review of the literature. *The Diabetes Educator*, 33(6), 962–988.

Kirk, A., Barnett, J., Leese, G., & Mutrie, N. (2009). A randomized trial investigating the 12-month changes in physical activity and health outcomes following a physical activity consultation delivered by a person or in written form in Type 2 diabetes: Time2Act. *Diabetic Medicine*, 26(3), 293–301.

Kyrou, I., Tsigos, C., Mavrogianni, C., Cardon, G., Van Stappen, V., Latomme, J., Kivela, J., Wikstrom, K., Tsochev, K., Nanasi, A., Semanova, C., Mateo-Gallego, R., Lamiquiz-Moneo, I., Dafoulas, G., Timpel, P., Schwarz, P. E. H, Iotova, V., Tankova, T., Makrilakis, K., Manios, Y.,

& on behalf of the Feel4Diabetes-study Group. (2020). Sociodemongraphic and lifestyle-related risk factors for identifying vulnerlabe groups for Type 2 diabetes: A narrative review with emphasis on data from Europe. *BMC Endocrine Disorders*, 20(suppl 1), 134. 10.1186/s12902-019-0463-3

Li, Y., Buys, N., Ferguson, S., Li, Z., & Sun, S. (2021). Effectiveness of cognitive behavioural therapy-based interventions on health outcomes in patients with coronary heart disease: A meta-analysis. *World Journal of Psychiatry*, 11(11), 1147–1166. 10.5498/wjp.v11.i11.1147

Loveman, E., Frampton, G. K., & Clegg, A. J. (2008). The clinical effectiveness of diabetes education models for Type 2 diabetes: A systematic review. *Health Technology Assessment*, 12(9), 1–136.

Marwick, T. H., Hordern, M. D., Miller, T., Chyun, D. A., Bertoni, A. G., Blumenthal, R. S., & Rocchini, A. (2009). Exercise training for Type 2 diabetes mellitus impact on cardiovascular risk: A scientific statement from the American Heart Association. *Circulation*, 119(25), 3244–3262.

NICE. (2015, updated 2022). Diabetes in Adults. NICE quality standard (QS6). Available at: www.nice.org.uk/guidance/ng28 (Accessed 2023).

Nolan, C. J., Damm, P., & Prentki, M. (2011). Type 2 diabetes across generations: From pathophysiology to prevention and management. *The Lancet*, 378(9786), 169–181.

Ogurtsova, K., da Rocha Fermamdes, J., Huang, Y., et al. (2017). IDF Diabetes Atlas: Global estimates for the prevalence of diabetes for 2015 and 2040. *Diabetes REsearh and Clinical Practice*, 128, 40–50.

Peel, E., Douglas, M., Parry, O., & Lawton, J. (2010). Type 2 diabetes and dog walking: Patients' longitudinal perspectives about implementing and sustaining physical activity. *The British Journal of General Practice*, 60(577), 570.

Pfaeffli Dale, L., Whittaker, R., Jiang, Y., Stewart, R., Rolleston, A., & Maddison, R. (2015). Text message and internet support for coronary heart disease self-management: Results from the Text4Heart randomised controlled trial. *Journal of Medical Internet Research*, 17(10). e237. 10.2196/jmir.4944

Qi, L., Liu, Q., Qi, X., Wu, N., Tang, W., & Xiong, H. (2015). Effectiveness of peer support for improving glycaemic control in patients with Type 2 diabetes: A meta-analysis of randomized controlled trials. *BMC Public Health*, 6, 15. 10.1186/s12889-015-1798-y

Richardson, C. R., Mehari, K. S., McIntyre, L. G., Janney, A. W., Fortlage, L. A., Sen, A., ... & Piette, J. D. (2007). A randomized trial comparing structured and lifestyle goals in an internet-mediated walking program for people with Type 2 diabetes. *International Journal of Behavioral Nutrition and Physical Activity*, 4(1), 59.

Scheumer, M. T., Sieverding, P., & Shekelle, P. G. (2008). Delivery of genomic medicine for common chronic adult diseases. A Systematic Review. *JAMA*, 299(11), 1320–1334

Shilts, M. K., Horowitz, M., & Townsend, M. S. (2004). Goal setting as a strategy for dietary and physical activity behavior change: A review of the literature. *American Journal of Health Promotion*, 19(2), 81–93.

Smith, S. M., Paul, G., Kelly, A., Whitford, D. L., O'Shea, E., & O'Dowd, T. (2011). Peer support for patients with Type 2 diabetes: Cluster randomised controlled trial. *BMJ: British Medical Journal*, 342. d715. doi/10.1136/bmj.d715

Song, J., Brown, M. K., Tan, M., MacGregor, M. T., Webster, J., Campbell, N. R. C., Trieu, K., Mhurchu, C. N., Cobb, L. K., & He, F. J. (2021). Impact of color-coded and warning nutrition labelling schemes: A systematic review and network meta-analysis. *PLOS Medicine*, 18(10), e1003765. 10.1371/journal.pmed.1003765

Steinsbekk, A., Rygg, L., Lisulo, M., Rise, M. B., & Fretheim, A. (2012). Group based diabetes self-management education compared to routine treatment for people with Type 2 diabetes mellitus. A systematic review with meta-analysis. *BMC Health Services Research*, 12(1), 213.

Stewart, R. A. H., Held, C., Hadziosmanovic, N., Armstrong, P. W. Cannon, C. P., Granger, C. B., Hagstrom, E., Hochman, J. S., Koenig, W., Lonn, E., Nicolau, J. C. Gabriel, P., Vedin, O.,

Wallentin, L., White, H. D., & on behalf of the STABILITY Investigators. (2017). Self-Reported Health and Outcomes in Patients With Stable Coronary Heart Disease. *Journal of the American College of Cardiology*, 70(14), 1689–1700. 10.1016/j.jacc.2017.08.017

Umpierre, D., Ribeiro, P. A., Kramer, C. K., Leitão, C. B., Zucatti, A. T., Azevedo, M. J., ... & Schaan, B. D. (2011). Physical Activity Advice Only or Structured Exercise Training and Association with HbA1c Levels in Type 2 Diabetes a Systematic Review and Meta-analysis. *JAMA: The Journal of the American Medical Association*, 305(17), 1790–1799.

United Kingdom Prospective Diabetes Study (UKPDS) Group. (1998). Intensive blood-glucose control with sulphonylureas or insulin compared with conventional treatment and risk of complications in patients with Type 2 diabetes (UKPDS 33). *Lancet*, 352, 837–853.

Upton, D., &Thirlaway, K. (2010). *Promoting healthy behaviour*. London: Pearson.

Valtorta, N. K., Kanaan, M., Gilbody, S., Ronzi, S., & Hanratty, B. (2016). Loneliness and social isolation as risk factors for coronary heart disease and stroke: Systematic review and meta-analysis of longitudinal observational studies. *Cardiac risk factors and prevention*, 102, 1009–1016. 10.1136/heartjnl-2015-308790

van der Wulp, I., de Leeuw, J. R. J., Gorter, K. J., & Rutten, G. E. H. M. (2012). Effectiveness of peer-led self-management coaching for patients recently diagnosed with Type 2 diabetes mellitus in primary care: A randomized controlled trial. *Diabetic Medicine*, 29(10), e390–e397.

Wei, M., Gibbons, L. W., Kampert, J. B., Nichaman, M. Z., & Blair, S. N. (2000). Low cardio respiratory fitness and physical inactivity as predictors of mortality in men with Type 2 diabetes. *Annals of Internal Medicine*, 132(8), 605.

Wheatley, S. D., Arjomandkhah, N. C., Murdoch, C., Whitaker, M. J. G., Evans, N. M., Hollinrake, P. B., Rees, T. E., Wellsted, D., & Deakin, T. A. (2021). Improved blood glucose control, cardiovascular health and empowerment in people attending X-PERT structured diabetes education. *Practical Diabetes*, 38(6), 31–35.

WHO. (2008). *Peer support programmes in diabetes: Report of a WHO consultation 5-7 November 2007*. Geneva, Switzerland: WHO.

WHO. (2020). *WHO guidelines on physical activity and sedentary behaviour*. Geneva: World Health organisation. 2020. Licence: CC BY-NC-SA 3.0 IGO.

Yates, T., Khunti, K., Troughton, J., & Davies, M. (2009). The role of physical activity in the management of Type 2 diabetes mellitus. *Postgraduate Medical Journal*, 85(1001), 129–133.

Coronary heart disease

Artinian, N. T., Fletcher, G. F., Mozaffarian D., Kris-Etherton, P., Van Horn, L., Lichtenstein, A. H., et al. (2010). Interventions to promote physical activity and dietary lifestyle changes for cardiovascular risk factor reduction in adults. A scientific statement from the American Heart Association. *Circulation*, 122, 406–441.

Barth, J., Schneider, S., & von Känel, R. (2010). Lack of social support in the etiology and the prognosis of coronary heart disease: A systematic review and meta-analysis. *Psychosomatic Medicine*, 72(3), 229–238.

Better Health. (Accessed 2023). www.nhs.uk

Blumenthal, J. A., Babyak, M. A., Doraiswamy, P. M., et al. (2007). Exercise and pharmacotherapy in the treatment of major depressive disorder. *Psychosomatic Medicine*, 69(7), 587–596.

British Heart Foundation. (2007). Cardiac Rehabilitation ... recovery or by-pass? National Campaign for Cardiac rehabilitation. The evidence. Available at: http://www.bhf.org.uk/publications/view-publication.

British Heart Foundation. (2010). Coronary Heart Disease Statistics 2010. Available at: www.heartstats.org

British Heart Foundation. (2011). *The National Audit of Cardiac Rehabilitation. The Annual Statistical Report 2011*. Available at: http://www.bhf.org.uk/publications/view-publication.

British Heart Foundation. (2022). UK Factsheet August 2022. (accessed 2023). Available at: BHF.org.uk

Burke, L. E., Sereika, S. M., Music, E., Warziski, M., Styn, M. A., & Stone, A. (2008). Using instrumented paper diaries to document self-monitoring patterns in weight-loss. *Contemporary Clinical Trials*, 29(2), 182–193.

Chow, C. K., Jolly, S., Rao-Melacini, P., Fox, K. A. A., Anand, S. S., & Yusuf, S. (2010). Association of diet, exercise, and smoking modification with risk of early cardiovascular events after acute coronary syndromes. *Circulation*, 121, 750–758.

Department of Health. (2000). *National Service Framework for Coronary Heart Disease*. Chapter 7. Cardiac Rehabilitation. Available at: www.dh.gov.uk/assetRoot/04/05/75/24/04057524.pdf

Department of Health. (2001). *Exercise Referral Systems: A National Quality Assurance Framework*. London: Department of Health.

Department of Health and Social Care, Llwodraeth Cymru Welsh Government, Department of Health Northern Ireland and the Scottish Government. (2019). UK chief medical officers physical activity guidelines. www.gov.uk/dhsc

Doherty, P., Petre, C., Onion, N., et al. (2018). National audit of cardiac rehabilitation (NACR): Annual statistical report 2017.

Farris, S. G., Abrantes, A. M., & Wu, W. (2019). anxiety and fear of exercise in cardiopulmonary rehabilitation: Patient and practitioner perspectives. *Journal of Cardiopulmonary Rehabilitation and Prevention*, 39(2), E9–E13.

Goldston, K., & Baillie, A. J. (2008). Depression and coronary heart disease: A review of the epidemiological evidence, explanatory mechanisms and management approaches. *Clinical Psychology Review*, 28, 288–306.

Goulding, L., Furze, G., & Birks, Y. (2010). Randomized controlled trials of interventions to change maladaptive illness beliefs in people with coronary heart disease: Systematic review. *Journal of Advanced Nursing*, 66(5), 946–961.

Gulliksson, M., Burell, G., Vessby, B., Lundin, L., Toss, H., & Svardsudd, K. (2011). Randomized Controlled Trial of Cognitive Behavioural Therapy vs. Standard Treatment to Prevent Recurrent Cardiovascular Events in Patients with Coronary Heart Disease. *Arch International Medicine*, 171(2), 134–140.

Held, C., Iqbal, R., Lear, S. A., Rosengren, A., Islam, S., Mathew, J., & Yusaf, S. (2012). Physical activity levels, ownership of goods promoting sedentary behaviour and risk of myocardial infarction: Results of the INTERHEART study. *European Heart Journal*, 33, 452–466.

Heran, B., Chen, J. M. H., Ebrahi. S., Moxham, T., Oldridge, N., Rees, K., Thompson, D. R., & Taylor, R. S. (2011). Exercise-based cardiac rehabilitation for coronary heart disease. *Cochrane Database of Systematic Reviews*, 7. 10.1002/14651858.CD001800.pub2

Hirst, D. (2020). Briefing paper 8615: Active Travel: Trends, policy and funding. www.parliament.uk/commons-library papers@parliament.uk @commonslibrary

Janssen, V., De Gucht, V., Dusseldorp, E., & Maes, S. (2012). Lifestyle modification programmes for patients with coronary heart disease: A systematic review and meta-analysis of randomized controlled trials. *European Journal of Preventive Cardiology*.

Jarrett, J., Woodcock, J., Griffiths, U. K., Chalabi, Z., Edwards, P., Roberts, I., & Haines, A. (2012). Effects of increasing active travel in urban England and Wales on costs to the national health service. *Lancet*, 379, 2198-205.

Kunz, S., Haasova, S., Rieb, J., & Florack, A. (2020). Beyond healthiness: The impact of traffic lifht labels on taste expectations and purchase intentions. *Foods*, 9(2), 134. 10.3390/foods9020134

Lavie, C. J., Thomas, R. J., Squires, R. W., Allison, T. G., & Milani, R. V. (2009). Exercise training and cardiac rehabilitation in primary and secondary prevention of coronary heart disease. *Mayo Clinic Proceedings*, 84(4), 373–383.

Lett, H. S., Blumenthal, J. A., Babyak, M. A., Sherwood, A., Strauman, T., Robins, C., & Newman, M. F. (2004). Depression as a risk factor for coronary artery disease: Evidence, mechanisms, and treatment. *Psychosomatic medicine*, 66(3), 305–315.

Mehra, V. M., Gaalema, D. E., Pakosh, M., & Grace, S. L. (2020). Systematic review of cardiac rehabilitation guidelines: Quality and scope. *European Journal of Preventative Cardiology*, 27(9), 912–928. 10.1177/2047487319878958

Morrato, E. H., Hill, J. O., Wyatt, H. R., Ghushchyan, V., & Sullivan, P. W. (2007). Physical activity in US adults with diabetes and at risk for developing diabetes, 2003. *Diabetes Care*, 30(2), 203–209.

Mozaffarian, D., Wilson, P., & Kannel, W. (2008). Beyond established and novel risk factors: Lifestyle risk factors for cardiovascular disease. *Circulation*, 117, 3031–3038.

NACR. (2010). British heart foundation. *The National Audit of Cardiac Rehabilitation: Annual Statistical Report*. Available at: http://www.cardiacrehabilitation.org.uk/nacr/docs/2010.pdf

National Institute for Health and Clinical Excellence. (2007a) *Behaviour Change at Population, Community and Individual Level* [NICE public health guidance 6]. Available at: http://www.nice.org.uk/nicemedia/live/11868/37987/37987.pdf

National Institute for Health and Clinical Excellence. (NICE, 2007b). *MI Secondary Prevention: NICE Clinical Guidance 48*.

NICE. (2020). *Behaviour Change: Digital and Mobile Health Interventions*. Public Health England. www.gov.uk

NICE. (2021). Impact cardiovascular disease management. Nice.org.uk.

Olivio, E. L., Dodson-Lavelle, B., Wren, A., Fang, Y., & Mehmet, C. O. (2009). Feasibility and effectiveness of a brief meditation-based stress management intervention for patients diagnosed with or at risk for coronary heart disease: A pilot study. *Psychology, Health and Medicine*, 14(5), 513–523.

Richards, S. H., Anderson, L., Jenkinson, C. E., Whalley, B., Rees, K., Davies, P., Bennett, P., Liu, Z., West, R., Thompson, D. R., & Taylor, R. S. (2018). Psychological interventions for coronary heart disease: Cochrane systematic review and meta-analysis. *European Journal of Preventive Cardiology*, 25(3), 247–259. 10.1177/2047487317739978

Riegel, B. J. (1993). Contributions to cardiac invalidism after acute myocardial infarction. *Coronary Artery Disease*, 4, 215–220.

Sigurgeirsdottir, J., Halldorsdottir, S., Arnardottir, R. H., Gudmundsson, G., & Bjornsson, E. H. (2022). Ethical Dilemmas in Physicians' Consultations with COPD Patients. *International Journal of Chronic Pulmonary Obstructive Disease*, 2(17), 977–991. 10.2147/COPD.S356107. eCollection 2022.

Sniehotta, F., Gorski, C., & Araujo-Soares, V. (2010). Adoption of community-based cardiac rehabilitation programs and physical activity following phase III cardiac rehabilitation in Scotland: A prospective and predictive study. *Psychology and Health*, 25(7), 839–854.

Tierney, P., Hughes, C., & Hamilton, S. (2011). Promoting health behaviour change in the cardiac patient. *British Journal of Cardiac Nursing*, 6(3), 126–130.

Vaccarino, V., Badimon, L., Bremmer, J. D., Cenko, E., Cubedo, J., Dorobantu, M., Duncker, D. J., Koller, A., Manfrini, O., Milicic, D., Padro, T., Pries, A. R., Quyyumi, A. A., Tousoulis, D., Trifunovic, D., Vasiljevic, Z., de Wit, C., & Bugiardini, R. (2020). Depression and coronary heart disease: 2018 position paper of the ESC working group on coronary pathophysiology and microcirculation. *European Heart Journal*, 41, 1687–1696. 10.1093/eurheartj/ehy913

Wellenius, G. A., Mukamal, K. J., Kulshreshtha, A., Asonganyi, S., & Mittleman, M. A. (2008). Depressive symptoms and the risk of atherosclerotic progression among patients with coronary artery bypass grafts. *Circulation*, 117(18), 2313–2319.

Wenzel, L. (2016). *Informal and flexible approaches to self-management education for people with diabetes*. London: The King's Fund.

WHO. (2021). *Fact sheet: Cardiovascular diseases*. World Health Organisation. (Accessed 2023). www.who.int

Whooley, M. A. (2006). Depression and cardiovascular disease: Healing the broken-hearted. *JAMA*, 295(24), 2874–2881.

Whooley, M. A., de Jonge, P., Vittinghoff, E., Otte, C., Moos, R., Carney, R. M., Ali, S., Dowray, S., Na, B., Feldman, M. D., Schiller, N. B., & Browner, W. S. (2008). Depressive symptoms, health behaviours, and the risk of cardiovascular events in patients with coronary heart disease. *JAMA, 300*(20), 2379–2388.

Yusuf, S., Hawken, S., Ounpuu, S., et al. (2004). Effect of potentially modifiable risk factors associated with myocardial infarction in 52 countries (the INTERHEART Study): Case-control study. *Lancet, 364*(9438), 937–952.

Common Mental Health Disorders

Azevedo Da Silva, M., Singh-Manoux, A., Brunner, E. J., Kaffashian, S., Shipley, M. J., Kivimäki, M., & Nabi, H. (2012). Bidirectional association between physical activity and symptoms of anxiety and depression: The Whitehall II study. *European Journal of Epidemiology, 27*, 537–546.

Barton, J., & Pretty, J. (2010). What is the best dose of nature and green exercise for improving mental health? A multi-study analysis. *Environmental Science & Technology, 44*(10), 3947–3955.

Cuijpers, P., Van Straten, A., & Warmerdam, L. (2007). Behavioral activation treatments of depression: A meta-analysis. *Clinical Psychology Review, 27*(3), 318–326.

Department of Health. (2001). *Exercise referral systems: A national quality assurance framework.* Available at: http://www.dh.gov.uk/en/Publicationsandstatistics/Publications/PublicationsPolicyAndGuidance/DH40096712001.

Fifth, J., Gangwisch, J. E., Borsini, A., Wootten, R. E., & Mayer, E. A. (2020). Food and mooed: How do diet and nutrition affect mental wellbeing? *British Medical Journal, 369*, m2382. 10.1136/BMS.m2382

Firth, J., Marx, W., Dash, S., Carney, R., Teasdale, S. B., Solmi, M., Stubbs, B., Schuch, F. B., Carvalho, A. F., Jacka, F., & Sarris, J. (2019). The effects of dietary improvement on symptoms of depression and anxiety: A meta-analysis of randomised controlled trials. *Psychosomatic Medicine, 81*, 265–280.

Flinders, S. (2022). *We are monitoring trends in the quality of mental health care.* London: Nuffield Trust. www.nuffieldtrust.org.uk

Forsyth, A., Deane, F. P., & Williams, P. (2009). Dietitians and exercise physiologists in primary care: lifestyle interventions for patients with depression and/or anxiety. *Journal of Allied Health, 38*(2), 63E–68E.

Jacka, F. N., & Berk, M. (2012). Depression, diet and exercise. *Medical Journal of Australia, 10*, 21.

Jacka, F. N., Mykletun, A., Berk, M., Bjelland, I., & Tell, G. S. (2011). The association between habitual diet quality and the common mental disorders in community-dwelling adults: The Hordaland Health Study. *Psychosomatic Medicine, 73*(6), 483–490.

Kandola, A., Ashdown-Franks, G., Hendrikse, J., & Sabiston, C. M. (2019). Physical Activity and depression: Towards understanding the antidepressant mechanisms of physical activity. *Neuroscience and Biobheavoural Reviews, 107*, 525–539.

Kazantzis, N., Deane, F. P., & Ronan, K. R. (2000). Homework assignments in cognitive and behavioural therapy: A meta-analysis. *Clinical Psychology: Science and Practice, 7*(2), 189–202.

Malone, V., Harrison, R., & Daker-White, G. (2018). Mental health service user and staff perspectives on tobacco addiction and smoking cessation: A meta-synthesis of published qualitative studies. *Journal Psychiatric Mental Health Nursing, 25*, 270–282. 10.1111/jpm.12458

McManus, S., Beddington, P., Jenkins, R., & Brugha, T. (eds) (2016). Mental health and wellbeing in England. *Adults Psychiatric Morbidity Survey 2014.* Leeds: NHS Digital.

Mead, G. E., Morley, W., Campbell, P., Greig, C. A., McMurdo, M., & Lawlor, D. A. (2009). Exercise for depression. *Cochrane Database of Systematic Reviews,* (3). 10.1002/14651858.CD004366.pub4

Mead, N., Lester, H., Chew-Graham, C., Gask, L., & Bower, P. (2010). Effects of befriending on depressive symptoms and distress: Systematic review and meta-analysis. *British Journal of Psychiatry, 196*(2), 96-101.

Mental Health Foundation. (2012). *Mental Health Statistics: Men and Women.* Available at: http://www.mentalhealth.org.uk/help-information/mental-health-statistics/men-women/?view= Standard (Accessed 5 November 2012).

Mental Health Foundation. (accessed 2023). Economic and social costs: Statistics. www.mentalhealth.org.uk

MIND. *How Common are Mental Health Problems?* http://www.mind.org.uk/help/research_and_policy/statistics_1_how_common_is_mental_distress#common

Mikolajczyk, R.T., Ansari, W.E., & Maxwell, A.E. (2009). Food consumption frequency and perceived stress and depressive symptoms among students in three European countries. *Nutrition Journal, 8*(31). 1186/1475-2891-8-31

NICE. (2004). National Institute of Health and Clinical Excellence. *Depression: Management of Depression in Primary and Secondary Care. National Clinical Practice Guideline Number 23.* Available at: http://www.nice.org.uk/cg023 (Accessed 14 November 2012)

NICE. (2009). National Institute of Health and Clinical Excellence. *The Treatment and Management of Depression in Adults. NICE Clinical Guideline 90.* Available at: http://www.nice.org.uk/nicemedia/live/12329/45888/45888.pdf (Accessed 14 November 2012)

NICE. (2014). Physical activity: Exercise referral schemes guidance Ph24. www.nice.org.uk.guidance/ph24

NICE. (2017). Depression in adults: Treatment and management. NICE Guidance. www.nice.org.uk

NICE. (2022). Health topics: Depression. http://www.nice.org.uk

Nystrom, M. B. T., Neely, G., Hassmen, P., & Carlbring, P. (2015). Treating Major Depression with physical activity: A systematic overview with recommendations. *Cognitive Behaviour Therapy, 44*(4), 341–352. 10.1080/16506073.2015.1015400

Oddy, W. H., Robinson, M., Ambrosini, G. L., de Klerk, N. H., Beilin, L. J., Silburn, S. R., ...& Stanley, F. J. (2009). The association between dietary patterns and mental health in early adolescence. *Preventive Medicine, 49*(1), 39–44.

Otto, M. W., Church, T. S., Craft, L. L., Greer, T. L., Smits, J. A., & Trivedi, M. H. (2007). Exercise for mood and anxiety disorders. *Primary Care Companion to the Journal of Clinical Psychiatry, 9*(4), 287–294.

Pedersen, W., & Von Soest, T. (2009). Smoking, nicotine dependence and mental health among young adults: A 13-year population-based longitudinal study. *Addiction, 104*(1), 129–137.

Prince, M., Patel, V., Saxena, S., Maj, M., Maselko, J., Phillips, M. R., & Rahman, A. (2007). No health without mental health. *The Lancet, 370*(9590), 859–877.

Rebar, A. L., Stanton, R., Geard, D., Short, C., Duncan, M. J., & Vandelanotte, C. (2015). A meta-meta-analysis of the effect of physical activity on depression and anxiety in non-clinical adult populations. *Health Psychology Review, 9*(3), 366–378. 10.1080/17437199.2015.1022901

Richardson, S., McNeill, A., & Brose, L. S. (2019). Smoking and quitting behaviours by mental health conditions in Great Britain (1993-2014). *Addictive Behaviours, 90*, 14–19.

Rimer, J., Dwan, K., Lawlor, D. A., Greig, C. A., McMurdo, M., Morley, W., & Mead, G. E. (2012). Exercise for depression. *Cochrane Database Syst Rev, 7*, CD004366.

Rosenbaum, S., Tiedemann, A., Stanton, R., Parker, A., Waterreus, A., Curtis, J., & Ward, P. B. (2016). Implementing evidence-based physical activity interventions for people with mental illness: An Australian perspective. *Australasian Psychiatry, 24*(1), 49–54.

Roshanaei-Moghaddam, B., Katon, W. J., & Russo, J. (2009).The longitudinal effects of depression on physical activity. *General Hospital Psychiatry, 31*(4), 306–315.

Sánchez-Villegas, A., Delgado-Rodriguez, M., Alonso, A., Schlatter, J., Lahortiga, F., Majem, L. S., & Martinez-Gonzalez, M. A. (2009). association of the mediterranean dietary pattern with the incidence of depression: The seguimiento universidad de Navarra/university of Navarra follow-up (sun) cohort. *Archives of General Psychiatry, 66*(10), 1090–1098.

Sarwer, D. B., & Polonsky, H. M. (2016). The Psychosocial burden of obesity. *Endocrinology and Metabolism Clinics of North America, 45*(3), 677–688.

Ströhle, A. (2009). Physical activity, exercise, depression and anxiety disorders. *Journal of Neural Transmission, 116*(6), 777–784.

Teychenne, M., Ball, K., & Salmon, J. (2008). Physical activity and likelihood of depression in adults: A review. *Preventive Medicine, 46*(5), 397–411.

Tolkien, K., Bradburn, S., & Murgatroyd, C. (2018). An anti-inflammatory diet as a potential intervention for depressive disorders: A systematic review and meta-analysis. *Clinical Nutrition, 38,* 2045–2052.

Tylee, A., Haddad, M., Barley, E., Ashworth, M., Brown, J., Chambers, J., ...& Walters, P. (2012). A pilot randomised controlled trial of personalised care for depressed patients with symptomatic coronary heart disease in South London general practices: The UPBEAT-UK RCT protocol and recruitment. *BMC Psychiatry, 12*(1), 58.

UK Chief Medical Officers. (2019). *UK Chief Medical Officers Physical Activity Guidelines 2019.* Department of Health and Social Care, Llwodraeth Cymru Welsh Government, Department of Health Northern Ireland and the Scottish Government (2019). www.gov.uk/dhsc

World Federation for Mental Health. (2018). Young people and mental health in a changing world. https://wfmh.global/world 2018.

World Health Organisation. (2005). Mental health facing the challenges, building solutions. Report from the WHO European Ministerial Conference. Copenhagen, Denmark:WHO Regional Office for Europe.

World Health Organisation. (2010). International Statistical Classification of Diseases and Related Health Problems 10th Revision (ICD-10) Version for 2010. Chapter V Mental and behavioural disorders (F00-F99). Available at: http://apps.who.int/classifications/icd10/browse/2010/en#/F30-F39 (Accessed 1 November 2012)

COPD

Bandura, A. (1997). *Self-efficacy: The exercise of control.* New York: Freeman.

Bourbeau, J. (2009). Activities of life: The COPD patient. *COPD: Journal of Chronic Obstructive Pulmonary Disease, 6*(3), 192–200.

British Lung Foundation. (Accessed 2023). Chronic Obstructive Pulmonary Disease (CPOD) statistics. www.statistics.blf.org.uk

Cochrane, W. J., & Afolabi, O. A. (2004). Investigation into the nutritional status, dietary intake and smoking habits of patients with chronic obstructive pulmonary disease. *Journal of Human Nutrition and Dietetics, 17*(1), 3–11.

Cox, K. (2011). Smoking cessation buddies in COPD. *Nursing Times, 107*(44), 22.

Department of Health. (2011). A strategic approach to prevention and early identification of COPD. Available at: http://www.improvement.nhs.uk (Accessed 15 November 2012)

Department of Health. (DH, 2012). Service Specification. Pulmonary Rehabilitation Service. London: DH. Available at: www.dh.gov.uk/publications (Accessed 25 November 2012)

Fromer, L. (2011). Diagnosing and treating COPD: Understanding the challenges and finding solutions. *International Journal of General Medicine, 4,* 729–739.

Galaviz, K. I., Narayan, K. M. V., & Weber, M. B. (2018). Lifestyle and the Prevention of Type 2 diabetes: A Status report. American. *Journal of Lifestyle Medicine, 12*(1), 4–20.

Gruffydd-Jones, K., & Loveridge, C. (2011). The 2010 NICE COPD Guidelines: How do they compare with the GOLD guidelines. *Primary Care Respiratory Journal, 20*(2), 199–204.

Guell, M., Cejudo, P., Ortega, F., Puy, M. C., Rodriguez-Trigo, G., Pijoan, J. I., Martinez-Indart, L., Gorostiza, A., Bdeir, K., Celli, B., & Galdiz, J. B. (2017). Benefits of Long-term Pulmonary Rehabilitation Maintenance Program in Patients with Severe Chronic Obstructive Pulmonary Disease. *American Journal of Respiratory and Critical Care Mdicine, 195*(5), 622–629. 10.1164/rccm201603-0602OC

Health and Safety Executive. (2012). *Chronic Obstructive Pulmonary Disease (COPD)*. Available from http://www.hse.gov.uk/statistics/index.htm (Accessed 27 November 2012).

Hogg, L., Grant, A., Garrod, R., & Fiddler, H. (2012). People with COPD perceive ongoing, structured and socially supportive exercise opportunities to be important for maintaining an active lifestyle following pulmonary rehabilitation: A qualitative study. *Journal of Physiotherapy, 58*(3), 189–195.

Hoogendoorn, M., Feenstra, T. L., Hoogenveen, R. T., & Rutten-van Mölken, M. P. (2010). Long-term effectiveness and cost-effectiveness of smoking cessation interventions in patients with COPD. *Thorax, 65*(8), 711–718.

Houghton, L. (2008). The Nutritional Management of Weight Loss in COPD. *BPJ, 15*, 16–17.

IMPRESS. (Improving and Integrating Respiratory Services, 2008). *Principles, definitions and standards for pulmonary rehabilitation*. Available at: http://www.impressresp.com/ServiceSpecifications/tabid/60/Default.aspx (Accessed 20 November 2012).

Løkke, A., Lange, P., Scharling, H., Fabricius, P., & Vestbo, J. (2006). Developing COPD: A 25 year follow up study of the general population. *Thorax, 61*(11), 935–939.

Maltais, F., Bourbeau, J., Shapiro, S., et al. (2008). Effects of home-based pulmonary rehabilitation in patients with chronic obstructive pulmonary disease: A randomised trial. *Ann International Medicine, 149*, 869–878.

Man, W., Kemp, P., Moxham, J., & Polkey, M. (2009). Skeletal muscle dysfunction in COPD: Clinical and laboratory observations. *Clinical Science, 117*, 251–264.

Matheson, L., O'Connor, J., Cartwright, T., Blunt, C. H., Clow, A., Lee, C., & Elkin, S. (2010). P44 COPD Patients derived benefits from attending PR: 'This has given me my life back'. *Thorax, 65*(Suppl 4), A95–A95.

Morris, J. F., & Temple, W. (1985). Spirometric "lung age" estimation for motivating smoking cessation. *Preventive Medicine, 14*, 655–662.

National Institute for Health and Clinical Excellence. (NICE 2010). Chronic obstructive pulmonary disease. Management of chronic obstructive pulmonary disease in adults in primary and secondary care. London (UK): National Institute for Health and Clinical Excellence (NICE); 2010 Jun. 61p. (Clinical guideline; no. 101).

NICE. (2011). Chronic Obstructive pulmonary disease in adults. Quality standard. www.nice.org.uk/qs10

NICE. (2018). Chronic obstructive pulmonary disease in over 16s: Diagnosis and management. www.nice.org.uk/guidance/ng115

O'Donnell, D. E., Hermandez, P., Kaplan, A., et al. (2008). Canadian Thoracic Society recommendations for management of chronic obstructive pulmonary disease - -2008 update – highlights for primary care. *Canadian Respiratory Journal, 15*(Supplement A), 1A–8A.

Office for Health Improvement and Disparities. (2021). Interactive health atlas of lung conditions in England (INHALE). November 2021 update. www.gov.uk

Parkes, G., Greenhalgh, T., Griffin, M., & Dent, R. (2008). Effect on smoking quit rate of telling patients their lung age: The Step2quit randomised controlled trial. *BMJ, 336*(7644), 598–600.

Polsky, M. B., & Moraveji, N. (2021). Early identification and treatment of COPD exacerbation using remote respiratory monitoring. *Respiratory Medicine Care Reports, 34*, 101475. 10.1016/j.rmcr.2021.101475

Price, D., Freeman, D., Cleland, J., Kaplan, A., & Cerasoli F. (2011). Earlier diagnosis and earlier treatment of COPD in primary care. *Primary Care Respiratory Journal, 20*(1), 15–22.

Rawal, G., & Yadav, S. (2015). Nutrition in chronic obstructive pulmonary disease: A review. *Journal of Translational Internal Medicine, 3*(4), 151–154.

Rochester, C. L. (2003). Exercise training in chronic obstructive pulmonary disease. *Journal of Rehabilitation Research and Development, 40*(5), 59–80.

Spruit, M. A., Pitta, F., McAuley, E., ZuWallack, R. L., & Nici, L. (2015). Pulmonary rehabilitation and physical activity in patients with chronic obstructive pulmonary disease. *American Journal of Respiratory and Critical Care Medicine, 192*(8), 924–933. 10.1164/rccm.201505-0929CL

Terzikhan, N., Verhamme, K. M. C., Hofman, A., Stricker, B. H., Brusselle, G., & Lahousse, L. (2016). Prevalence and incidence of CPOD in smokers and non-smokers: The rotterdam study. *European Journal of Epidemiology, 31*(8), 785–792.

van Eerd, E. A. M., van der Meer, R. M., van Schayck, O. C. P., & Kotz, D. (2016). Somking cessation for people with chronic obstructive pulmonary disease (review). *Cochrane Database of Systematic Reviews*, (8). www.cochranelibrary.com

van Wetering, C. R., Hoogendoorn, M., Mol, S. J. M., Rutten-van Molken, M. P. M., & Schols, A. M. (2010). Short and long-term efficacy of a community-based COPD management programme in less advanced COPD: A randomised controlled trial. *Thorax, 65*, 7–13.

van Wetering, C. R., Van Nooten, F. E., Mol, S. J. M., et al. (2008). Systemic impairment in relation to disease burden in patients with moderate COPD eligible for a lifestyle program. *International Journal of COPD, 3*, 443–451.

WHO. (2023). Factsheet: Chronic obstructive pulmonary disease (COPD). Www.who.int

Wigal, J. K., Creer, T. L., & Kotses, H. (1991). The COPD Self-efficacy Scale. *Chest, 95*, 1193–1196.

ZuWallack, R. (2007). How Are You Doing? What Are You Doing? Differing Perspectives in the Assessment of Individuals with COPD. *COPD: Journal of Chronic Obstructive Pulmonary Disease, 4*, 293–297.

ZuWallack, R. L. (2009). How do we increase activity and participation in our patients? In *Seminars in Respiratory and Critical Care Medicine, 30*(6), 708.

11 Special populations

LEARNING OBJECTIVES

At the end of this chapter, you will be able to:

- identify groups of individuals who may have specific health needs.
- understand the challenges faced by health care professionals in working with these groups.
- identify and understand the use of psychology in promoting health to individual populations.
- recognise how specific and community-level interventions can help a range of individuals from across the population.
- appreciate how multidisciplinary teams can be effective in promoting health across the population.

Introduction

Hard-to-reach populations provide challenges for health professionals and the health service. As outlined in Chapter 3, health inequalities exist between various groups and the key to tackling and reducing these is to target the health behaviours of specific groups. This may encompass a whole swathe of individuals across from the population. Older people, drug users, people with learning disabilities and individuals in prison are examples of distinct sections of the population, or as we have termed them, 'Special Groups', that may require specific interventions. They are special groups since they require thought, application and commitment, along with potentially special support and intervention methods. In successfully reaching these groups, it is imperative to understand what strategies for health promotion are effective while understanding that this can be challenging and require different skill sets; however, ultimately, it can be both rewarding and fruitful for all concerned.

In reaching these groups and attempting to maximise health status, interventions must adopt individualised strategies tailored towards the individual group's specific health needs. Adopting a 'blanket approach' to health care or health promotion is inappropriate, given the variety of individuals within the population. For example, older individuals will have different views, opinions, and needs from individuals within the prison population or those with learning difficulties (and, of course, there may be crossover between these

DOI: 10.4324/9781003471233-11

groups). Health promotion schemes need to occur in various settings, including nursing homes, prisons and other locations, to reach these populations, and they require different and unique approaches.

The health needs of individuals vary according to a range of demographic factors (see, for example, Chapter 3), and these may be a consequence of a wealth of factors. Some health needs can result from risky behaviours; for example, those individuals who take drugs (including those in the prison population) may have impaired health. It goes without saying that individuals who engage in risky behaviours, for example, taking illicit drugs, face potentially significant health risks—the drug taking may not be controlled or supervised by professionals, and drugs that are sold 'on the streets' are of variable quality, strength and origin. Alternatively, it may be because the environment is not conducive to positive health—living conditions may be harmful or cultural norms may influence behaviour negatively (e.g., in prison).

Assessing the needs of special populations

Health needs assessments are a methodological approach to identifying the health needs of specific and special groups, such as those in prison, individuals with learning disabilities and older people. This chapter will consider several groups within the population and the specific health issues that arise in these groups, the skills needed to tackle them and the techniques that work best for health promotion in the specific groups. The groups presented in this chapter are, to a certain extent, randomly selected, and a host of others could have been included (e.g., pregnant women and teenagers). However, we ultimately selected those in prison, those who take illicit drugs, those with a learning disability and those who are older. These groups were chosen to reflect the diversity of people with whom professionals have to work, the specific issues of these populations and the range of skills needed by those trying to promote health.

Prison population

Case study

Julie is a 49-year-old woman who has been in and out of prison all her life. She has recently been released from a 6-month prison sentence for shoplifting and resisting arrest. Her continued offences are a result of her drug habit—she needs to steal to pay for the costs of the heroin. However, on this occasion, Julie has committed herself to stopping the drugs and said she never wants to return to prison again.

Julie's history is of previous significant social and psychological difficulties. As a child, she suffered violence and abuse from her father (who was also addicted to drugs). As a result, and in an attempt to hide visible bruises, Julie often skipped school throughout her childhood. She subsequently gained no qualifications and does not work. In addition, she would often shoplift from local shops and occasionally get caught. She also engaged in sex work to obtain money and drugs.

When Julie was 21, she became pregnant and safely delivered a baby girl (although she was born preterm and had to spend some months in the Special Baby Care Unit). Having a daughter made Julie change her ways, and she became more responsible and tried to stay out of trouble, although with little success. Her criminal behaviour has increased since her daughter moved out of the family home 8 years ago: Julie has resorted to her old ways and started taking drugs, shoplifting and engaging in sex work again. As a result of her theft and possession of illicit substances, Julie was sent back to prison.

Julie's daughter has recently given birth to a baby daughter, and consequently, Julie wants to change her behaviour as she wants to be an active part of her granddaughter's life. She feels that she needs help and support in prison to address several issues, including her mental health and the impact of her childhood and drug taking, to move forward. This is important to her as she wants to be a good Nan and role model for her new grandchild.

Introduction

According to the latest prison population figures, an estimated 82,538 individuals are currently in United Kingdom (UK) prisons (GOV.UK, 2023). Health care within prisons has been previously criticised, which has led to the reform of services for prisoners over the last two decades. This reform enabled the prison health services to become part of the NHS in 2006 and to be commissioned by local PCTs (Primary Care Trusts). In enabling this, health care and health promotion within prisons will be at the same standard as the general population. However, due to the nature of incarceration within a secure facility, delivering NHS health services does not necessarily translate to inmates receiving treatment. Thus, health disparities continue to prevail despite the reform (Otudeko, 2020). For example, due to limits on their personal autonomy, health-seeking behaviours are not often facilitated in prisons.

Prisoners often express complex and diverse health needs, with a high percentage of individuals smoking, taking drugs and having mental health problems (see Table 11.1). Mortality rates in prisons are 50% higher than the general public (Otudeko, 2020). Research has also identified that prison inmates are more likely to suffer from such mental health issues and to a greater extent compared to the rest of the population, with minority ethnic groups, women (Nowotny, Rogers & Boardman, 2017), young offenders (Barnet et al., 2017) and older inmates (Garrido & Frakt, 2020) having the most diverse health needs of the entire prison population. In a health context, prisons level the playing field in several ways; for example, nutrition, physical activity and access to health care are relatively controlled. In this regard, they provide an important context from a public health perspective. However, disparities exist even within this equal-access system.

Table 11.1 Prisoners suffering from anxiety and depression

	No anxiety and depression		Anxiety and depression	
	N	%	N	%
Male	1,004	77	299	23
Female	68	52	64	49
Total	1,072	75	363	25

Source: Ministry of Justice (2012).

Table 11.2 Opportunities and challenges faced by health workers in prisons

Opportunities	Challenges
Provides access to individuals who would not consider health care and health promotion in the outside world	Risky behaviours such as smoking and taking drugs can be more prevalent in prison due to boredom of inmates
The complex health issues that prisoners possess make them a key target for health promotion	The complex needs and variety of needs within each prison means health care staff need to have a vast knowledge base
Provides a constant unchanging environment for the individual while tackling health issues. This environment may not have been possible outside of prison.	Constraints of the prison environment in providing health care
Potentially, the prisoner will not be exposed to external cues that may trigger risky behaviour.	

The prison population is a specific closed community, providing opportunities and challenges in delivering health care services and health promotion (Table 11.2). Initiatives that consider these must be implemented and work at both an individual and community level within the prison to improve health and wellbeing. In addition, health promotion within prisons will impact the prisoners, their families and the prison staff.

Interventions to tackle prisoners' health

When aiming to improve the health of prisoners and reduce the prevalence of risky behaviours, it is important to consider the environment and personal factors that may contribute to the individual's health. In doing so, it is important that any intervention is based on multicomponent models and uses both medical and psychological methods. This will treat symptoms and change lifestyle behaviours for a lasting effect once the prisoner is released.

Individual level interventions—individual prisoners

Prison healthy living centre

Conducted by the charity Rethink, healthy living centres provide a 12-week course for young offenders while in custody. The course aims to improve prisoners' general health and mental wellbeing by providing them with the skills and the ability to understand the implications of their behaviour on their health and realise how they can change their health behaviours.

The course, which has been successfully undertaken at Swinfen Hall Prison, takes a holistic approach and involves several aspects:

- regular physical exercise
- participation in education, working or training
- access to art and music
- antibullying strategies
- relationship and team building
- depression prevention

- cognitive behavioural therapies (CBT)
- spiritual reflection
- aromatherapy
- relaxation and meditation skills

By considering these aspects, the offenders are encouraged to consider their motivation, potential barriers and actions, which will be needed to maintain good mental health.

This individual-level intervention uses psychological-based theories such as CBT. CBT emphasises the importance of internal thoughts on our behaviour, and it is widely recognised that CBT can benefit individuals who suffer from mental health conditions. This therapy is recognised as adaptable to the prison setting and can be used as an effective treatment for common mental health problems in prison (Yoon, Slade & Fazel, 2017). Many interventions within the prison setting use CBT for rehabilitation programmes as it helps the individual resolve their personal problems, increase their self-efficacy and, therefore, achieve inner goals and expectations. Beyond the issue of mental health, using CBT in prisons to help inmates quit smoking is one example that has been effective in improving physical health, particularly when used in conjunction with nicotine replacement therapy (Andrade & Kinner, 2017).

With CBT, prisoners can be made aware of the consequences of their behaviour and how it will affect their life and health. They learn to retrain the relationship between thoughts and behaviour (Figure 11.1). The importance of using psychological-based models in the prison population can have many advantages, such as reducing recidivism (Beaudry et al., 2021). Psychological models such as risk, need and responsivity can make valuable contributions to understanding and managing criminal behaviour (Douglas & Otto, 2020).

The importance of considering psychological variables concerning the prison population's health, such as those acknowledged within CBT, has been demonstrated. Much research has considered the link between health and psychological factors in the general population; however, less is known about such relationships within the prison community. Research has explored the relationship between the physical health of

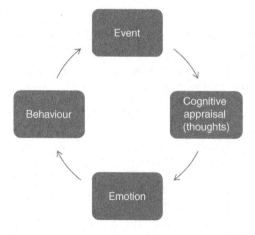

Figure 11.1 Basic cognitive behaviour model.

prisoners and optimism. In doing so, it was discovered that prisoners' optimism levels are related to physical health concerns—the higher the optimism, the fewer physical health concerns (Heigel et al., 2010). Likewise, more recent research on Australian prisoners has shown that poor self-rated mental health status is a significant predictor of poor physical health (Ross et al., 2019). The researchers note that despite including specific measures of suicidal ideation/self-harm (PHQ-9 and GAD-7), only the single-item question asking 'in general, how would you rate your mental health?' was a significant predictor of poor physical health. Research has yet to define the specific aspect of psychological distress associated with reduced physical health. Nevertheless, in the context of Heigel et al. (2010) findings, this highlights the importance of considering optimism as a psychological variable within interventions that aim to improve the health of prisoners.

Smoking in prisons

In many countries, the leading causes of death and disease in prisons are conditions related to smoking (World Health Organization, 2021). Within the UK, prisoners can smoke within their cells, and inmates who smoke do not share cells with inmates who do not smoke. There is a debate on introducing a smoking ban in UK prisons. This would reflect current smoke-free legislation of English young offender institutes, which introduced the ban in 2007. Currently, prisons in the USA, Canada, Sweden, New Zealand and the Isle of Man are all smoke-free (ASH, 2010). It is believed that introducing smoke-free prisons would benefit in many ways, such as:

- helping prisoners to quit
- reducing inmates' and prison officers' exposure to second-hand smoke
- improving health and safety within prisons by reducing the chances of fires
- reducing costs.

Public Health England has highlighted its work as a World Health Organization Collaborating Centre and reflected on its efforts to meet the United Nations Minimum Standard Rules for the Treatment of Prisoners in its annual review. Public Health England was asked to present evidence on prison health care by the National Partnership Agreement in England. One of the achievements highlighted in the review was the delivery of smoke-free prisons in England and Wales, with the final two prisons becoming smoke-free in April 2018. This achievement was reached with a partnership approach between the HM Prison and Probation Service, NHS England and Public Health England. The use of e-cigarettes and vaping devices in prisons has significantly reduced tobacco-smoking behaviour among prisoners, with over 65,000 vaping products sold weekly in prison canteens. The programme can potentially reduce harmful tobacco-smoking behaviour in prison and in the community as people return from prison. However, as seen in Chapter 8, using e-cigarettes as a smoking cessation device is controversial because there is no conclusive evidence regarding their long-term safety and efficacy in helping individuals quit smoking.

As this is still a relatively new area of research, evaluation of total smoke-free legislation in prisons is scarce. Research conducted among prisoners who have been part of smoke-free legislation provides promising and concerning results. A smoke-free prison policy (SFPP) was introduced in Scottish prisons in 2018 to address concerns about occupational exposure to second-hand smoke and tobacco-related harm among people in custody (PiC). A study by Brown et al. (2001) aimed to evaluate the SFPP from the perspectives of people living and working in prisons. Focus groups and interviews were conducted with staff (n = 99) and PiC (n = 23) 6 to 9 months post-implementation of the SFPP, and data were analysed using the framework approach. The study found that the new smoking restrictions were widely accepted by PiC, with benefits for the safety and comfort of staff, PiC who were no longer exposed to second-hand smoke and the health of PiC who were now smoking-abstinent. However, difficulties managing without tobacco and using alternatives were reported as drawbacks of the SFPP. Contraband tobacco was not reported as a major problem after prisons became smoke-free. The study highlights the need for careful planning, partnership working and support for smokers when implementing SFPPs. Overall, the findings suggest that SFPPs can be implemented without causing major disruption and may interest jurisdictions considering smoke-free rules in prisons. Although introducing this to the UK may have many positive results, the potential consequences must also be considered. These consist of the possibility of disorder between inmates and the rise in contraband. In Australian prisons, smoking bans are becoming the norm. However, there are concerns that enforced bans could lead to black markets in tobacco and other smokable substances and an escalation of violence (Butler & Yap, 2015). Moreover, banning smoking outright has been ineffective in reducing smoking rates among this population, as relapse rates are high after release. The conflicting views highlight the need for future research that addresses the health, behavioural and managerial implications of abiding by a ban.

Applying this to Julie

As a result of her childhood experiences, Julie has a very negative view of herself and suffers from depression. Julie would benefit from undertaking CBT in an attempt to help her with the depression and understanding how her childhood experiences have impacted her behaviour.

Community level interventions—the prison as a whole

In 2002, a whole-prison approach to health promotion in prisons was considered necessary (Department of Health, 2002). The whole-prison approach incorporated three main aims:

- Impacting the mental, physical and social health of prisoners and staff.
- Helping prevent any deterioration in prisoners' health while in custody or as a result of being in custody.
- Helping prisoners adopt healthy behaviours that can be translated to the community upon release.

The issues to be addressed under this approach can vary from healthy eating to drug abuse and include a basis of five key areas (mental health promotion and wellbeing, smoking, healthy eating and nutrition, healthy lifestyles [including sex and relationships] and active living, and drug and other substance misuse). In implementing this approach, it is possible to address prisoner's physical needs and important psychological issues related to their behaviour. These can stem from classic behaviourism and can have implications for future behaviour. One such influence on behaviour is thought to be self-efficacy. As previously outlined in Chapter 4, self-efficacy is individuals' beliefs regarding their ability to perform specific behaviours. This is considered an important factor to consider concerning health behaviours (Farley, 2020).

Research has supported the notion of self-efficacy amongst prisoners and concluded that the prison population has varying levels of self-efficacy in managing their health while in prison. In addition, correlations were found between high levels of self-efficacy and engagement in health-promoting and health-monitoring behaviour (Loeb et al., 2011). This research highlights the importance of considering self-efficacy in relation to the prison population's health.

Inmates must understand the importance of health and health management in prison and for transference to the community setting upon release. Therefore, prisons may need to consider assessing self-efficacy upon detention or using health-related self-efficacy scales when attempting to tackle health issues. In applying a whole-system, community approach that acknowledges self-esteem, it is possible that all the work will help improve individuals' health-related behaviour inside and outside of prison.

A whole-systems approach in prison helps create a supportive environment for that specific behavioural change. An evaluation of a whole-systems community approach towards oral health was undertaken in a Scottish prison. The project being evaluated (The Oral Health Improvement Project) aimed to influence knowledge, attitudes and behaviours concerning oral health. It was also hoped that the project would benefit the inmates and transfer to the families of the inmates and the prison staff. Mixed results were seen, and it was concluded that some staff gained knowledge, whereas the prisoners were seen to gain knowledge and a change in attitude as a result of the intervention. However, this did not result in a change in oral health-related behaviours (Akbar et al., 2012). Whole-system approaches must be developed that result in behaviour change if health is to be influenced.

Applying this to Julie

Julie may have low self-efficacy concerning changing her behaviour. In addition, there is a suggested link between low self-efficacy and depression. Therefore, improving her self-efficacy could impact Julie's mental health.

Working effectively with others

A multidisciplinary team must be employed to have a healthy prison; this will enable all the health needs of the prisoners to be addressed in the best possible way. One way of bringing different agencies together to impact prisoners' health is to conduct a health care needs assessment for the prison. As a result, various professionals, such as psychologists, GPs, nurses and health care staff, work effectively together to assess and impact health needs. In doing so, new strategies to address health issues can be implemented (Norris et al., 2022). The fusion of care and custody can often be complex, with goals often being met by crossing professional boundaries; however, effective communication and an effective multidisciplinary relationship can ensure stability and suitable care for prisoners (Mullins, 2012).

Mentors

Mentoring can provide individuals who are either in prison or newly released with much-needed support. This support could help impact crime rates, incarceration rates and health. Mentors can be used as a support mechanism to help prisoners adapt to life in the community while providing support throughout the transition from prison to the community. The mentoring system has been set up in various areas within the UK and is considered invaluable in changing the lives of offenders. A systematic review by Bagnall et al. (2015) examined the effectiveness and cost-effectiveness of peer education and peer support interventions in prisons. The authors conducted a comprehensive search of relevant studies and found that peer education and support programmes in prisons can improve various health outcomes for prisoners, including mental health, substance use and human immunodeficiency virus prevention. Peer-led interventions were also found to be more cost-effective than interventions led by professionals. The authors concluded that peer education and support can be a valuable strategy for promoting health and wellbeing among prisoners and recommended further research to explore the best ways to implement and sustain these programmes in correctional settings.

Nacro is the biggest crime reduction charity in the UK and supports vulnerable individuals who are likely to resort to crime if unsupported. The service has several focus areas, including prevention, offender management and resettlement. Tackling these three main areas is thought to impact both the individual and community levels by, for example, reducing crime rates and improving the health and wellbeing of offenders and the general public (http://www.nacro.org.uk/).

Mentors can be a member of a public agency such as Nacro, a family member or a peer. In addition to providing individuals with general support, mentors can also help to influence individuals' cognitive processes. This can include impacting personal attributes such as self-esteem and interpersonal traits, which are thought to contribute to criminal behaviour.

Applying this to Julie

It would be helpful for Julie to receive health care interventions while in prison, considering that she has been struggling with psychological issues and has not prioritised her physical health in the past. It is important to support her in maintaining good health and ultimately encouraging a change in attitude towards her health. This change could include attending regular health and dental check-ups to ensure she has a healthy future with her daughter and grandchild.

Illicit drug use

Case study

Duane is a 20-year-old man who lives with his girlfriend in their shared flat. Currently, he is working as a dustbin man for the local council. His parents had high hopes for him as he achieved 11 GCSEs at A* level. However, following this success, he became more involved in cannabis (he had previously been involved in glue sniffing and some alcohol abuse) and was eventually expelled from school for attempting to sell cannabis to his peers. Since his days at school, he has always used cannabis, drunk alcohol regularly and been a heavy smoker; he has also developed a cocaine habit. Despite his assurances, his girlfriend feels his drug habit affects his job and their social life. She has threatened to leave him and has given him a final ultimatum.

Duane has started acting strangely and is under investigation at work for some recent bizarre behaviour and poor timekeeping. However, Duane is struggling to deal with the pressures of working regularly and has started increasing his drug intake. Further, he has started selling drugs at a local drug haunt, as he is finding it difficult to fund his drug taking on his current salary. He goes to the local pub most nights, where he meets his mates before returning to either their flat or his own to take drugs into the early hours. Although this is a habit that Duane has tried to manage on several occasions, he always seems to be drawn back to the same circle of friends and ends up on a downward spiral. His girlfriend has come to you in tears and wants support and advice—how can she help Duane?

Introduction

In a 2020/22 survey, 35.3% of UK adults reported having taken illegal drugs during their lifetime and 2.7% in the last year (ONS, 2022). The proportion of people aged between 16 and 24 who had taken drugs in the last year was 18.6%, the lowest level since measurement began in 1996. In addition, the use of Class A drugs in the last year among the same age group has remained stable since 1996 and stands at around 3%. Other figures indicate that the most frequently used drug by adults is cannabis (ONS, 2022).

Although drug use has either remained stable or decreased over recent years, there has been a reported rise in hospital admissions in England as a result of drug poisoning in the 10 years between 2008 and 2018, with figures rising by 48.9% (see Table 11.3; Friebel & Maynou, 2022). In addition, it is also estimated that the highest number of drug-related hospital admissions in 2011/12 was seen in the 25–34 age group, and almost three times as many males were admitted to hospitals with drug-related mental health or behavioural disorders than females (Health and Social Care Information Centre, 2012). Australian statistics between 2019 and 2020 saw 62,757 drug-related hospitalisations (172 per day), with males accounting for 52% of incidences. The highest number of drug-related hospital admissions was seen in the 20–39 age group. Sadly, the majority of drug-related poisonings (62%) were intentional. This suggests a concerning trend of intentional harm related to

Table 11.3 Drug poisoning hospital related admissions

Year	Total (1000s)
2012/13	15.580
2013/14	17.864
2014/15	17.658
2015/16	18.128
2016/17	16.791
2017/18	17.031
2018/19	18.053
2019/20	16.994

Source: NHS: Statistics on Drug Misuse, England 2020.

drug use, which may require a different approach to prevention and intervention efforts than if most cases were accidental.

It goes without saying that individuals who take illicit drugs face potentially significant health risks—the drugs taken are often not controlled or supervised by professionals, and those that are sold 'on the streets' are of variable quality, strength and origin. As well as the immediate health risks, drugs can lead to long-term addiction, health damage and death.

Drug-related deaths often attract significant political and media attention. The ONS (ONS) produces mortality statistics for drug-related deaths based on information on death certificates (see Table 11.4), and these indicate 4,393 deaths related to substance misuse in 2019 in England and Wales.

These deaths are, of course, relatively low and significantly less than those caused by either alcohol or smoking (see Chapters 7 and 8). Nonetheless, they are avoidable and significant to individual families and friends. Obviously, the consequences of substance misuse are not restricted to death, and health may be impacted differently depending on the drugs being used (see Table 11.5). However, what is clear is that all illicit drug use is associated with significant morbidity.

In addition to the link between substance use, mortality and morbidity, it is also important to recognise the relationship between illicit drug use and other risky health behaviours. For example, associations have been identified between drug use and risky sexual behaviours (Hines et al., 2020). Consequently, it is understood that drug use can harm the cessation of additional risky behaviours, such as smoking (González-Roz et al., 2019). Acknowledging the associations between drug use and other risky health behaviours challenges reducing drug use and other risky behaviours in complex ways.

Interventions to reduce illicit drug use and subsequent risky health behaviours

The UK Government's 10-year drug plan to cut crime and save lives is built upon previous strategies and aims to reduce overall drug use to a 30-year low by reducing drug supply and increasing the number of people receiving addiction treatment. The plan is supported by £900 million of funding and is the government's response to the independent reviews of drugs led by Dame Carol Black. The plan focuses on three priorities: breaking drug supply chains, building a world-class treatment and recovery system, and reducing the demand for recreational drugs (GOV.UK, 2022).

Table 11.4 Number of drug-related poisonings, England and Wales, deaths 2010–2021

Substance	2021	2020	2019	2018	2017	2016	2015	2014	2013	2012	2011	2010
All drug poisoning deaths	4,859	4,561	4,393	4,359	3,756	3,744	3,674	3,346	2,955	2,597	2,652	2,747
New psychoactive substances	258	137	125	126	62	123	114	82	63	56	31	23
Cathinones	16	6	14	16	7	31	49	27	26	18	6	6
Mephedrone	4	3	1	2	1	15	44	22	18	12	5	6
GHB	14	28	27	27	17	30	26	20	18	13	20	12
Benzodiazepine analogues	171	62	26	9	9	10	11	14	3	4	2	0
Methiopropamine	0	0	0	1	0	10	6	7	4	2	0	0
Alpha-methyltryptamine	0	0	0	0	0	0	5	6	7	4	0	0
Benzofurans	0	0	0	0	0	3	2	5	7	3	0	0
Novel amphetamines	0	7	1	3	0	1	1	4	3	1	0	0
Novel opiates	3	1	1	13	2	3	2	4	0	0	0	0
Piperazine derivatives	0	1	0	0	0	0	0	2	1	9	2	6
NBOMes	0	0	0	0	0	1	1	2	0	0	0	0
Synthetic cannabinoids	69	53	56	60	25	27	8	5	0	1	0	0
Other specified NPS	8	2	2	0	2	19	14	5	5	7	1	0

Source: ONS (2022).

Table 11.5 Illicit drug use and health consequences

Drug	Consequences
Heroin and morphine	Short-term effects include a surge of euphoria followed by alternately wakeful and drowsy states and cloudy mental functioning. Associated with fatal overdose and, particularly in users who inject the drug, infectious diseases such as HIV/AIDS and hepatitis
Cocaine (including crack)	A powerfully addictive drug, cocaine usually makes the user feel euphoric and energetic. Common health effects include heart attacks, respiratory failure, strokes and seizures. Large amounts can cause bizarre and violent behaviour. In rare cases, sudden death can occur on the first use of cocaine or unexpectedly thereafter
Club drugs (the most common club drugs include GHB, Rohypnol, ketamine, methamphetamine)	Chronic use of MDMA may lead to changes in brain function. GHB abuse can cause coma and seizures. High doses of ketamine can cause delirium, amnesia and other problems. Mixed with alcohol, Rohypnol can incapacitate users and cause amnesia
Cannabis	Short-term effects include memory and learning problems, distorted perception, and difficulty thinking and solving problems
LSD	Unpredictable psychological effects. With large enough doses, users experience delusions and visual hallucinations. Physical effects include increased body temperature, heart rate and blood pressure; sleeplessness; and loss of appetite
Ecstasy	Short-term effects include feelings of mental stimulation, emotional warmth, enhanced sensory perception and increased physical energy. Adverse health effects can include nausea, chills, sweating, teeth clenching, muscle cramping and blurred vision
PCP/Phencyclidine	Many PCP users are brought to emergency rooms because of overdose or because of the drug's unpleasant psychological effects. In a hospital or detention setting, people high on PCP often become violent or suicidal

Consequently, the strategy aims to reduce the prevalence of drugs on our streets and the number of current drug users using effective treatment and support in a whole-system approach. Although a whole-system approach is adopted, the relationship between drug use and other risky health behaviours is not addressed. Addressing other risky health behaviours to stop or prevent their uptake can be important when considering treatments. The following sections will address how interventions can be used with individuals taking drugs to ensure that other health behaviours are not increased.

Assessment of drug use

The most effective way to assess a potential client is through an interview (or self-administered tool). One survey employs a mnemonic that refers to attempts to Cut down on drinking, Annoyance with criticisms about drinking, Guilt about drinking and using alcohol as an Eye-opener. Although several questionnaires are available, the CAGE questionnaire (Ewing, 1984) is the most practical for health care professionals to use as a screening tool.

The CAGE questionnaire consists of four questions that examine the respondent's *own feelings* regarding their drinking habits to make a diagnosis. The health practitioner asks the respondents if they have ever *felt* that they should cut down on the amount they regularly drink, been annoyed by other people's criticisms of their drinking habits, felt guilty about how much they drink or felt the need to have a drink first thing in the morning to face the day. Each question has a score of 0 for no and 1 for yes. A score of 2 or more is considered clinically significant and worthy of further investigation.

Although initially designed for alcohol, the CAGE questionnaire has been adapted for other drugs (see Table 11.6) and individuals with substance abuse (Couwenbergh et al., 2009). The CAGE-AID questionnaire is a screening tool to identify potential substance abuse and dependence, including illicit and prescription drug use. The questionnaire includes four questions about cutting down drug use, annoyance from criticism, guilt about drug use and use of drugs first thing in the morning (Edwards et al., 2023). Patients who answer yes to two or more of these questions should be further assessed for substance use problems. As this tool can be used with both drug and alcohol concerns, it is useful when considering other risky behaviours that may increase or develop while drug use and abuse are being addressed. The questionnaire takes approximately 1 minute to complete and can be a screening tool to ensure the health care professional is prompted to look further at the client's behaviour and develop appropriate therapies based on psychological principles (see Table 11.7).

The normal cut-off for the CAGE is two positive answers, although if one is positively responded to, then this may suggest the health care professional should review behaviour. The problem's severity can be assessed using the Drug Abuse Screening Test, and screening for the risk of harm to oneself or others is recommended (Assanangkornchai & Edwards, 2021). It is also advised to assess injecting behaviour to determine health risks.

The CAGE questionnaire does not differentiate between current and former problems, and it detects alcoholism more accurately than problem drinking. However, it is reported as being 60–90% sensitive when two or more questions are positive and 40–60% specific for excluding substance abuse (Mersy, 2003).

Table 11.6 CAGE questions adapted to include drugs (CAGE-AID)

1.	Have you ever felt you ought to cut down on your drinking or drug use?
2.	Have people annoyed you by criticising your drinking or drug use?
3.	Have you felt bad or guilty about your drinking or drug use?
4.	Have you ever had a drink or used drugs first thing in the morning to steady your nerves or to get rid of a hangover (eye-opener)?

Source: Brown and Rounds (1995).

Table 11.7 A brief summary of the main psychological therapies used in treating substance misuse

Behavioural therapy (BT)	A structured therapy focusing on changing behaviour and the environmental factors that trigger maladaptive behaviour. *Includes:*
Cue exposure treatment (CET)	A structured treatment involving exposure to drug-related cues that have been associated with past drug use without consumption of the drug. This is intended to lead to a reduction (or habituation) of reactivity to drug cues and hence to a reduced likelihood of relapse
Community reinforcement approach (CRA)	A behavioural approach that focuses on what the client finds rewarding in their social, occupational and recreational life. It aims to help them change their lifestyle and social environment to support long-term changes in behaviour whereby using substances is less rewarding than not using them
Contingency management (CM)	Also known as voucher-based therapy, this aims to encourage adaptive behaviour by rewarding the client for attaining agreed goals (e.g., no use of illicit drugs as checked by urine screens) and not rewarding them when these goals are unmet (e.g., illicit drug use). Vouchers can usually be exchanged for consumer goods
Cognitive therapy (CT)	A structured therapy using cognitive techniques (e.g., challenging a person's negative thoughts) and behavioural techniques (e.g., behavioural experiments; activity planning) to change maladaptive thoughts and beliefs. *Includes:*
Cognitive behavioural therapy (CBT)	A combination of both cognitive and behavioural therapies
Relapse prevention (RP)	Uses several CBT strategies to enhance the client's self-control and prevent relapse. It highlights problems that the client may face and develops strategies they can use to deal with high-risk situations
Motivational interviewing (MI)	A focused approach aiming to enhance motivation for changing substance use by exploring and resolving the individual's ambivalence about change
Motivational enhancement therapy (MET)	A brief intervention based on MI which also incorporates a 'check-up' assessment and feedback
Twelve-step approaches	Interventions used by self-help organisations like Alcoholics Anonymous. They are based on a philosophy that adopts an illness model and sees substance use as stemming from an innate vulnerability. An individual must acknowledge their addiction and the harm it has caused to themselves and others; they must also accept their lack of control over use and thus the only acceptable goal is abstinence
Other approaches	The involvement of partners and family through marital and family therapy builds on the known social context of substance use. There are also various forms of counselling, group therapy and milieu therapy

If needed, an even shorter questionnaire is the conjoint screening test, which involves only two questions:

- In the past year, have you ever drunk or used drugs more than you meant to?
- Have you felt you wanted or needed to cut down on your drinking or drug use in the past year? (Brown et al., 2001)

At least one positive response detects current substance use disorders with nearly 80% sensitivity and specificity.

If the patient denies use, you can acknowledge their wise choice by abstaining from drugs. However, it is necessary to continue to screen, ideally at each encounter. In some situations, patients may deny use, but a constellation of signs and symptoms suggests abuse. In this case, it may be prudent to rescreen frequently or conduct specific blood/urine/hair testing.

Individual level interventions

Stages of change model

On an individual basis, if a patient has shared with you that they are abusing illicit drugs (after you have asked them) but are not ready to take the next step of comprehensive assessment and treatment through a professional programme, then it is useful to turn to the Stages of Change (SoC) model developed by Prochaska et al. (1992). As discussed in previous chapters (e.g., how the SoC can be applied to smoking interventions in Chapter 8), the five SoCs can be used to guide both the patient and the practitioner, and these will be discussed in the intervention section after we have first explored why people take drugs. It is useful in both the Assessment and the Advise sections. Although this model has been discussed extensively elsewhere in this book, it is worth recapping this and demonstrating how it can be applied to drug misuse:

1 *Pre-contemplation*: the patient is not considering change during the pre-contemplation stage.

- They do not believe it is necessary.
- They do not know or understand the risks involved.
- They have unsuccessfully tried many times to quit, so they have given up and do not want to try again.
- They have gone through withdrawal before and fear the process or its effects on their body.
- They feel strongly that no one is going to tell them what to do with their body.
- They have a mental illness and do not have a good grasp of what using drugs and alcohol means, even when information is given to them.
- They have family members or partners whom they depend on who use. They may not contemplate changing when everyone else continues to use.

The individual in pre-contemplation may present as resistant, reluctant, resigned or rationalising.

Presentation	What the patient is saying	Health care professional response
Resistant	Don't tell me what to do.	Work with the resistance. Avoid confrontation by giving facts about what drugs and alcohol will do to them. Ask what they know about the effects, ask permission to share what you know and ask their opinion of the information. This

(Continued)

		exchange often leads to reduced resistance and allows for a more open dialogue.
Reluctant	I don't want to change; there are reasons.	Empathise with the real or possible results of changing. It is possible to give strong medical advice to change and still empathise with possible negative outcomes. Guide them towards problem-solving.
Resigned	I can't change, I've tried.	Instil hope and explore barriers to change. Increase self-efficacy and confidence. Provide small steps with achievable goals.
Rationalising	I don't use that much.	Decrease discussion. Listen rather than responding to the rationalisation. Respond to the patient by empathising and reframing their comments to address the conflict of wanting to be healthy and not knowing whether using is causing harm.

2 *Contemplation:* The patient is ambivalent about changing their behaviour. They can think of the positive reasons to change but are also very aware of the negative aspects of change. In this stage, it is important to provide the health benefits of changing their behaviour (as discussed earlier in the chapter). There is a need to help the patient explore goals for health and problem-solve how to deal with the negative aspects of abstinence.

3 *Preparation:* Patients are exploring options to assist their process of change. They may be experimenting by cutting down or have been able to quit for one or more days. Although their ambivalence is lessening, it is still present and may increase when they are challenged by those around them, triggered by the environment or under other types of stress they have handled by using in the past. The health care professional should acknowledge the individual's strengths in reaching this stage but simultaneously anticipate problems and pitfalls to change and assist the patient in generating their plan for obtaining abstinence. Health care professionals should problem-solve with patients regarding barriers to success.

4 *Action:* The patient has stopped using drugs and/or alcohol, and their success needs to be celebrated. Offer to be available for assistance if they feel that they want to use drugs/alcohol again.

5 *Relapse:* Relapse is common and should not be thought of as failure but as part of the recovery process. At this stage, the health care professional must discuss triggers, stressors and social pressures that may lead to relapse and help the patient plan for them. At future visits, if relapse has occurred, guide the patient towards identifying what steps they used to quit before. Offer hope and encouragement and allow the patient to explore the negative side of quitting and what they can do to deal with those issues. Offer to help find resources to help the patient return to abstinence.

Applying this to Duane

Duane is at the pre-contemplation stage of change and presents as resigned. Therefore, his self-efficacy and confidence must be improved, and any barriers impacting behaviour change must be discussed. In addition, it is also important that Duane is made aware of the consequences of his risky health behaviours, including drug taking, smoking and drinking alcohol. This is a good opportunity for the health care professional to monitor the impact of any change in Duane's drug-taking behaviour upon his other risky behaviours, such as smoking. It is important to be aware that as Duane ceases taking drugs, other risky health behaviours may be undertaken and increased.

An alternative to the SoC model is the behaviour change wheel (BCW). The BCW is a more circular approach that emphasises the multiple factors and complexities that can influence behaviour change, including social, psychological and environmental factors. The BCW is a framework for designing effective behaviour change interventions. It has three layers, with the COM-B (capability, opportunity and motivation) model at the centre. The middle layer of the BCW includes seven policy categories, including communication, regulation and environmental/social planning, which can support intervention implementation. The outer layer of the BCW consists of nine intervention functions, including education, training and environmental restructuring, which can be used to modify behaviour. Rather than a linear progression, the wheel of change model suggests that individuals may move back and forth between stages and that behaviour change is influenced by factors such as self-efficacy, social support and coping strategies. The reliability of the BCW has been examined in two domains of behaviour change, tobacco control and obesity, and it was found to be reliable in characterising interventions in both domains (Michie et al., 2011). However, the BCW is likely useful for other behaviours, such as substance abuse and related behaviours (e.g., Gilchrist et al., 2021; Nielsen & Olsen, 2021).

In terms of illicit drug use, both the SoC and wheel of change models can be useful for understanding the complex behaviour change process. However, the SoC model may be more helpful for identifying an individual's readiness for change, while the wheel of change model may be more useful for understanding the various factors that can influence behaviour change over time.

One of the most important things an individual health care professional can do for someone abusing drugs is to provide some information and education. Although it is a safe assumption that most individuals will have some knowledge of the effects of alcohol and other drugs, it is important to assess this. Ask the patient what they know, fill in the missing pieces and clarify misconceptions. This process is an excellent opportunity to educate the patient about the adverse effects of alcohol/drugs and any other risky health behaviours, and the benefits of stopping them at any time.

Numerous cognitive behavioural approaches have developed an evidence base for treating substance misuse, including the interventions described below.

Contingency management therapies

Contingency management is one form of behavioural therapy in which patients receive incentives for achieving specific behavioural goals. These approaches are based on operant conditioning whereby appropriate behaviour is rewarded with positive consequences and, therefore, more likely to be repeated. Contingency management can be applied to any behaviour that needs to be changed, from drug use to smoking and alcohol use (e.g., Ainscough et al., 2017). These interventions have particularly strong and robust empirical support (Dutra et al., 2008). For example, Petry et al. (2017) demonstrated the efficacy of earning chances to win prizes for adherence to the intervention in addition to longer abstinence rates.

Of course, there are some limitations to contingency management interventions. For example, the intervention's effects tend to reduce after the contingencies are reduced. Second, illicit drug users are responsive to contingency management, and there is, consequently, a need to explore differences in individual responses to behavioural treatment. For example, differences in the effectiveness of contingency management between younger and older drug users have been discovered (Weiss & Petry, 2011). Further, there are some ethical considerations, such as a potential increase in the risk of a gambling relapse, the potentially deceptive nature of prize-based contingency management, the emphasis on individual behaviours over social and structural determinants of health and the failure to address vulnerability and power dynamics (see Gagnon et al., 2021).

Cognitive behaviour and skills-training therapies

Cognitive behaviour approaches, such as relapse prevention, are grounded in social learning theories and principles of operant conditioning. Several meta-analyses and literature reviews have established the value of cognitive behavioural approaches in substance-using populations (e.g., Magill et al., 2019).

Motivational interviewing

Motivational interviewing (MI) approaches have strong empirical support for use in treating alcohol users and smokers (see Chapters 7 and 8). Further, a systematic review by Calomarde-Gómez et al. (2021) found MI effective in achieving abstinence from cannabis in both adult and adolescent populations. It also effectively reduced the frequency and quantity of use in adults but not in adolescents. The review concluded that MI should be included as an essential psychological intervention in treating cannabis use, especially among adults and patients with no prior history of psychotic disorders. In a study on heavy cocaine users, motivational intervention was shown to reduce days of cocaine use by 30%, even amongst those who were not actively seeking help (Brown University, 2009), illustrating the potential benefits of this treatment with individuals who undertake multiple risky health behaviours as the approach is adaptive to other behaviours. However, the research has not always been positive and equivocal results have been found. For example, McCambridge et al. (2008) found no differences in outcome between MI and offering drug information and advice among over 300 adolescents.

The National Institute for Health and Clinical Excellence (NICE, 2007) issued guidelines for psychosocial drug misuse interventions. They recommended using psychosocial interventions to treat people who misuse opioids, stimulants and cannabis in the health care and criminal justice systems. There were several key priorities for implementation:

- *Brief interventions:* Opportunistic brief interventions focused on motivation should be offered to people in limited contact with drug services (e.g., those attending a needle and syringe exchange or primary care settings) if concerns about drug misuse are identified by the service user or staff member.

- *Self-help:* Staff should routinely provide people who misuse drugs with information about self-help groups. These groups should normally be based on 12-step principles.
- *Contingency management:* Drug services should introduce contingency management programmes. The programme should offer incentives (usually vouchers that can be exchanged for goods or services of the service user's choice, or privileges such as take-home methadone doses) contingent on each presentation of a drug-negative test (e.g., free from cocaine or non-prescribed opioids).
- *Contingency management to improve physical health care:* For people at risk of physical health problems (including transmittable diseases) resulting from drug misuse, material incentives (e.g., shopping vouchers of up to £10 in value) should be considered to encourage harm reduction.

It should be noted that NICE has published guidelines on drug misuse since 2007, with an updated version released in 2017. However, the updated version does not cover psychosocial interventions. The 2017 NICE guidelines on drug misuse recommend that pharmacological treatments, such as methadone and buprenorphine, should be considered as first-line options for opioid detoxification. However, the guidelines also highlight the importance of psychosocial interventions as an integral part of managing drug dependence. Overall, the 2017 guidelines reflect a shift towards a more person-centred approach to managing drug dependence, with a greater focus on recovery-oriented care and the use of evidence-based pharmacological treatments.

Community level interventions

The Theory of Planned Behaviour

The Theory of Planned Behaviour and Theory of Reasoned Action (TRA) have been applied to using illicit drugs, as have other such models. The TRA proposes that an individual's substance abuse behaviours are based on intentions determined by attitudes and perceived social norms regarding substance use (see Chapter 4). Further, the TRA suggests that attitudes are determined by perceived costs and benefits and the affective value placed on those consequences (Petraitis et al., 1995). Intervention campaigns that have targeted key TRA variables have proven successful in preventing substance use (Flynn et al., 1994). On this basis, media campaigns that influence attitudes and perceived norms regarding substance misuse have been developed.

Such approaches have used psychological models in a social marketing context, and it is worth exploring the social marketing techniques used for illicit drug taking. Social marketing is the application of commercial sector marketing tools to resolve several social and health problems. The idea dates back to 1951 when Wiebe asked, 'Can brotherhood be sold like soap?' (Wiebe, 1951–1952.) Social marketing thinking is now at the centre of many government health improvement programmes, including reducing illicit drug use. A distinguishing feature of social marketing is that it goes beyond education and awareness-raising and focuses on behaviour. Although outcomes have traditionally been conceptualised in terms of behaviour change, more recent work has expanded this conceptualisation to include preventing certain behaviours, such as using illicit substances (Andreasen, 2006).

'FRANK'

The UK's attempt at reducing drug taking through social marketing is 'Project FRANK', which has been widely advertised using traditional media and the more informal advanced methods preferred by the target audience (i.e., teenagers). The evaluation of such prevention programmes is currently 'very poor' (McGrath et al., 2006). Although no formal evaluation of the FRANK programme's effectiveness in drug reduction has been published, Sumnall and Bellis (2007) suggest that it may be little different from the other social marketing campaigns in the United States and the UK. Although there is evidence that FRANK is well-known, the overall impact on drug taking appears more limited.

In one study, however, researchers adapted an effective peer-led smoking prevention intervention, the Alcohol, Smoking and Substance Involvement Screening Test (ASSIST), to prevent drug use using information from the UK national drug education website *Talk to FRANK*. The ASSIST model is a peer-led smoking prevention intervention that has been adapted for use in preventing illicit drug use. ASSIST stands for 'A Stop Smoking in Schools Trial'. It involves training young people to act as peer supporters or mentors who support and inform their peers about the risks of smoking and how to avoid it. The ASSIST model is based on the idea that young people are more likely to listen to and be influenced by their peers than by adults or authority figures. The study by White et al. (2017) developed two peer-led drug prevention interventions, ASSIST + FRANK and FRANK friends, which were refined and tested in 12 high schools in South Wales. The schools were randomly assigned to receive ASSIST + FRANK, FRANK friends, ASSIST or no intervention. A survey was conducted to measure drug use, and interviews were conducted with school staff, parents and young people to explore their views on the interventions. The results showed that both interventions were feasible and acceptable, with FRANK friends being viewed more positively than ASSIST + FRANK. Although the study was not designed to prove whether either intervention prevented drug use, the research suggested that a larger study should be conducted to examine the effectiveness of FRANK friends in preventing illicit drug use in young people.

Moreover, Sumnall and Bellis (2007) suggested that such campaigns may harm health. They implied that since the campaigns regularly suggest that taking cannabis results in mental health difficulties and affects the 'brain' or 'mind' individuals may begin to believe that they are experiencing such effects. Consequently, Sumnall and Bellis (2007) suggested that cannabis users may suffer 'a motivational, memory loss or even paranoia, not as a direct result of the drug, but through psychological mechanisms induced through high-profile social marketing campaigns that effectively 'sell' such negative 'effects'. Although there is no clear evidence of this, policy makers and health care professionals must be aware of such concerns to deal appropriately with such cases individually.

In addition to the concerns above, it is important to consider the potential harm of using social stigma to deter drug use. Social marketing campaigns that focus on the negative effects of drug use may unintentionally stigmatise individuals who use drugs, leading to further marginalisation and discrimination (Zwick et al., 2020). This approach can also create a barrier to accessing health care services and support essential for promoting positive health outcomes among drug users (Aronowitz & Meisel, 2022). Therefore, policy makers and health care professionals should be mindful of the potential harmful effects of using social stigma to deter drug use and work to implement evidence-based approaches that prioritise harm reduction and support for individuals who use drugs.

Community-level interventions aimed at reducing and preventing the uptake of drug use focus predominantly on these aspects and do not consider the implications of other risky behaviours when promoting behaviour change. It may be considered necessary for such campaigns to acknowledge the potential relationship between risky behaviours. Providing such information to the public might enable individuals to reduce the prevalence of risky behaviour rather than replace their drug-taking behaviour with a different risky behaviour.

Applying this to Duane

Community-level campaigns can make Duane more aware of the potential health consequences of his drug-taking habits. In addition, they could help him realise that he needs some help with his risky health behaviours and that it is okay to seek support.

Working effectively with others

Couples and family treatments

The defining feature of couples and family treatments is that they treat drug-using individuals in the context of family and social systems in which substance use may develop or be maintained. Engaging the individual's social networks in treatment can be a powerful predictor of change, and thus, including family members in treatment may help reduce attrition (particularly among adolescents) and address multiple problem areas (Liddle et al., 2001) (see Box 11.1; also see Horigian et al., 2016 for a more recent study on family-based treatments for adolescent substance use). Reviews of such treatments, including meta-analyses, indicated that these approaches are effective (e.g., Deas & Thomas, 2001). The Department of Education reported that intensive, multi-agency family interventions resulted in 597 families no longer being involved in substance misuse, a 50% success rate (Dixon et al., 2010). Further, according to studies on multidimensional family therapy (MDFT), between 64% and 93% of adolescents who receive this type of therapy report abstinence from substance use at the 1-year mark (Rowe, 2010). In addition, MDFT has been shown to reduce the severity of substance-related impairment at the 1-year post-intake mark, with 93% of young adolescents in MDFT reporting no substance-related problems at the 12-month follow-up. These findings highlight the effectiveness of MDFT in addressing substance misuse and its potential to produce positive outcomes for young people and their families (Liddle et al., 2018).

When abstinence is not possible, harm reduction assists patients in taking steps to reduce use and harm to themselves. Strategies for preventing further harm may include:

- evaluating and referral for any underlying problems (e.g., alcohol use)
- encouraging the patient to keep track of substance use
- decreasing use
- reducing dosage and frequency of use
- recommending reducing their use by one-half each day; if this is not possible, any decrease in use is beneficial

- interspersing use with periods of abstinence
- using a safer drug administration route
- finding a substitute for the substance, for example, a prescribed, safer alternative (methadone)
- avoiding friends who use.

Whichever method is used, it is important to be vigilant to ensure no relapse. Relapse prevention is often based on psychological principles (Menon & Kandesamy, 2018). Relapse prevention is a treatment intervention designed to teach clients a wide range of cognitive and behavioural coping skills to avoid or deal with a brief return to substance use (lapse) or a protracted return to previous levels of use (relapse) following a period of moderation or abstinence.

Applying research in practice

A longitudinal analysis of some risk and protective factors in marijuana use by adolescents receiving child welfare services (Cheng & Lo, 2011). This study examined risk and protective factors in marijuana use by adolescents involved with child welfare services. Records of 1,797 adolescents were extracted from the National Survey of Child and Adolescent Well-Being data set. The results showed that 1 out of 10 adolescents reported using marijuana in the past 30 days. An adolescent's likelihood of being a current marijuana user increased with prior lifetime use of the drug. The findings also demonstrated that among adolescents, parental monitoring and closeness to parents, engagement with school environment and out-of-home services deterred current marijuana use.

Applying this to Duane

Duane's support system must come together and involve themselves in any methods used to help him overcome his drug use. Having the support of loved ones could be crucial in his recovery journey, and it is important for everyone involved to work together towards his wellbeing.

Learning disabilities

Case study

Nathan is a 33-year-old man who has Down's syndrome. His mother and father are now older, and he lives in sheltered housing with a warden. Although this is the case, he is very independent and likes to go to the shops and care for himself. He does all of his own shopping, cleaning and general household jobs.

Nathan is hard of hearing and has a heart complaint, which requires regular medication and monitoring. Although Nathan is very independent, he occasionally forgets to take his medication and attend his check-ups at the hospital. He is also classed as obese and does not eat a healthy diet.

His parents are increasingly worried that Nathan needs support to help him with daily activities, as each time they visit him, his flat appears ill-kept. They are also concerned about his health, as he has admitted not taking his medicine regularly. His parents are too old and frail to take on the role, even though they want to support him. His parents have come to you for support for Nathan, which will put their minds at ease as they will know that he is looking after himself properly.

Introduction

It is estimated that there are approximately 1.5 million individuals living in England who have learning disabilities (See Table 11.8, Emerson et al., 2011). It is well recognised that individuals who have learning disabilities suffer from poorer health (NICE, 2021). As a result, such individuals are expected to have a life expectancy reduced by up to 25 years (Emerson et al., 2011). This is partly due to difficulties identifying ill health among people with learning disabilities and gaining timely access to appropriate services (Emerson et al., 2011; Turner, 2013). Consequently, introducing annual health checks for people with learning disabilities living in England was suggested (Disability Rights Commission, 2006).

In addition to individuals with learning disabilities having poorer health, it is also thought that an estimated 21% of individuals are known to learning disabilities services. It goes without saying that if such individuals do not make themselves known, they will not be able to get the help and assistance they may need. This fact alone can impact the health outcomes of individuals with learning disabilities.

Emerson and Baines (2011) identified the factors contributing to health inequalities for people with learning disabilities. They are thought to be:

1 increased risk of exposure to social factors affecting our health (social determinates of health), such as unemployment and poorer living conditions
2 increased risk of developing genetically based health problems linked to the learning disability
3 communication difficulties, including poor communication skills
4 poor understanding of and adherence to healthy lifestyle guidelines
5 problems accessing health care and high-quality health care

It is important to understand an individual's views and barriers towards health services alongside the impacts of interventions or policies to improve the health of individuals

Table 11.8 Estimated number of individuals with learning disabilities by gender

Age	Male	Female	Total
0-17	180,487	105,818	286,305
18-80+	529,507	375,249	904,756

Source: Adapted from Emerson et al., 2011.

with learning disabilities. Codling and Macdonald (2011) suggested that the impact of health education was minimal in people with learning disabilities. The authors suggested that although health education was effective, transferring this knowledge to an individual's health was more problematic.

Interventions to improve the health of individuals with learning disabilities

Government policies have acknowledged the importance of providing a fair society for individuals with learning disabilities. Each of the four UK countries has its policies on how the needs of people with learning disabilities should be met. These policies describe a holistic approach to supporting people with learning disabilities to reach their potential and take their place in the community.

The policies aim to improve quality of life and are based on broad themes:

- citizenship
- empowerment
- having choices and making decisions
- having the same opportunities as other people
- having the same rights as other people
- social inclusion.

The UK policies concerning people with learning disabilities are:

England: Department of Health and Social Care (2022): The *National Disability Strategy* outlines the measures that the government will implement to enhance the daily experiences of individuals with disabilities.

Northern Ireland: The aim of the announcement made by the Minister for Communities on 24 September 2020 was to commence work on a suite of new social inclusion strategies, including the Disability Strategy. The Disability Strategy will be developed through a co-design approach, with the department proactively seeking input from deaf and disabled individuals and their representative organisations.

Scotland: Legislation to protect the rights and welfare of disabled people in Scotland has been introduced, including the *Social Care (Self-directed Support) Act 2013*, the *Disabled Persons' Parking Badges (Scotland) Act 2014*, the *Children and Young People (Scotland) Act 2014*, the *Welfare Funds (Scotland) Act 2015*, the *Education (Scotland) Act 2016*, and the *Carers (Scotland) Act 2016*. Equality considerations are integrated into everyday work, and statistics and research evidence on disability are used to identify issues that must be addressed.

Wales: In 2013, the Welsh Government's *Framework for Action on Independent Living* aimed to reduce or eliminate social barriers to promote inclusivity and equality for disabled individuals. The framework identified key priority areas for action, including advice and information, personal care and support, person-centred technology, employment, housing, transport and access to places.

Each policy addresses health needs in various ways but focuses on similar issues:

- promoting collaborative working
- accessing general health services with specialist support
- providing access to information, advocacy, personal care and support, person-centred technology, employment, housing, transport and access to places

- delivering specialist training to general health care staff
- registering individuals with GPs
- offering a personalised health care plan with, in England and Northern Ireland, a specialised health action plan
- completing regular health checks
- creating accessible health promotion materials
- enhancing daily experiences
- promoting inclusivity and equality
- protecting the rights and welfare of disabled people through legislation
- integrating equality considerations into everyday work

This policy will enable such individuals to have the same opportunities as others. Thus, it could be assumed that the health of this population will benefit as government targets work towards this. This assumption is, of course, optimistic.

Individual level interventions

Health checks

Annual health checks for individuals with learning disabilities were recommended in 2006. It is suggested that these health checks benefit the individual in two ways. First, they detect new health concerns, and second, they result in actions to address health needs (Wigham et al., 2022). Although these consultations are potentially beneficial, their uptake is less than 50% (Emerson et al., 2011). More must be done to encourage the uptake of this service to improve the health of individuals with learning disabilities and reduce health inequalities in this group. Research should consider the effectiveness of promoting such services to increase attendance.

Social learning theory

As previously mentioned in chapters throughout this book, social learning theory can improve individuals' health irrespective of whether the individual has a learning disability or not. In people with a learning disability, carers and family surrounding the individual must positively model healthy lifestyle behaviours. It is suggested that modelling these behaviours can impact behaviour change (Shoneye, 2012). Conversely, family members and carers can impede healthy living. Individuals with intellectual disabilities may feel pressured to consume unhealthy foods offered by their family, for instance (O'Leary et al., 2018).

Mentors have been shown to be effective in influencing the mentees' lives in many settings, such as foster care (see Poon et al., 2021 for a review). It is suggested that matching the personality traits of individuals with learning disabilities to their mentor enhances the mentor's success in changing or influencing behaviour (Glomb et al., 2006). The effectiveness of peer mentoring as an intervention for enhancing socio-emotional wellbeing and mental health in youth with learning disabilities and attention deficit hyperactivity disorder has also shown promise (Haft et al., 2019). This evidence highlights the significance of fostering robust interpersonal relationships as a protective measure. Mentors could be used to apply social learning theory to health and health-related behaviours for individuals with learning disabilities. This could help promote healthy lifestyles at an individual level.

Person-centred planning

Person-centred planning (PCP) takes a bottom-up approach by placing control with the individual. It enables the patient or client to address the needs they feel are important to them. PCP prioritises individuals with intellectual disabilities in service and support planning, considering their desires and needs to live their lives to the fullest. This approach can potentially increase social inclusion and community involvement and may also improve characteristics such as self-esteem. A study in Dublin analysed the impact of PCP on community participation for adults with severe-profound intellectual disabilities using mixed methods. Results suggest that PCP may improve community participation with appropriate support, including familiar staff and family. However, the lack of these supports can undermine the success of PCP for individuals with complex needs. Regarding health promotion and improving the health of individuals with learning disabilities, it could be suggested that taking an individual stance on health outcomes may be appropriate. Carers and families can work with individuals to develop a PCP approach to their health, which could include goal setting.

Applying this to Nathan

Nathan could benefit from having some support to help him in his daily activities. A mentor could help devise a health action plan and encourage him to have healthy lifestyle behaviours.

Community level interventions

Wellbeing

It has been suggested that promoting wellbeing rather than traditional health promotion could be more effective in improving the health of individuals with learning disabilities (Cardell, 2015). This approach would involve addressing multiple aspects of life, such as skill development and inclusion in the community through positive social networks. These health characteristics are particularly relevant for meeting daily needs, utilising talents, acknowledging goals and promoting a sense of purpose in daily activity. By shifting the focus to wellbeing promotion, direct health benefits could be observed, such as physical and psychological improvements from participation in activity groups like swimming, and a more comprehensive assessment of the needs of this population could be realised. Therefore, there is a need to reassess how health promotion addresses the needs of individuals with learning disabilities.

Learning disability community nurses

Learning disability community nurses provide many services, from health checks to health advice and promotion. It is their role to ensure individuals with learning difficulties within their community receive all the health care they need. They can also assist with routine screening (e.g., health checks) with this population.

> **Applying this to Nathan**
>
> Nathan could make use of local support groups for individuals with learning disabilities. These will not only help improve his weight and overall fitness but also improve his self-esteem.

Working effectively with others

This population is considered more vulnerable than most; therefore, addressing health and wellbeing effectively is important, whether by supporting individuals with learning disabilities within the community or successfully promoting healthy behaviours. Various professionals can provide ongoing support for these individuals regarding health and wellbeing. These may be part of a multidisciplinary Community Learning Disability Team, including:

- doctors
- psychologists
- occupational therapists
- nurses
- dieticians
- physiotherapists
- speech and language therapists.

With access to these professionals, individuals with learning disabilities can receive the best support to live independent, healthy lives. The approach takes the individual through an assessment to discover their needs and then provides the required treatment and support. As the approach is multidisciplinary, it enables the individual to gain access to any service they may need, whether for a physical or mental health problem.

Social workers

Social workers have a wide range of skills and can provide advice on health-related issues in addition to general support. The social work profession aims to enhance the quality of life for individuals, families, groups, communities and society as a whole. This is underpinned by the belief that the wellbeing of individuals and society depends on creating socially inclusive communities that uphold principles of social justice, human dignity and human rights. Social workers aim to impact the general wellbeing of specific groups within the community, such as those with learning disabilities. After completing an assessment, the social worker can work with the individual and their family to suggest services or organisations that may be useful (Sims and Cabrita Gulyurtlu, 2014).

> **Applying this to Nathan**
>
> It may be an appropriate time for Nathan's parents to arrange an assessment with the Community Learning Disability Team. They will enable Nathan to get all the help and support he needs to remain independent.

Turner (2013) stressed the importance of working in partnerships for people with learning disabilities and highlighted the importance of working with:

- the Learning Disability Partnership Board
- self-advocates
- the family carers group
- public health
- social care providers
- local involvement networks.

Older age

Case study

Grace is an 86-year-old woman living in a semidetached house in a small village. She has two children in their 60s, and her husband of 65 years has recently died due to a stroke.

Now that Grace lives alone, her children increasingly worry about her health and safety around the house. They have set up a downstairs bedroom for her so she does not have to climb the stairs, which she now finds nearly impossible. Grace's mobility has rapidly declined, and she now uses a Zimmer frame in the house and an electric wheelchair when she goes out. In addition, her confidence in her ability to go out of the house and even just into her garden has declined. As she now lives alone, she is worried that she could fall while in the garden and there would be nobody to help her.

Grace and her late husband had always been sociable people who regularly met with friends, went on holiday and attended their local bowls club. However, since Grace's husband passed away and her mobility has deteriorated, she is less able to see her friends and spends much time alone at home. Her children are worried about her and would like advice on improving her health and social life.

Introduction

The UK has an ageing population, with the number of individuals over 85 in the UK continually rising. In the most recent census, the population of individuals who were at least 65 years old was over 11 million, which accounts for 18.6% of the total population. This is an increase from the previous census in 2011, where this age group made up only 16.4% of the population. Among those aged 65 or older, more than 527,900 individuals were at least 90 years old (ONS, 2022). The rise in this population creates challenges for the health service and government from both an equality and financial point of view.

The ONS reported that the leading cause of death in individuals aged over 65 is ischaemic heart disease. The number of deaths resulting from ischaemic heart disease in males aged 65 to 79 has decreased from 26.0% in 2001 to 14.8% in 2018, although it remains the leading cause of death in this age group. In females aged 65 to 79 years, ischaemic heart disease was the leading cause of death until 2013, when malignant neoplasm of the trachea, bronchus and lung became the leading cause, accounting for 10.4% of female deaths in this age group in 2018 (ONS, 2020). As people are now living longer, it is even more important to have effective health promotion strategies that address this population's most prominent health issues. Effective health promotion methods that acknowledge this particular group's physical and psychological needs must be used. Interventions and policies should target this specific group and the whole population to increase the healthy living years of all of society. This will ensure productive and healthy years in later life for all.

Interventions to improve the health of older people

Many interventions that target older people are effective (Beswick et al., 2008). If interventions are seen to be effective in improving older people's health and wellbeing, knock-on effects can be seen in relation to nursing home admissions, hospital admissions and individual wellbeing. Below, different types of interventions will be identified and explored.

According to a systematic review by Buyl et al. (2020), e-health interventions could potentially support the wellbeing of ageing populations by empowering older individuals to manage their health by providing them with access to information, resources and tools to help them make informed decisions about their health. The review explores how specific e-health interventions and their characteristics impact healthy ageing. Fourteen studies comparing e-health interventions to controls were included, and the results show that e-health interventions could improve physical activity, healthy behaviours, psychological outcomes and clinical parameters. However, given the low certainty of the evidence related to most outcomes, these results should be interpreted with caution. The article concludes that better quality evidence is needed to determine the effects of e-health on the different dimensions of healthy ageing.

Individual level interventions

Fall prevention

A large proportion of individuals over 65 suffer from falls. These can have serious health implications, such as broken and fractured bones and even mortality. This impacts individuals' health and wellbeing and the economy through hospital and NHS expenditure. Falls present a significant public health concern. Almost a third of those over 65 who live in the community fall at least once a year, with this figure rising to 66.6% for people 80 and over (ONS, 2022). A hip fracture is one of the most serious consequences of a fall. Hip fractures alone result in 1.8 million hospital bed days and cost £1.1 billion annually, not including the substantial cost of social care. Patients who suffer from hip fractures have poor short- and long-term outlooks, with an increased 1-year mortality rate ranging between 18% and 33%. In addition to this, hip fractures also harm daily living activities like walking and shopping. For these reasons, interventions for fall prevention are of utmost importance to older people.

A review by Guirguis-Blake et al. (2018) considered the effectiveness of fall prevention interventions and concluded that benefits can be seen from these interventions. The study encompassed a range of intervention types, including exercise, vitamin D supplementation, modifications to the environment, psychological interventions, medication management, and education and knowledge. These interventions could be delivered singly, as a combination or as a personalised combination of interventions tailored to an individual's baseline assessment results, known as a multifactorial approach. Multifactorial interventions showed a reduction in falls but did not affect other fall-related outcomes. Exercise interventions were associated with a reduction in falls and injuries. Vitamin D supplementation had mixed results, with a high dose associated with increased fall-related outcomes. Overall, exercise interventions had the most consistent evidence for fall-related benefits. One form of exercise that has become increasingly popular with the older generation is Tai Chi. This exercise involves slow movements, which build muscle and aid balancing techniques. Evidence suggests that the benefits of Tai Chi on cognitive functioning may provide a better approach to reducing falls than other types of interventions (Nyman, 2021). In addition to interventions that address the prevention of falls from a physical stance, it is also important to address the psychological components contributing to falls and the fear of falling. As highlighted elsewhere, CBT can effectively treat psychological issues and lifestyle behaviours. As CBT addresses the cognitive thought processes associated with a behaviour, it can be considered useful for addressing the fear of falling in this population. Interventions combining physical and psychological therapy have been shown to be effective in preventing falls and improving quality of life (Tzu-Ting et al., 2011). A protocol is currently under development with the Cochran Database of Systematic Reviews to evaluate the latest research surrounding the benefits and potential harms of CBT in reducing fear of falling among older adults living in the community, either as a standalone treatment or when combined with exercise (Lenouvel et al., 2021).

Fall assessments

In addition to interventions being rolled out, effective assessments are also necessary to consider the individual's risk of falling. The NICE (2013) guidelines states that every individual aged 65 or over who is in contact with a health professional should be assessed (Matarese & Ivziku, 2016). Tools thought to impact the individual successfully have also been developed, enabling fall prevention strategies to be implemented before an incident happens. For instance, Robinson et al. (2019) discuss the development of 'React to Falls' training resources to assist care home staff in managing falls among their residents. Care home residents are more prone to falls than older people living in their own homes, making it a crucial area for care home staff to address. The resources were developed with fall prevention researchers, expert clinicians, care home staff and residents. The objective was to create a freely accessible online and paper-based resource that would cater to the needs of different care home settings.

Applying this to Grace

As Grace is worried about falling in her home and garden, it is necessary to undertake a fall and risk assessment in her home. This will enable potential risks to be identified and managed. In turn, this could help improve Grace's confidence and reduce her fear of falling.

Community level interventions

Public services

To reduce the prevalence of falls, the local council can ensure that public services are kept in the best condition and easily accessible to the older population. This could include ensuring that roads and footpaths are in good condition and level, ensuring transport services are available and taking measures to ensure older people feel safe in their community. An example of one of these measures is introducing tilting buses. These buses can lower the step up to the bus to make it more accessible for older people and individuals who use wheelchairs.

Day centres

These are used to provide social and general support for older people in addition to providing breaks for careers and family members. The centres can provide a range of activities such as arts, crafts, games and physical exercise sessions. In addition to providing social activities, most also provide older people with a meal. In supplying such facilities, the older generation will potentially benefit physically and psychologically.

Physical health can be improved by the activities undertaken; for example, exercise classes to improve muscle strength. Data from the National Institutes of Health-AARP Diet and Health Study found that racquet sports, running and walking for exercise were associated with the greatest relative risk reductions for all-cause mortality among 59–82-year-olds. The social aspect of the event can influence psychological health in addition to the mental stimulation of the brain through games and activities. Psychologically, it is thought that participation in such games and activities is associated with improved subjective wellbeing, even in individuals with notable mental illness (Dobbins et al., 2018). Overall, the sessions provide a vast range of stimulation that may not otherwise be possible. Indeed, participating in exergames as a group can benefit older adults in terms of their recovery and overall health as it can enhance their social integration, boost their confidence and improve their physical wellbeing through exercise.

In addition to these benefits, this time can also be used to educate participants on health awareness and general wellbeing. Sessions could be used to inform older people of any help and resources that may benefit them. Conjointly, day centres can contribute towards individuals' health and wellbeing and can be a useful means of health promotion.

Applying this to Grace

Grace would benefit from finding a local day centre to attend once a week. There, she would have the opportunity to interact and meet new people as she spends a lot of her time alone.

Working effectively with others

NHS falls clinic

Parts of the UK have specific NHS falls clinics. These clinics comprise a multidisciplinary team working with the individual to assess, advise and rehabilitate them either after a fall or to prevent a fall. The teamwork with the individual to understand why they are suffering from falls and how they can prevent them. This can have long-term implications on their health and independence, alongside reducing admissions to accident and emergency departments. The team of professionals can include:

- nurses
- occupational therapists
- physiotherapists
- fall consultants
- doctors
- therapists.

Fall clinics are evident in many countries and have been evaluated to determine their effectiveness. It can be suggested that such clinics successfully prevent falls and injuries related to falls, in addition to improving balance, strength and confidence. A study at the Falls and Fracture Clinic in Nepean Hospital (Penrith, NSW, Australia) assessed a novel combined-care model for preventing osteoporosis and falls among outpatients. The study found that, after a 6-month follow-up, there was a significant reduction of over 80% in falls and recurrent falls, as well as a 50% decrease in fractures (Gomez et al., 2019).

Home fire and safety visits

Older people are entitled to a free home fire and safety visit by the fire service to improve their health and safety. The fire service assesses the individual's home and suggests ways to make it safer. This may mean installing smoke alarms or pointing out any potential fire hazards.

Gym sessions/personal trainers

As the chapter on healthy eating shows, personal trainers can provide a valuable service for the whole population. Older people can have many benefits from exercise sessions; as previously mentioned, this can include strengthening muscles and improving posture, which can influence fall rates. Physical exercise effectively stimulates bone osteogenesis in osteoporotic patients. In a study by Bendetti et al. (2018), the most appropriate exercise features for increasing bone density in these patients were reviewed. Two types of exercises emerged as effective. First, weight-bearing aerobic exercises, such as walking, stair climbing, jogging and Tai Chi, which must reach a mechanical intensity to establish the important ground reaction force. Second are strength and resistance exercises carried out with or without loading to increase muscle mass and bone mineral density in specific body regions. Multicomponent exercises, which combine aerobics, strengthening, progressive resistance, balancing and dancing, seem particularly appropriate for older patients. Whole-body vibration exercises, performed with dedicated devices, have shown promising results in improving balance and reducing the risk of falling. Still, their effects on bone mineral density are controversial, and contraindications typical of senility should be considered. Once again, in addition to the physical benefits, it is also suggested that benefits can be seen in individuals' psychological wellbeing as a result of exercise. Undertaking gym sessions at either an individual or group level can provide a good opportunity to improve and influence the health and wellbeing of the older generation.

> **Applying this to Grace**
>
> Grace may benefit from some form of light physical exercise/training. This could work on strengthening her muscles, impacting her ability to carry out day-to-day activities.

Conclusion

The complex needs of individual segments of the population challenge health care professionals. This chapter has considered some ways in which health promotion can be conducted effectively to promote change in a small review of different population segments. It is apparent, of course, that different groups will not only have different health needs but will also require different approaches and different methods of engagement.

Key points

- It is essential to adapt health interventions to make them effective for all members of the population.
- Understanding the impact of psychological variables within these populations is important in the development and implementation of interventions.
- CBT is a useful tool for behaviour change, especially for psychological issues.
- Working with offenders in prisons offers advantages (e.g., easy access) and disadvantages (e.g., environmental constraints) when attempting behaviour change.
- Illicit drug use has increased recently and has caused numerous potential health concerns.
- Applying the SoC Model and/or MI can change illicit drug use.
- Social marketing programmes for reducing illicit drug use show variable success rates.
- People with learning disabilities have specific health concerns and have greater health issues than others.
- Improving the access and availability of health check-ups for people with a disability would prove beneficial.
- Working with older people to prevent falls can benefit the individual overall.
- Multi-faceted and multidisciplinary approaches to fall prevention in older people can be very effective.

Points for discussion

- Critically discuss the arguments for and against health promotion in the prison setting.
- What health promotion could be delivered to older people in day centres?
- Consider the advantages and disadvantages of targeting special groups for health promotion.
- What psychological variables do you consider important in health promotion within special groups?

Further resources

Talk to Frank—Advise on drugs http://www.talktofrank.com
Improving Health and Lives – IhaL: https://www.ndti.org.uk/projects/improving-health-and-lives-ihal
Age UK—http://www.ageuk.org.uk

References

Ainscough, T. S., McNeill, A., Strang, J., Calder, R., & Brose, L. S. (2017). Contingency management interventions for non-prescribed drug use during treatment for opiate addiction: A systematic review and meta-analysis. Drug Alcohol Dependence, *178*, 318–339. 10.1016/j.drugalcdep.2017.05.028

Akbar, T., Turner, T., Themessl-Huber, M., & Freeman, R. (2012). The evaluation of HMP Shotts' oral health improvement project. Retrieved from http://www.sps.gov.uk

Andrade, D., & de Kinner, S. A. (2017). Systematic review of health and behavioural outcomes of smoking cessation interventions in prisons. Tobacco Control, *26*, 495–501. 10.1136/tobaccocontrol-2016-053297

Andreasen, A. R. (Ed.). (2006). Social marketing in the 21st century. London: Sage.

ASH. (2010). Smokefree prisons. London: ASH.

Aronowitz, S., & Meisel, Z. F. (2022). Addressing stigma to provide quality care to people who use drugs. JAMA Network Open, *5*, e2146980. 10.1001/jamanetworkopen.2021.46980

Assanangkornchai, S., & Edwards, J. G. (2021). Clinical screening for illegal drug use, prescription drug misuse and tobacco use. In N. el-Guebaly, G. Carrà, M. Galanter & A. M. Baldacchino (Eds.), Textbook of addiction treatment: International perspectives (pp. 619–635). Cham, Switzerland: Springer International Publishing. 10.1007/978-3-030-36391-8_43

Bagnall, A. M., South, J., Hulme, C., Woodall, J., Vinall-Collier, K., Raine, G., ... & Wright, N. M. (2015). A systematic review of the effectiveness and cost-effectiveness of peer education and peer support in prisons. BMC Public Health, *15*(1), 1–30.

Barnert, E. S., Dudovitz, R., Nelson, B. B., Coker, T. R., Biely, C., Li, N., & Chung, P. J. (2017). How does incarcerating young people affect their adult health outcomes?. Pediatrics, *139*(2), e20162624. 10.1542/peds.2016-2624

Beaudry, G., Yu, R., Perry, A. E. & Fazel, S. (2021). Effectiveness of psychological interventions in prison to reduce recidivism: A systematic review and meta-analysis of randomised controlled trials. The Lancet Psychiatry, *8*(9), 759–773. 10.1016/S2215-0366(21)00170-X

Benedetti, M. G., Furlini, G., Zati, A., & Letizia Mauro, G. (2018). The effectiveness of physical exercise on bone density in osteoporotic patients. BioMed Research International, *2018*, 4840531. 10.1155/2018/4840531

Beswick, A., Rees, K., Dieppe, P., Ayis, S., Gooberman-Hill, R., Horwood, J., & Ebrahim, S. (2008). Complex interventions to improve physical function and maintain independent living in elderly people: A systematic review and meta-analysis. Lancet, *371*(9614), 725–735.

Brown University (2009). Brief motivational intervention reduces drug use in community-based heavy Cocaine users. London: Wiley Periodicals, Inc.

Brown, R. L., Leonard, T., Saunders, L. A. & Papasouliotis, O. A. (2001). A two item conjoint screen for alcohol and other drug problems. Journal of the American Board of Family Practice, *14*, 95–106.

Brown, R. L., & Rounds, L. A. (1995). Conjoint screening questionnaires for alcohol and other drug abuse: criterion validity in a primary care practice. Wisconsin Medical Journal, *94*(3), 135–140.

Buyl, R., Beogo, I., Fobelets, M., Deletroz, C., Van Landuyt, P., Dequanter, S., Gorus, E., Bourbonnais, A., Giguère, A., Lechasseur, K., & Gagnon, M. P. (2020). e-Health interventions for healthy aging: A systematic review. Systematic Reviews, *9*(1), 128. 10.1186/s13643-020-01385-8

Butler, T. G., & Yap, L. (2015). Smoking bans in prison: Time for a breather? The Medical Journal of Australia, *203*(8), 313. 10.5694/mja15.00688

Calomarde-Gómez, C., Jiménez-Fernández, B., Balcells-Oliveró, M., Gual, A., & López-Pelayo, H. (2021). Motivational interviewing for cannabis use disorders: A systematic review and meta-analysis. European Addiction Research, *27*(6), 413–427. 10.1159/000515667

Cardell, B. (2015). Reframing health promotion for people with intellectual disabilities. Global Qualitative Nursing Research, 2. doi:10.1177/2333393615580305

Cheng, T., & Lo, C. (2011). A longitudinal analysis of some risk and protective factors in marijuana use by adolescents receiving child welfare services. Children & Youth Services Review, *33*(9), 1667–1672.

Codling, M., & Macdonald, N. (2011). Sustainability of health promotion for people with learning disabilities. Nursing Standard, *25*(22), 42–47.

Couwenbergh, C., van der Gaag, R. J., Koeter, M., De Ruiter, C., & Van den Brink, W. (2009). Screening for substance abuse among adolescents validity of the CAGE-AID in youth mental health care. Substance Use & Misuse, *44*(6), 823–834.

Deas, D., & Thomas, S. E. (2001). An overview of controlled studies of adolescent substance abuse treatment. American Journal of Addiction, *10*(2), 178–189.

Department of Health and Social Care. (2022).

Department of Health. (2002). Health-promoting prisons: A shared approach. London, UK: Department of Health.

Disability Rights Commission. (2006). Equal treatment: Closing the gap. Stratford upon Avon, UK: Disability Rights Commission.

Dixon, J., Schneider, V., Lloyd, C., Reeves, A., White, C., Tomaszewski, W., …Ireland, E. (2010). Monitoring and evaluation of family interventions: Information on families supported to March 2010 (Research report DFE-RR044). London, UK: Department of Education.

Dobbins, S., Hubbard, E., Flentje, A., Dawson-Rose, C., & Leutwyler, H. (2018). Play provides social connection for older adults with serious mental illness. Aging & Mental Health, *24*(4), 596–603. 10.1080/13607863.2018.1544218

Douglas, K. S., & Otto, R. K. (Eds.). (2020). Handbook of violence risk assessment (2nd ed.). Camebridge: Routledge. 10.4324/9781315518374

Dutra, L., Stathopoulou, G., Basden, S., Leyro, T., Powers, M., & Otto, M. (2008). A meta-analytic review of psychosocial interventions for substance use disorders. American Journal of Psychiatry, *165*(2), 179–187.

Edwards, T., Arthur, J., Joy, M., Lu, Z., Dibaj, S., Bruera, E., & Zhukovsky, D. (2023). Assessing risk for nonmedical opioid use among patients with cancer: Stability of the CAGE-AID questionnaire across clinical care settings. Palliative & Supportive Care, 1–5.

Emerson, E. and Baines, S. (2011), Health inequalities and people with learning disabilities in the UK. Tizard Learning Disability Review, *16*(No. 1), 42–48. 10.5042

Farley, H. (2020). Promoting self-efficacy in patients with chronic disease beyond traditional education: A literature review. Nursing Open, 7, 30–41. 10.1002/nop2.382

Emerson, E., Copeland, A., & Glover, G. (2011). The uptake of health checks for adults with learning disabilities: 2008/9 to 2010/11. Stockton on Tees, UK: Improving Health and Lives: Learning Disabilities Observatory.

Ewing, J. A. (1984). Detecting alcoholism: The CAGE questionnaire. Journal of the American Medical Association, *252*, 1905–1907.

Flynn, B. S., Worden, J. K., Secker-Walker, R. H., Pirie, P. L., Badger, G. J., Carpenter, J. H., & Geller, B. M. (1994). Mass-media and school interventions for cigarette smoking prevention: Effects 2 years after completion. American Journal of Public Health, *84*, 1148–1150.

Friebel, R., & Maynou, L. (2022). Trends and characteristics of hospitalisations from the harmful use of opioids in England between 2008 and 2018: Population-based retrospective cohort study. Journal of the Royal Society of Medicine, *115*(5), 173–185. 10.1177/01410768221077360

Gagnon, M., Payne, A., & Guta, A. (2021). What are the ethical implications of using prize-based contingency management in substance use? A scoping review. Harm Reduction Journal, *18*, 82. 10.1186/s12954-021-00529-w

Garrido, M., & Frakt, A. B. (2020, February). Challenges of aging population are intensified in prison. In JAMA Health Forum (Vol. 1, No. 2, pp. e200170- e200170). American Medical Association.

Gilchrist, E., Johnson, A., McMurran, M., Stephens-Lewis, D., Kirkpatrick, S., Gardner, B., ... Gilchrist, G. (2021). Using the behaviour change wheel to design an intervention for partner abusive men in drug and alcohol treatment. Pilot and Feasibility Studies, *7*, 191. 10.1186/s4 0814-021-00911-2

Glomb, N. K., Buckley, L. D., Minskoff, E. D., & Rogers, S. (2006). The learning leaders mentoring program for children with ADHD and learning disabilities. Preventing School Failure, *50*(4), 31–35.

Gomez, F., Curcio, C. L., Brennan-Olsen, S. L., Boersma, D., Phu, S., Vogrin, S., ...Duque, G. (2019). Effects of the falls and fractures clinic as an integrated multidisciplinary model of care in Australia: A pre-post study. BMJ Open, *9*, e027013. 10.1136/bmjopen-2018-027013

González-Roz, A., Ruano, L., Aonso-Diego, G., García-Pérez, Á., Weidberg, S., & Secades-Villa, R. (2019). Smoking cessation interventions in substance use treatment facilities: Clinical implications and recommendations for implementation. Adicciones, *31*, 327–328. 10.20882/ adicciones.1270

GOV.UK (2023), Prison population figures. https://www.gov.uk/government/publications/prison-population-figures-2023. Accessed 21st October 2023

GOV.UK (2022). From Harm to Hope: A 10-year drugs plan to cut crime and save lives. https:// www.gov.uk/government/publications/from-harm-to-hope-a-10-year-drugs-plan-to-cut-crime-and-save-lives/from-harm-to-hope-a-10-year-drugs-plan-to-cut-crime-and-save-lives. Accessed 21st October 2023

Guirguis-Blake, J. M., Michael, Y. L., Perdue, L. A., Coppola, E. L., & Beil, T. L. (2018). Interventions to prevent falls in older adults: updated evidence report and systematic review for the US Preventive Services Task Force. JAMA, *319*(16), 1705–1716.

Heigel, C., Stuewig, J., & Tangney, J. (2010). Self-reported physical health of inmates: Impact of incarceration and relation to optimism. Journal of Correctional Health Care, *16*(2), 106–116.

Haft, S. L., Chen, T., LeBlanc, C., Tencza, F., & Hoeft, F. (2019). Impact of mentoring on socio-emotional and mental health outcomes of youth with learning disabilities and attention-deficit hyperactivity disorder. Child and Adolescent Mental Health, *24*(4), 318–328.

Health and Social Care Information Centre. (2012). Statistics on drugs misuse: England, 2012. London: NHS Digital.

Hines, L. A., Trickey, A., Leung, J., Larney, S., Peacock, A., Degenhardt, L., ... Lynskey, M. (2020). Associations between national development indicators and the age profile of people who inject drugs: Results from a global systematic review and meta-analysis. The Lancet Global Health, *8*, e76–e91. 10.1016/S2214-109X(19)30462-0

Horigian, V. E., Anderson, A. R., & Szapocznik, J. (2016). Family-based treatments for adolescent substance use. Child and Adolescent Psychiatric Clinics of North America, *25*, 603–628. 10.1016/ j.chc.2016.06.001

Lenouvel, E., Novak, L., Wirth, T., Denkinger, M., Dallmeier, D., Voigt-Radloff, S., & Klöppel, S. (2021). Cognitive behavioural interventions for reducing fear of falling in older people living in the community. Cochrane Database of Systematic Review, *3*, CD014666. 10.1002/1465185 8.CD014666

Liddle, H. A., Dakof, G. A., Parker, K., Diamond, G. S., Barrett, K., & Tejeda, M. (2001). Multidimensional family therapy for adolescent drug abuse: Results of a randomized clinical trial. The American Journal of Drug and Alcohol Abuse, *27*, 651–688.

Liddle, H. A., Dakof, G. A., Rowe, C. L., Henderson, C., Greenbaum, P., Wang, W., & Alberga, L. (2018). Multidimensional family therapy as a community-based alternative to residential treatment for adolescents with substance use and co-occurring mental health disorders. Journal of Substance Abuse Treatment, *90*, 47–5610.1016/j.jsat.2018.04.011

Loeb, S. J., Steffensmeier, D., & Kassab, C. (2011). Predictors of self-efficacy and self-rated health for older male inmates. Journal of Advanced Nursing, *67*(4), 811–820.

Magill, M., Ray, L., Kiluk, B., Hoadley, A., Bernstein, M., Tonigan, J. S., & Carroll, K. (2019). A meta-analysis of cognitive-behavioral therapy for alcohol or other drug use disorders: Treatment efficacy by contrast condition. Journal of Consulting Clinical Psychology, *87*, 1093–1105. 10.1037/ccp0000447

Matarese, M., & Ivziku, D. (2016). Falls risk assessment in older patients in hospital. Nursing Standard, *30*(48).

McCambridge, J., Slym, R. L., & Strang, J. (2008). Randomized controlled trial of motivational interviewing compared with drug information and advice for early intervention among young cannabis users. Addiction, *103*(11), 1809– 1809.

McGrath, Y., Sumnall, H., Edmonds, K., McVeigh, J., & Bellis, M. (2006). Review of grey literature on drug prevention among young people. London, UK: NICE.

Menon, J., & Kandasamy, A. (2018). Relapse prevention. Indian Journal of Psychiatry, *60*, S473–S478. 10.4103/psychiatry.IndianJPsychiatry_36_18

Mersy, D. J. (2003). Recognition of alcohol and substance abuse. American Family Physician, *67*, 1529–1532.

Michie, S., van Stralen, M. M., & West, R. (2011). The behaviour change wheel: A new method for characterising and designing behaviour change interventions. Implementation Science, *6*, 42. 10.1186/1748-5908-6-42

Mullins, J. (2012). A multidisciplinary approach to mental health care for prisoners. Mental Health Practice, *15*(10), 30–31.

National Institute for Health and Care Excellence. (2013). Falls: Assessment and prevention of falls in older people. NICE Clinical Guideline 161. London: NICE.

NICE. (2007). Drug misuse: Psychosocial interventions. London, UK: NICE.

NICE. (2021). NICE impact people with a learning disability. Retrieved from https://www.nice.org.uk/about/what-we-do/into-practice/measuring-the-use-of-nice-guidance/impact-of-our-guidance/nice-impact-people-with-a-learning-disability

Nielsen, S., & Olsen, A. (2021). Using the behaviour change wheel to understand and address barriers to pharmacy naloxone supply in Australia. International Journal of Drug Policy, *90*, 103061. 10.1016/j.drugpo.2020.103061

Norris, W. K., Allison, M. K., Fradley, M. F., & Zielinski, M. J. (2022). 'You're setting a lot of people up for failure': What formerly incarcerated women would tell healthcare decision makers. Health & Justice, *10*(1), 1–10.

Nowotny, K. M., Rogers, R. G., & Boardman, J. D. (2017). Racial disparities in health conditions among prisoners compared with the general population. SSM—Population Health, *3*, 487–496. 10.1016/j.ssmph.2017.05.011

Nyman, S. R. (2021). Tai chi for the prevention of falls among older adults: A critical analysis of the evidence. Journal of Aging and Physical Activity, *29*, 343–352. 10.1123/japa.2020-0155

O'Leary, L., Taggart, L., & Cousins, W. (2018). Healthy lifestyle behaviours for people with intellectual disabilities: An exploration of organizational barriers and enablers. Journal of Applied Research in Intellectual Disabilities, *31*, 122–135. 10.1111/jar.12396

ONS. (2020). Leading causes of death, UK: 2001 to 2018. London, UK: ONS. Retrieved from https://www.ons.gov.uk/peoplepopulationandcommunity/healthandsocialcare/causesofdeath/articles/leadingcausesofdeathuk/2001to2018.

ONS. (2022). Drug misuse in England and Wales: Year ending June 2022. London, UK: ONS. Retrieved from https://www.ons.gov.uk/peoplepopulationandcommunity/crimeandjustice/articles/drugmisuseinenglandandwales/yearendingjune2022#cite-this-article

ONS. (2022). Voices of our ageing population: Living longer lives. London, UK: ONS. Available from https://www.ons.gov.uk/peoplepopulationandcommunity/birthsdeathsandmarriages/ageing/articles/voicesofourageingpopulation/livinglongerlives

Otudeko, D. T. (2020, 21 August). Mind the gap—Healthcare disparities in UK prisons. Medact. Retrieved from https://www.medact.org/2020/blogs/mind-the-gap-healthcare-disparities-in-uk-prisons/

Petraitis, J., Flay, B. R., & Miller, T. Q. (1995). Reviewing theories of adolescent substance use: Organising piece in the puzzle. Psychological Bulletin, *117*, 67–86.

Petry, N. M., Alessi, S. M., Olmstead, T. A., Rash, C. J., & Zajac, K. (2017). Contingency management treatment for substance use disorders: How far has it come, and where does it need to go? Psychology of Addictive Behaviors, *31*, 897–906. 10.1037/adb0000287

Poon, C. Y. S., Christensen, K. M., & Rhodes, J. E. (2021). A meta-analysis of the effects of mentoring on youth in foster care. Journal of Youth Adolescence, *50*, 1741–1756. 10.1007/s10964-021-01472-6

Prochaska, J. O., DiClemente, C. C., & Norcross, J. C. (1992). In search of how people change: Applications to addictive behaviours. American Psychologist, *47*, 1102–1114.

Robinson, K. R., Jones, K., Balmbra, J., Robertson, K., Horne, J., & Logan, P. A. (2019). Developing the react to falls resources to support care home staff in managing falls. Journal of Frailty, Sarcopenia and Falls, *4*, 1–10. 10.22540/JFSF-04-001

Ross, J., Field, C., Kaye, S., & Bowman, J. (2019). Prevalence and correlates of low self-reported physical health status among prisoners in New South Wales, Australia. International Journal of Prisoner Health, *15*(2), 192–206. https://doi.org/10.1108/IJPH-06-2018-0039

Rowe, C. L. (2010). Multidimensional family therapy: Addressing co-occurring substance abuse and other problems among adolescents with comprehensive family-based treatment. Child and Adolescent Psychiatric Clinics of North America, *19*, 563–576. 10.1016/j.chc.2010.03.008

Shoneye, C. (2012). Prevention and treatment of obesity in adults with learning disabilities. Learning Disability Practice, *15*(3), 32–37.

Sims, D., & Cabrita Gulyurtlu, S. S. (2014). A scoping review of personalisation in the UK: Approaches to social work and people with learning disabilities. Health & social care in the community, *22*(1), 13–21.

Turner, S. (2013). Improving the uptake of health checks for adults with learning disabilities (Evidence into practice report no. 6). London, UK: DoH.

Stephens, R. S., Roffman, R. A., & Curtain, L. (2000). Comparison of extended versus brief treatments for marijuana use. Journal of Consulting and Clinical Psychology, *68*, 898–908.

Sumnall, H. R., & Bellis, M. A. (2007). Can health campaigns make people ill? The iatrogenic potential of population-based cannabis prevention. Journal of Epidemiology and Community Health, *61*, 930–931.

Tzu-Ting, H., Lin-Hui, Y., & Chia-Yih, L. (2011). Reducing the fear of falling among community-dwelling elderly adults through cognitive-behavioural strategies and intense tai chi exercise: A randomized controlled trial. Journal of Advanced Nursing, *67*(5), 961–971.

Weiss, L. M., & Petry, N. M. (2011). Interaction effects of age and contingency management treatments in cocaine-dependent outpatients. Experimental and Clinical Psychopharmacology, *19*(2), 173–181.

White, J., Hawkins, J., Madden, K., Grant, A., Er, V., Angel, L., ... & Moore, L. (2017). Adapting the ASSIST model of informal peer-led intervention delivery to the talk to FRANK drug prevention programme in UK secondary schools (ASSIST+ FRANK): intervention development, refinement and a pilot cluster randomised controlled trial. Public Health Research, *5*(7), 1.

Wiebe, G. D. (1951–1952). Merchandising commodities and citizenship on television. Public Opinion Quarterly, *15*, 679–691.

Wigham, S., Bourne, J., McKenzie, K., Rowlands, G., Petersen, K., & Hackett, S. (2022). Improving access to primary care and annual health checks for people who have a learning disability: A multistakeholder qualitative study. BMJ Open, *12*(12), e065945. 10.1136/bmjopen-2022-065945

World Health Organization. (2021). WHO global report on trends in prevalence of tobacco use 2000–2025.

Yoon, I. A., Slade, K. & Fazel, S. (2017). Outcomes of psychological therapies for prisoners with mental health problems: A systematic review and meta-analysis. Journal of Consulting and Clinical Psychology, *85*, 783–802. 10.1037/ccp0000214

Zwick, J., Appleseth, H., & Arndt, S. (2020). Stigma: How it affects the substance use disorder patient. Substance Abuse Treatment, Prevention, and Policy, *15*, 50. 10.1186/s13011-020-002 88-0

12   Conclusion

Public health arose from the ambition to reduce the toil of infectious diseases and, until the middle of the last century, focused on preventing the spread of infectious diseases such as smallpox, measles and influenza using a range of medical and social interventions, including vaccination and improving sanitation and nutrition. Public health attention in most developed nations has moved from protection to prevention, with a particular focus on lifestyle behaviours and individual responsibility for health and wellbeing. Definitions of health started to shift from an absence of disease and/or illness towards a concept of wellness and investment in health through lifestyle choices. Although there is a significant history of pandemics (Piret & Boivin, 2021), the COVID-19 global pandemic is the most recent and possibly the most far-reaching in its impact on populations and health services. The COVID-19 pandemic undoubtedly instigated serious protective measures from most governments, including lockdowns, masks and, eventually, vaccination. However, the pandemic did not shift the focus away from prevention as much as might have been expected. In July 2020, the then United Kingdom (UK) Prime Minister Boris Johnson said he was overweight when he was hospitalised with COVID-19, and that there was consistent evidence that people who are overweight have a higher risk of being hospitalised, entering intensive care or dying after contracting COVID-19 than those in weight ranges considered healthy. The UK government launched 'Our Better Health Strategy' to cut the country's obesity rates as part of its pandemic response. Boris Johnson went on to say, 'If we all do our bit, we can reduce our health risks and protect ourselves against the coronavirus—as well as taking pressure off the NHS' (Nugent, 2020).

The *Better Health* strategy (NHS, n.d.) to encourage people to make healthy choices is not radically different from previous health strategies. Its new selling point was that it

DOI: 10.4324/9781003471233-12

was no longer to protect you from a chronic condition that may occur in the future but was to protect you from the consequences of an infectious disease in the present. In this way, the government returned to the fear-drive behavioural change model, hoping that fear of dying from COVID-19 would motivate the overweight to take action.

This concluding chapter will explore the role of psychological interventions within a political and social context. Although the techniques, research and evidence presented in this book will be useful to the individual health care professional, the policy framework must be recognised. While it is beyond the scope of this text to explore all of these elements, and other books adopt a more socio-political perspective on lifestyle (e.g., Thirlaway & Upton, 2009), the health care professional must appreciate the context in which they work. Consequently, this chapter will outline the lifestyle policy in the UK since the 1990s and how this has impacted the ethics of intervention and individual practice.

Health professionals promoting evidence-based strategies (and we have tried to concentrate on these research—or evidence-based methods) for lifestyle change face criticism and competition from many sources, many of which base their critiques and alternative solutions on personal experience. For example, Janet Street-Porter (2008) in the *Independent on Sunday* claimed that 'Obesity is a result of wilful self-abuse' rather than offering any coherent psychological explanation. Boris Johnson, in 2020, was more sympathetic and recognised that he was overweight but still proposed that individuals, armed with advice and guidance from health professionals, should lose weight to protect themselves and the NHS. In January 2023, Eluned Morgan, a minister in the Labour government of Wales, adopted a similar position when asking people to try to live more healthily to help with the ongoing NHS crisis. It seems that regardless of political viewpoint, the belief that health is the responsibility of individuals is the accepted position, and this position has not altered throughout the differing editions of this book.

Conservative politicians such as Boris Johnson are often opposed to any strategy that limits personal choice and have accused previous governments of building a 'nanny state'. Nevertheless, a minimum price of alcohol is being implemented in some countries, and the debates around a sugar tax continue. The latter is a good example of political considerations crashing into research evidence. There is considerable evidence that increased consumption of sugar-sweetened drinks increases the risk of significant morbidity, including Type 2 diabetes, cardiovascular disease, dental caries and obesity (Malik & Hu, 2022; Valenzuela et al., 2021). Further, epidemiological evidence suggests that introducing the 'sugar tax' on soft drinks in April 2018 by the then UK government resulted in an 8% relative reduction in obesity levels in Year 6 girls (Rogers et al., 2023). Despite this, the subsequent Conservative leader and Prime minister, Boris Johnson, railed against this to arrest the 'creep of the nanny state'. As such, he launched a review into the effectiveness of such taxes while making clear that he is a sceptic. As Purdie et al. (2019) write, 'Johnson's headline-grabbing comments are effective not because of their implications for health, but because they appeal to the public's ideals of freedom, autonomy, and choice' and conclude that 'Using "nanny state" language serves to deflect from or attempt to conceal issues of how choice is manufactured and shaped by a range of industries and institutions'. Once again, the confusion between the libertarian, individual decision-based approach and the evidential policy-based structural interventions is laid bare.

Of course, it is encouraging that lifestyle diseases and lifestyle behaviours are receiving media coverage and that the health problems that arise from unsafe sex, binge drinking and so on are front-page news. Not long ago, Harrabin et al. (2003) voiced concern at the media's lack of interest in lifestyle diseases. What is concerning, however, is that everybody now sees themselves as an expert on lifestyle, and alongside the columnists creating controversy are many lay persons offering health and lifestyle advice ranging from the ill-advised to the positively dangerous. Consequently, this text offers sensible advice based on psychological principles supported by consistent, high-quality research.

Of course, the health care professional does not operate within a vacuum, and there is a need for the health care professional to appreciate the socioeconomic and policy environment in which their practice occurs. Preventing lifestyle diseases through promoting healthy lifestyle choices has been a central tenet of health policy in the UK since 1999 (Department of Health, 1999). The government faces two interrelated challenges. First, they need to change the established lifestyle habits of the current generation of adults. Second, they must prevent the next generation of adults from establishing similar or worse lifestyle habits. Lifestyle policy in the UK addresses these two issues first by attempting to modify cultural norms. For example, the policy to promote sensible drinking has been to shape the environment—to change the cultural norms to sensible and safe drinking rather than characterised by binge drinking (HM Government, 2007). Similar efforts have also been made for exercise, sexual health and diet. However, what has to be recognised is that this will be a long and generational process; for example, 'cultures exist where being active or eating "healthy" foods are not top priorities' (Jones et al., 2007, p. 38). Further, it is important to appreciate that culture is difficult to change, especially if people do not have the resources to change: 'The behaviour of these individuals may be the most difficult to modify due to both the difficulties in reaching them and overcoming their norms' (Jones et al., 2007, p. 38), irrespective of the facilities and support available to them. As Alan Johnson (the UK's then health secretary) stated: 'The causes of poor health are not so much about the choices people make, *but the choices they are able to make*' (A. Johnson, speech, 19 March 2009).

Changing cultural norms could establish healthy lifestyle habits from the outset and make it easier for individuals to change established unhealthy lifestyles, and there would no longer be a need for this book. Lifestyle policy aims to direct cultural trends (Department of Health, 1999; HM Government, 2007; Jones et al., 2007) but is itself a product of our history and culture. For instance, there is no clear scientific rationale for a drug like cannabis to be illegal while a drug like alcohol is not. Alcohol is an integral part of our history and culture, and banning it in Britain has never been considered a viable response to the problems that arise from drinking. The opening statement of 'Safe. Sensible. Social' (HM Government, 2007) made it clear that alcohol is seen as a primarily positive aspect of society despite its severe behavioural and health consequences. The same document then reports that 'Alcohol can play an important and positive role in British culture' (HM Government, 2007). This position was not significantly changed when the UK Chief Medical Officers launched their new safe drinking guidelines in 2016 (UK Chief Medical Officers, 2016). However, some governments are recognising the significant costs of alcohol consumption and in 2023, Canada reduced its weekly guidelines to fewer than six standard drinks a week (Paradis et al., 2023).

A population-level approach to public health interventions has always been assumed to be the most cost-effective and efficient way to change behaviour. It is cheaper and can get the message to more individuals than clinical measures can, and it will result (hopefully) in developing cultural changes. The most significant population-level smoking intervention in recent years has been legislation restricting smoking in public places. Since March 2006 in Scotland, April 2007 in Northern Ireland and Wales and July 2007 in England, all public places and workplaces have been smoke-free. Introducing this change was not particularly controversial—the proportion of the population supporting such a change was high. Of course, commentators such as Rod Liddle have argued strongly against the ban. For example, when commenting on the smoking ban introduced by Sir Liam Donaldson, the Chief Medical Officer, Liddle asserted:

> Sir Liam is the chap who believes today's unjust and draconian smoking ban is 'only a start' and wishes to pursue smokers into the family home. Despite evidence to the contrary, Donaldson believes passive smoking kills millions of people; but then his career has been built upon scaring people.
>
> (Liddle, 2007)

However, it appears that this 'draconian ban' has already reduced the number of heart attacks in the UK. Indeed, this legislation has resulted in substantial population health gain, including reductions in workplace exposure to second-hand smoke (Semple et al., 2010), increased smoking quit rates (Hackshaw et al., 2010) and decreased hospital admissions for acute myocardial infarction (Mackay et al., 2010; Sims et al., 2010) along with improvements in childhood asthma rates (Millett et al., 2013). It may be draconian, but it is effective and more effective than decades of antismoking promotion activities (Pell & Haw, 2009). Indeed, the Tobacco Control Scorecard (based on collated evidence to aggregate estimated impacts of different policies) suggested that the biggest impact was regulations and taxes. The best policy, which was expected to reduce smoking rates by 10%, was smoking bans (Levy et al., 2018).

An interesting perspective and debate were raised by the Nuffield Council on Bioethics (2007), who argued that public health policies should include enforcement. They proposed an 'intervention ladder' as a useful way of conceptualising public health interventions and their impact on an individual's choice (see Table 12.1). How does smoking fit into the ladder? It can be seen that currently, the government 'guides by disincentives' and 'restricts choice' to a certain extent. The ban on smoking in public places is significant as it is the first legislative attempt to alter lifestyle choices made by governments for many years. However, surely it can be argued that the government should eliminate choice; that is, we should ban smoking. On the one hand, smoking is an avoidable behaviour—society and civilisation would not suffer considerably if it were banned nationwide. Certainly, the Nuffield Council on Bioethics (2007) would argue that this would be important, that enforcement should be used, and that this curtailment of individual freedom would be ethically justified. Their argument concerns proportionality—can the enforcement benefits outweigh the interference in people's lives? Smoking is a dangerous lifestyle behaviour rooted in social, physiological and psychological elements. Its dangers are obvious to most, and it can kill the individual and the innocent bystander. Is this sufficient to 'eliminate choice' (to use the phrasing of the Nuffield Council, aka 'ban', 'coerce' or 'outlaw')? Obviously, libertarians would argue that smoking is an individual right, and if individuals want to choose this behaviour, then this is their right. Consequently, it is up to health promoters, health psychologists and health care professionals to promote smoking cessation and not to severely curtail

Table 12.1 The intervention ladder

Level	Description	Example
Eliminate choice	Introduce laws that entirely eliminate choice	Compulsory isolation of those with an infectious disorder
Restrict choice	Introduce laws that restrict the options available to people	Remove unhealthy foods from shops
Guide through disincentives	Introduce financial or other disincentives to influence behaviour	Increase taxes on cigarettes
Guide through incentives	Introduce financial or other incentives to influence people's behaviour	Tax breaks for bicycle purchases
Guide choices	Changing the default policy	Change the standard side dish from chips to salad
Enable choice	Help individuals to change their behaviour	Free stop-smoking programmes
Provide information	Inform and educate public	Encourage people to eat five portions of fruit/veg a day
Do nothing	Or monitor situation	

Source: Nuffield Council on Bioethics (2007).

our freedoms. An editorial in *The Times* ('A Sugared Pill', 2007) argues that 'John Stuart Mill held that the only justification for state coercion was to prevent harm, or "evil", being done to others. It is a stretch to say that ... smoking at home meets this definition'. However, others have argued that the ladder provides an ethical framework for public health interventions that can be applied to other lifestyle behaviours, such as alcohol use and poor diet (Walton & Megwasser, 2012).

The Nuffield Ladder has its critics: Griffiths and West (2015) suggest that it fails to reflect the extent to which protecting people's health can enhance their autonomy. However, it has been widely used in the literature. For example, Theis and White (2021) used this framework to analyse government obesity strategies in England between 1992 and 2000, finding that no policies entirely eliminated choice. In contrast, most policies either attempted to inform (e.g., media campaigns) or enable choice (e.g., provide vouchers for healthy foodstuffs). In other words, to quote Bhattacharya (2023), 'Policymakers have been far more comfortable towards the bottom of the ladder of intervention' (p. 5).

Laws that eliminate or restrict lifestyle choices are generally implemented to protect others from harm, not the individuals themselves. Consequently, people can no longer smoke in public places to protect others, and driving under the influence of alcohol is illegal. Critics of such interventionist policies have argued that such measures are 'nanny state-ist' (Jochelson, 2006) and an unnecessary intrusion into people's personal lives. The current government and the official opposition distance themselves from such interventionist attitudes, although the current health secretary did teasingly ask, 'Is it too great a leap to assume that what works today for smoking will also work for obesity, or for that matter alcohol?' (Johnston, 2009). However, this debate about the limits to state freedom and public health is not new. Libertarians have long argued that minimal state intervention is the way to protect individual freedom. For example, a commentator suggested that the original *Public Health Act* (1848) was 'paternalistic' and 'despotic', and 'a little dirt and freedom' was 'more desirable than no dirt at all and slavery' (Porter, 1999).

At the other end of the intervention ladder (Table 12.1), the government remains committed to a policy of guiding choice despite the irrefutable evidence across all lifestyle behaviours that educational and risk communication messages do not have any significant effect on lifestyle choices (Blue, 2007; Floyd et al., 2000; Milne et al., 2000; Ruiter, 2004; Taubman Ben-Ari & Findler, 2005). However, cultural norms can be modified: drink-driving is no longer acceptable, and drink-related road accidents have been reduced. Smoking in public places is no longer acceptable, and the move to this position was not nearly as contentious as feared (Office for National Statistics, 2005). However, these cultural shifts have been supported by clear legislation; it is unlikely that health promotion alone will change lifestyle culture (Bhattacharya, 2023).

In the context of this social and policy background, the health care practitioner has to promote healthy behaviour and behaviour change. The government has set many targets around reducing the incidence of lifestyle diseases, and their main strategy to achieve these goals is to increase healthy and decrease unhealthy lifestyle choices. However, although health care professionals have a fundamental role, they are not the only ones responsible for improving health and behavioural choices. Many different government policies task a range of public servants—the police, local authorities, the NHS, schools and voluntary organisations—with delivering the government's public health strategies. Further, the government also identifies the alcohol industry, the wider business industry, the media and local communities as having a role in delivering their strategy. There has been increasing recognition that people tasked with delivering behavioural change messages need training in effective ways to intervene (Public Health England [PHE], 2016). Consequently, National Institute for Health and Clinical Excellence (NICE, 2010) recommends that health care professionals could deliver brief behavioural change messages during routine appointments but recommend training (NICE, 2010). Feedback from public health practitioners who had a role in supporting the implementation of brief behavioural change messages (or *Making Every Contact Count*) in the UK suggests that standardising training for health care professionals may enhance implementation (Chisholm et al., 2019). A recent narrative review suggested barriers to and enablers of delivering brief behaviour change interventions (Keyworth et al., 2020). Barriers and enablers included the perceptions of the knowledge and skills required to deliver interventions, professional roles, resources and support needed.

Thus, the principal candidates for delivering behavioural change interventions remain primary care practitioners: general practitioners, practice nurses, health visitors and other associated health care professionals (PHE, 2016). Primary care has been central in the delivery of individual lifestyle advice for some time, and there is conflicting evidence about whether merely advising patients to change their lifestyle can lead to lifestyle change (Ashenden et al., 1997; Moyer et al., 2002). However, it is clear that a psychology-based intervention is more likely to be successful (Biddle et al., 1997; Connor & Norman, 2015, 2017; Moyer et al., 2002) and that appropriate training can provide primary care professionals with the skills necessary to change behaviour (PHE, 2016; Simkin-Silverman & Wing, 1997). To give health care professionals the best chance of delivering psychology-based lifestyle interventions, they will need more than a copy of this book. Here, we simply introduce the key concepts and ideas. health care professionals will need training and resources to deliver the behaviour changes that governments are seeking (Keyworth et al., 2020).

Health practitioners will need various resources and skills to deliver effective preventative lifestyle interventions. First, they will need to be able to measure current lifestyle behaviours quickly and reliably and recognise individuals with severe problems that need referral to a specialist. We presented assessment information within each chapter of this book, and there may be many such techniques. Importantly, the individual health care professional needs to be able to recognise the limits of their expertise and make referrals as appropriate. Thus, for example, they need to be able to recognise the difference between substance use, misuse and addiction and refer for specialist help as appropriate.

Health professionals who wish to enable their patients to change their lifestyles first and foremost need to recognise that simply providing people with information about the risks of unhealthy lifestyles will not result in lifestyle change. If health professionals wish to encourage lifestyle change, they should seek to increase self-motivation and self-regulatory skills, set achievable goals and increase self-efficacy in their clients. Although reading this text is a start, it is not a finishing point: there are additional seminars, courses and resources available that health care professionals need to make use of.

We are at a turning point in health promotion. The ineffectiveness of the previous decades of educational interventions is irrefutable, and policymakers and health professionals are starting to recognise the importance of psychological processes in lifestyle change (PHE, 2016; Thirlaway & Upton, 2009). Fortunately, psychology is a discipline with a strong record of high-quality research, and we are already able to provide evidence-based advice about appropriate psychological interventions. Lifestyle behaviours are extremely varied, but the same psychological constructs are relevant to promoting change. The potential opportunity to develop training and protocols for interventions that can be applied across all lifestyle behaviours should not be ignored.

Conclusion

This final chapter has attempted to place the material presented throughout this text within a social and policy context. The healt hcare professional must recognise the key role of public policy in promoting healthy lifestyles and their individual practice. This chapter stresses the tension between the libertarian perspective currently predominant in our society and the evidence that a more interventionist approach to public health policy can significantly impact health and wellbeing.

Motivation, self-efficacy and self-regulation have been established as key cognitive factors in successful lifestyle change. For now, the health care professional needs to maximise intervention-based knowledge and develop and enhance self-efficacy as a key route for lifestyle change. However, we need to explore the role of non-cognitive factors such as habitual responses and enjoyment in establishing lifestyle choices. We must develop research protocols, evidence-based interventions and strategies that can extend our understanding and implementation of successful lifestyle change. People do not usually make initial lifestyle choices based on future health implications, and by the time they wish to protect their health, they need to overcome well-established bad habits. Ultimately, we hope that the material in this text becomes redundant and the focus alters from changing unhealthy behaviours to maintaining healthy ones.

Summary points

- Everyone is an expert on lifestyle change, and often, advice is based on personal experience of change rather than research evidence.
- There is a tension between libertarian and interventionist approaches to public health.
- Restricting lifestyle choices through legislation can significantly contribute to changing cultural norms and individual behaviour and improving long-term health.
- Health care professionals play a key role in promoting behaviour change.
- A psychological approach to lifestyle change can be central to developing a healthy society.

References

Ashenden, R., Silagy, C., & Weller, D. (1997). A systematic review of the effectiveness of promoting lifestyle change in general practice. Family Practice, *14*, 160–174.

A Sugared Pill: The Nuffield Council tries, but fails, to justify the nanny state (2007, 13 November). The Times. Retrieved from http://www.timesonline.co.uk/tol/comment/leading_article/article2859367.ece

Bhattacharya, A. (2023, 27 July). Carrots and sticks: Can governments do without public health regulation? Social Market Foundation. Retrieved from https://www.smf.co.uk/publications/carrots-and-sticks-public-health/

Biddle, S., Edmunds, L., Bowler, I. & Killoran, A. (1997). Physical activity promotion through primary health care in England. British Journal of General Practice, *47*(419), 367–369.

Blue, C. L. (2007). Does the theory of planned behaviour identify diabetes-related cognitions for intention to be physically active and eat a healthy diet? Public Health Nursing, *24*(2), 141–150.

Chisholm, A., Ang-Chen, P., Peters, S., Hart, J., & Beenstock, J. (2019). Public health practitioners' views of the 'Making Every Contact Count' initiative and standards for its evaluation. Journal of Public Health, *41*(1), e70–e77. 10.1093/pubmed/fdy094

Conner, M., & Norman, P. (2015). Predicting and changing health behaviour: Research and practice with social cognition models (3rd ed.). Berkshire, United Kingdom: Open University Press.

Conner, M., & Norman, P. (2017). Health behaviour: Current issues and challenges. Psychology & Health, *32*(8), 895–906. 10.1080/08870446.2017.1336240

Department of Health. (1999). Saving lives: Our healthier nation. London, United Kingdom: The Stationery Office.

Floyd, D. L., Prentice-Dunn, S., & Rogers, R. W. (2000). A meta-analysis of protection motivation theory. Journal of Applied Social Psychology, *30*, 407–429.

Griffiths, P. E., & West, C. (2015). A balanced intervention ladder: Promoting autonomy through public health action. Public Health, *129*(8), 1092–1098.

Hackshaw, L., McEwen, A., West, R., & Bauld, L. (2010). Quit attempts in response to smoke-free legislation in England. Tobacco Control, *19*(2), 160–164.

Harrabin, R., Coote, A., & Allen, J. (2003). Health in the news: Risk, reporting and media influence. London, United Kingdom: King's Fund.

HM Government. (2007). Safe, sensible, social. The next steps in the national alcohol strategy. London, United Kingdom: Department of Health and The Home Office.

Jochelson, K. (2006). Nanny or steward? The role of government in public health. Public Health, *120*, 1149–1155.

Johnston, A. (2009, 19 March). 'Nanny state, Nudge State or No state?' Royal Society of Arts, London.

Jones, A., Bentham, G., Foster, C., Hillsdon, M., & Panter, J. (2007). Tackling obesities: Future choices—obesogenic environments—evidence review. London, United Kingdom: Foresight.

Keyworth, C., Epton, T., Goldthorpe, J., Calam, R., & Armitage, C. (2020). Delivering opportunistic behavior change interventions: A systematic review of systematic reviews. Prevention Science, *21*(3), 319–331. 10.1007/s11121-020-01087-6

Levy, D. T., Tam, J., Kuo, C., Fong, G., & Chaloupka, F. (2018). Research full report: The impact of implementing tobacco control policies: The 2017 tobacco control policy scorecard. Journal of Public Health Management and Practice, *24*(5), 448.

Liddle, R. (2007, 1 July). So that's his real NHS priority—a £2 billion stealth cut in England. Sunday Times.

Mackay, D. F., Irfan, M. O., Haw, S., & Pell, J. P. (2010). Metaanalysis of the effect of comprehensive smoke-free legislation on acute coronary events. Heart, *96*(19), 1525–1530.

Malik, V. S., & Hu, F. B. (2022). The role of sugar-sweetened beverages in the global epidemics of obesity and chronic diseases. Nature Reviews Endocrinology, *18*(4), 205–218.

Millett, C., Lee, J. T., Laverty, A. A., Glantz, S. A., & Majeed, A. (2013). Hospital admissions for childhood asthma after smoke-free legislation in England. Pediatrics, *131*, e495.

Milne, S., Sheeran, P., & Orbell, S. (2000). Prediction and intervention in health-related behaviour: A meta review of protection motivation theory. Journal of Applied Social Psychology, *30*, 106–143.

Moyer, A., Finney, J. W., Swearingen, E., & Vergun, P. (2002). Brief interventions for alcohol problems: A meta-analytic review of controlled investigations in treatment seeking and non-treatment seeking populations. Addiction, *97*, 279–292.

NHS. (n.d.). Better health. London, United Kingdom: NHS. Retrieved from https://www.nhs.uk/better-health/

NICE (2010). Alcohol-use disorders: Preventing harmful drinking (NICE public health guidance 24). London, United Kingdom: NICE.

Nuffield Council on Bioethics. (2007). Public health ethical issues. London, United Kingdom: Nuffield Council. Retrieved from www.nuffieldbioethics.org

Nugent, C. (2020, 27 July). 'I Was Too Fat' Prime Minister Boris Johnson says Brits must lose weight to fight coronavirus. TIME. Retrieved from https://time.com/5872175/boris-johnson-weight-loss-coronavirus/

Office for National Statistics. (2005). Smoking-related behaviour and attitudes, 2005. London, United Kingdom: HMSO.

Paradis, C., Butt, P., Shield, K., Poole, N., Wells, S., Naimi, T., ... The Low-Risk Alcohol Drinking Guidelines Scientific Expert Panels (2023). Canada's guidance on alcohol and health: Final report. Ottawa, Ontario: Canadian Centre on Substance Use and Addiction.

Pell, J. P., & Haw, S. (2009). The triumph of national smoke free legislation. Heart, *95*, 1377–1380.

Piret, J., & Boivin, G. (2021). Pandemics throughout history. Frontiers in Microbiology, *11*, 631736.

Porter, D. (1999). Health, civilisation and the state. A history of public health from ancient to modern times. London, United Kingdom: Routledge.

PHE. (2016). The public health burden of alcohol and the effectiveness and cost-effectiveness of alcohol control policies: An evidence review. London: UK Government.

Purdie, A., Buse, K., & Hawkes, S. (2019, 17 July). Syntax and the 'sin tax': The power of narratives for health. The BMJ Opinion. Retrieved from https://blogs.bmj.com/bmj/2019/07/17/syntax-and-the-sin-tax-the-power-of-narratives-for-health/

Rogers, N. T., Cummins, S., Forde, H., Jones, C. P., Mytton, O., Rutter, H. ... Adams, J. (2023). Associations between trajectories of obesity prevalence in English primary school children and the UK soft drinks industry levy: An interrupted time series analysis of surveillance data. PLoS Med, *20*(1), e1004160. 10.1371/journal.pmed.1004160

Ruiter, R. A. C. (2004). Effecten van angstaanjagende tv-spotjes [Effects of fear-arousing TV commercials; Final report]. Maastricht, Netherlands: Maastricht University, Department of Experimental Psychology.

Semple, S., van Tongeren, M., Galea, K. S., MacCalman, L., Gee, I., Parry, O., ... Ayres, J. G. (2010). UK smoke-free legislation: Changes in PM2.5 concentrations in bars in Scotland, England, and Wales. Annals of Occupational Hygiene, *54*(3), 272–280.

Simkin-Silverman, L. R., & Wing, R. R. (1997). Management of obesity in primary care. Obesity Research, *5*, 603–612.

Sims, M., Maxwell, R., Bauld, L., & Gilmore, A. (2010). Short term impact of smoke-free legislation in England: Retrospective analysis of hospital admissions for myocardial infarction. BMJ, *340*, c2161.

Street-Porter, J. (2008, 27 January). Let the adult fatties eat themselves to death. The kids we can save. Independent on Sunday.

Taubman Ben-Ari, O., & Findler, L. (2005). Proximal and distal effects of mortality salience on willingness to engage in health promoting behavior along the life span. Psychology & Health, *20*, 303–318.

Theis, D. R. Z., & White, M. (2021). Is obesity policy in England fit for purpose? Analysis of government strategies and policies, 1992–2020. The Milbank Quarterly, *99*(1), 126–170.

Thirlaway, K., & Upton, D. (2009). The psychology of lifestyle: Promoting healthy behaviour. London, United Kingdom: Routledge.

UK Chief Medical Officers (2016). UK chief medical officers' low risk drinking guidelines. London: UK Government.

Valenzuela, M. J., Waterhouse, B., Aggarwal, V. R., Bloor, K., & Doran, T. (2021). Effect of sugar-sweetened beverages on oral health: A systematic review and meta-analysis. European Journal of Public Health, *31*(1), 122–129.

Walton, M., & Megwasser, E. (2012). An ethical evaluation of evidence: A stewardship approach to public health policy. Public Health Ethics (2012), *5*(1), 16–21.

Index

Note: *Italicized*, **bold** and ***bold italics*** refer to figures, tables and boxes.